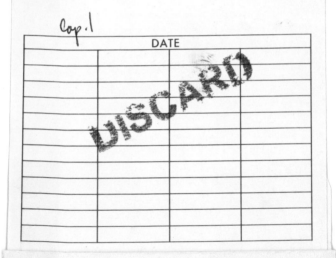

COMMUNITY PSYCHOLOGY IN TRANSITION

THE SERIES IN CLINICAL AND COMMUNITY PSYCHOLOGY

CONSULTING EDITORS:

CHARLES D. SPIELBERGER and IRWIN G. SARASON

Averill	• Patterns of Psychological Thought: Readings in Historical and Contemporary Texts
Becker	• Depression: Theory and Research
Brehm	• The Application of Social Psychology to Clinical Practice
Cattell and Dreger	• Handbook of Modern Personality Theory
Endler and Magnusson	• Interactional Psychology and Personality
Friedman and Katz	• The Psychology of Depression: Contemporary Theory and Research
Iscoe, Bloom, and Spielberger	• Community Psychology in Transition
Janisse	• Pupillometry: The Psychology of the Pupillary Response
Kissen	• From Group Dynamics to Group Psychoanalysis: Therapeutic Applications of Group Dynamic Understanding
Klopfer and Reed	• Problems in Psychotherapy: An Eclectic Approach
Manschreck and Kleinman	• Renewal in Psychiatry: A Critical Rational Perspective
Reitan and Davison	• Clinical Neuropsychology: Current Status and Applications
Spielberger and Diaz-Guerrero	• Cross-Cultural Anxiety
Spielberger and Sarason	• Stress and Anxiety, volume 1
Sarason and Spielberger	• Stress and Anxiety, volume 2
Sarason and Spielberger	• Stress and Anxiety, volume 3
Spielberger and Sarason	• Stress and Anxiety, volume 4
Ulmer	• On the Development of a Token Economy Mental Hospital Treatment Program

IN PREPARATION

Bermant, Kelman, and Warwick	• The Ethics of Social Intervention
Cohen and Mirsky	• Biology and Psychopathology
London	• Strategies of Personality Research
Olweus	• Aggression in the Schools

COMMUNITY PSYCHOLOGY IN TRANSITION

Proceedings of the
National Conference on Training
in Community Psychology

EDITED BY

IRA ISCOE
The University of Texas at Austin

BERNARD L. BLOOM
University of Colorado, Boulder

CHARLES D. SPIELBERGER
University of South Florida, Tampa

HEMISPHERE PUBLISHING CORPORATION
WASHINGTON   LONDON

A HALSTED PRESS BOOK

JOHN WILEY & SONS
NEW YORK   LONDON   SYDNEY   TORONTO

Hemisphere Publishing Corporation
1025 Vermont Ave., N.W., Washington, D.C. 20005

Distributed solely by Halsted Press, a Division of John Wiley & Sons, Inc.,
New York.

1 2 3 4 5 6 7 8 9 0   D O D O   7 8 3 2 1 0 9 8 7

Library of Congress Cataloging in Publication Data

Main entry under title:

Community psychology in transition.

    (The Series in clinical and community psychology)
    "Based on the proceedings . . . held in Austin, Texas,
in April 1975."
    Includes indexes.
    1. Community psychology—Congresses.   I. Iscoe, Ira.
II. Bloom, Bernard L.   III. Spielberger, Charles
Donald, 1927–   IV. National Conference on Training
in Community Psychology, Austin, Tex., 1975.
RA790.A1C54   362.2'2   77-5882
ISBN 0-470-99172-0

Printed in the United States of America

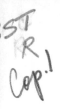

Contents

VII EPILOGUE

APPENDIXES

Preface

The present volume is based on the proceedings of the National Conference on Training in Community Psychology held in Austin, Texas, in April 1975. This conference was sponsored by the Division of Community Psychology (Division 27) of the American Psychological Association. Founded in 1967, the Division of Community Psychology is composed of psychologists with a strong commitment to the promotion of mental health through proactive approaches to the design, delivery, and evaluation of mental health and other human services.

The past decade has witnessed a remarkable increase in the number of educational programs centrally concerned with community psychology. Expanding interest in the field and the development of new community psychology training programs has stimulated the search for appropriate training models, and provided the impetus for the Division of Community Psychology to seek support from the National Institute of Mental Health for a National Conference on Training.

The primary goal of the National Conference on Training in Community Psychology was to examine systematically the many questions and issues that have arisen with regard to appropriate models for doctoral training in community psychology. Analyses of current training models and approaches, discussions of central training issues, commentaries on critical training problems, and efforts to clarify future direction and trends are reported in these conference proceedings. Background factors leading to the convening of the conference and organization and planning activities are also described.

In a very real sense, this volume reflects the work of the participants at the National Conference on Training in Community Psychology. These proceedings were organized and planned by the editors in consultation with the Executive Committee of the Division of Community Psychology. To facilitate the preparation of this volume, the responsibility for developing background materials and summaries for the several parts were divided among the editors. Part I provides information about the historical context in which the conference developed and the planning and monitoring activities of the Conference Planning Committee. We have endeavored to identify significant background factors leading up to the conference and to share with the reader some of the excitement that was associated with the planning process.

Part II consists of the texts of three invited keynote position papers presented at the conference by senior statesmen in community psychology. Each of these papers sets forth new directions for community psychology with direct and important implications for future training programs.

Part III is concerned with different models and approaches to training in community psychology. The initial chapter in this section is based on an invited keynote position paper providing an analysis of training models that was submitted to the Conference Planning Committee in response to a call for descriptions of community psychology training programs. The remaining chapters of Part III reflect the intense deliberations that took place during the conference as these were elaborated and refined in postconference meetings and correspondence. More than any other section of these proceedings, the contents of Part III reflect the main thrust of the conference.

Part IV is concerned with critical issues encountered in different models and approaches to training in community psychology. Prior to the conference, five younger community psychologists were recruited (some say conscripted) and assigned the task of evaluating issues considered central in all approaches to training in community psychology. Drawing on their personal observations and the discussion of these issues by special interest groups, these psychologists presented preliminary summaries of their evaluations at the conference, and subsequently participated in a three-hour symposium at the 1975 APA meetings in Chicago. In general, the papers reported in Part IV highlight current thinking with regard to central training issues in community psychology and identify problems that will require intensive consideration in the future.

The results of four studies concerned with current training needs and trends in community psychology are reported in Part V. In order to provide input on a number of issues that were touched on but not considered in depth at the conference, participants who indicated special concern with these issues were invited to contribute papers expressing their personal reviews. These papers are included in Part VI. Finally, in Part VII, some reflections on *Community Psychology in Transition* are offered by the editors.

In the words of one veteran community psychologist whose contributions to the development of the discipline span the quarter-century between the Boulder and Austin conferences, "The view from the mountain is clouded in places but patches of sunshine are glimpsed from time to time." Salient issues with regard to the current status of training in community psychology and the relationship between community psychology and other subspecialties are considered in depth in this volume along with training needs and future prospects. While community psychology is still quite young as an area of specialization, there is much evidence in these proceedings that it has earned its place as a substantive field within the discipline of psychology.

ACKNOWLEDGMENTS

A successful conference requires a strong commitment and considerable investment of time by many people. The willingness to attend to the many details, large and small, that require attention is also essential. The Executive Committee of the Division of Community Psychology, through its continuing support, encouragement, and early commitment of funds, furnished the necessary impetus to initiate planning for the conference and to transform these plans into reality.

On behalf of the Division of Community Psychology, we would like to express appreciation to the National Institute of Mental Health for the initial and supplementary grants (MH 13849 and MH 13849-01S1) that provided the funds needed to plan and convene the conference and to prepare these proceedings, and for the dedicated consultation and flexibility of the staff of the Psychology Training Branch who worked with us. The Division of Community Psychology is also deeply grateful to the Hogg Foundation for Mental Health for contributing funds to support the conference, and to its President, Wayne H. Holtzman, for his early and continuing encouragement and participation in the conference program. We are also indebted to the president of the University of Texas at Austin and the director and staff of the Thompson Conference Center for their cooperation and material assistance.

The editors of these proceedings wish to express their thanks to each of the contributors to this volume and, especially, to the chairpersons of the training models and special interest groups. We would also like to express our personal thanks and the appreciation of the Division of Community Psychology to the graduate students and staff of the Community Psychology Program at the University of Texas at Austin. In enthusiastically undertaking numerous planning activities and local arrangement responsibilities at the Conference, Bertha Holiday, Meg Meyer, and Bryan Wilcox typify those qualities in community psychology graduate students which ensure that the future of the field is in very good hands. Our colleagues, Charles Holahan,

Karl Slaikeu, and Tim Kuehnel, provided wise counsel and support in planning the conference and in making the conference itself a success. They, too, typify the new breed of dedicated community psychologists.

Hidden from public view in the planning and the conduct of the conference were a number of persons on whom we could rely not to panic, and to make those judicious decisions that contributed in so many ways to the success of the conference and the preparation of these proceedings. Sheryl Kelly and Renee Beauchamp worked for many months before, during and after the conference in corresponding with participants and ensuring accurate communications and reports. As general supervisor and administrative field general for both the conference and the preparation of these proceedings, the sincere thanks of the Division of Community Psychology and the editors are expressed to Bertha Shanblum.

In this volume, we have endeavored to provide an accurate and complete description of the proceedings of the National Conference on Training in Community Psychology and the immediate postconference followup activities. It is our hope that these proceedings will serve as a useful guide for training programs in community psychology as we face the challenge of transition from our present status to implementation of the exciting new directions and approaches to training that were articulated by the participants at the Austin Conference.

Ira Iscoe
Bernard L. Bloom
Charles D. Spielberger

I PLANNING FOR THE NATIONAL CONFERENCE

1 Community Psychology

The Historical Context

Ira Iscoe and Charles D. Spielberger

Over the past 25 years, there has been a dramatic shift in emphasis within professional psychology, from an exclusive concern with intrapsychic phenomena to growing recognition of the influence of social systems on human behavior. It has also become increasingly evident that traditional clinical approaches to the treatment of mental illness are limited in their effectiveness, and that psychology must turn to other disciplines in the social and behavioral sciences for the basic knowledge that is needed to understand the impact of communities on people.

Within the past decade, the needs of society have created many new and different roles for psychologists in community settings, and community psychology has emerged as a viable specialty within the discipline of psychology. Rather than changing people or helping them to adjust to community pressures, many psychologists are now involved in efforts to change communities to meet human needs. As has been previously suggested, "community psychology represents a new frontier in the study of human behavior, which is broadly concerned with clarifying the complex interrelationships between individuals and their environment" (Spielberger & Iscoe, 1970, p. 244).

Psychologists who work in community settings are now being called upon to engage in service, research, and consultation activities for which they were not prepared in their graduate training, and community psychologists associated with graduate education programs are hard pressed to keep up with the many new developments in the field. As a consequence, practitioners and academicians alike have experienced increasing frustration, tension, and feelings of inadequacy. Given the rapid and continuing changes in the demands that are being made on psychologists who work in community settings, the need for corresponding modifications in graduate education programs in psychology has become increasingly evident.

In the spring of 1975, Division 27 (Community Psychology) of the American Psychological Association organized and convened a National Conference on Training in Community Psychology. Preliminary planning for this conference was begun eight years earlier at an informal symposium held at the University of Texas at Austin in the spring of 1967. Intensive planning for the conference was initiated by the Executive Committee of the Division of Community Psychology at its midwinter meeting in Chapel Hill, N.C., in

January 1974. The National Conference on Training in Community Psychology was held at the University of Texas at Austin, April 27–May 1, 1975.

The proceedings of The National Conference on Training in Community Psychology are reported in this volume. This chapter examines the historical context within which plans for the conference developed. Details of the planning process and preparation for the conference are described in chapter 2. Keynote addresses that were presented at the conference are reported in part II, approaches to training in community psychology are described in part III, and recurring issues in community psychology are discussed in part IV. Current trends in training and practice are reported in part V, and solicited reflections on the Austin Conference are given in part VI. Finally, some thoughts about the future of community psychology are noted in part VII.

FROM BOULDER TO VAIL: NATIONAL CONFERENCES ON TRAINING IN PSYCHOLOGY

A brief review of previous national conferences on training in psychology will provide a useful frame of reference for evaluating this report of the proceedings of The National Conference on Training in Community Psychology. More detailed descriptions of general historical trends that have influenced the evolution and development of clinical and community psychology are provided in the introductory chapters of books by Sarason, Levine, Goldenberg, Cherlin, and Bennett (1966), Cowen, Gardner, and Zax (1967), Iscoe and Spielberger (1970), and Zax and Specter (1974).

The first national conference on graduate education in clinical psychology was held in 1949 in Boulder, Colo. (Raimy, 1950). Stimulated by requests from the Veterans Administration and the U.S. Public Health Service for authoritative information with regard to the quality of doctoral training programs in clinical psychology (Lloyd & Newbrough, 1966), the Boulder Conference took place in an atmosphere of increased demands for clinical services during the post–World War II era. Some 15 general issues were considered during this two-week conference, including background preparation for clinical psychologists; core curriculum in graduate education programs; modes of training in assessment, psychotherapy, and research; the selection and evaluation of students; staff development and training; and problems related to the accreditation of doctoral programs and the certification and licensing of clinical psychologists.

Most of the 72 participants at the Boulder Conference were academically based clinical psychologists. The dominant theoretical orientation of the participants was psychoanalytic, and diagnostic testing was generally regarded as one of the main justifications for the training of clinical psychologists. Psychotherapy and research functions were also stressed. The scientist-professional model for graduate education in clinical psychology, with its joint emphasis on both professional training and research, was first articulated at the Boulder Conference. It seemed evident at the time that most graduates of clinical psychology training programs would enter service-related positions, but there were also substantial demands for faculty in existing, expanding, and newly formed doctoral programs.

In 1955, a national conference on "Psychology and Mental Health" was held at Stanford University (Strother, 1956). The convening of this conference was influenced by many forces, among them the rapid growth of the mental health movement in the early 1950s and the recommendation of the Boulder Conference for a systematic review and follow-up of training developments. Although the Stanford Conference was not specifically concerned with the training of psychologists, the issues that were considered, and the opinions, views, and recommendations of the 66 participants, had important implications for graduate education programs. Since more than 80% of the participants were clinical psychologists, the fact that there was substantial agreement that training should be provided in a number of approaches to behavior change, in addition to psychotherapy, makes the Stanford Conference a milestone in the evolution of community psychology. Specific alternatives to psychotherapy that were suggested included mental health education, the utilization of therapeutic environments, and preventive intervention to counteract adverse environmental influences.

A third national conference, concerned with "Graduate Education in Psychology," was held in 1958 in Miami Beach (Roe, Gustad, Moore, Ross, & Skodak, 1959). In contrast to the earlier conferences, fewer than half of the participants at the Miami Conference were clinical psychologists, and this conference did not focus on training in any single psychological specialty. Instead, broad issues of graduate education, pressing manpower demands and shortages, new roles for psychologists, and issues with regard to certification and licensing laws were examined.

The prevailing manpower shortages at the time of the Miami Conference served to focus the concerns of the participants on alternative roles for psychologists and on training experiences that would help prepare graduate students for work in a rapidly changing society. While the need for more efficient and widely applicable techniques for meeting mental health service requirements was recognized, the demand for psychologists of all types was very strong, and such conditions tended to reinforce the status quo in training.

In 1965, a fourth national conference on the "Professional Preparation of Clinical Psychologists" was held in Chicago (Hoch, Ross, & Winder, 1966). Although the scientist-professional training model was reaffirmed at this conference, it was conceded with some regret that the graduates of APA-accredited doctoral training programs in clinical psychology were not very active in research. The development of new methods in clinical psychology were noted at the Chicago Conference, and alternate models of doctoral training were encouraged to produce PhDs who would be better prepared to deal with the diverse service demands that were now clearly on the horizon. Surprisingly, there was relatively little emphasis on the community, but this was perhaps understandable since a great majority of participants were academic psychologists or traditionally oriented clinical field supervisors. The pressures and issues then facing clinical psychology, as noted by the participants in the Chicago Conference, are well described by Hoch et al. (1966):

1. On the other hand, clinical psychology is still busily putting its own house in order. There is the painful and urgent problem of identity. There is widespread concern that ours be a fully independent profession. There is need to produce enough PhDs to meet the social need which even now outstrips the numbers being trained.
2. Quite apart from internal pressures, developments in the community are already creating newer, bigger problems to be confronted. (a) A live concern with mental health keeps demands for psychological services mounting. (b) An even new concern—the prevention of psychological disorders—has added further problems and opportunities. (c) Now it turns out that the newest concern of all—that of "community psychology," the more effective utilization of human potential—calls for clinical psychologists to fill still newer and more unaccustomed roles while not yet having resolved some of the present dilemmas. (p. 42)

The Chicago Conference recognized an identity crisis in clinical psychology and urged that field training be better integrated with academic training. The need for psychology to address pressing social problems such as crime, racial integration, and unrest on college campuses was also recognized. Unfortunately, most of the Chicago Conference recommendations were never implemented. The reasons for this may be found in the prosperity of the times and the fact that jobs were plentiful. New PhDs in clinical psychology, often with very limited knowledge of community processes, were being hired to staff the newly created comprehensive community mental health centers, and clinical psychology faculties saw little need for modification of their training programs. They were well supported by the National Institute of Mental Health (NIMH) and the Veterans Administration, and there was understandable reluctance to initiate changes in training models that had proved successful since 1946.

A national conference on "Levels and Patterns of Professional Training in Psychology" was convened in 1973 at Vail, Colo. (Korman, 1974). The Vail Conference reflected the increasing malaise that had developed in professional psychology because deficiencies in academic training programs that had been identified at the Chicago Conference were not being resolved. This dissatisfaction with doctoral training programs was noted by Korman (1974) in his preliminary report on the Vail Conference:

Many professional psychologists continued, even after the Chicago Conference, to express strong dissatisfaction with the apparent lack of appropriateness of training provided by many doctoral programs, their low responsivity to social issues, and their uncritical allegiance to the traditional scientist-professional model. Some of this dissatisfaction led to the formation of the National Council on Graduate Education in Psychology and found expression in new training ventures such as the Doctor of Psychology Program at the University of Illinois and the founding of the California School of Professional Psychology. (p. 441)

The Vail Conference represented a marked departure from previous national conferences in that participation was deliberately weighted toward the representation of ethnic minority groups, women, and graduate students, and there was substantially less representation of departmental heads and directors of training programs. The Vail Conference recommended a variety of patterns and locations for professional training in psychology. The expansion of Doctor of Psychology (PsyD) programs for psychologists who wanted to be practitioners was encouraged, as were the development of free-standing schools of psychology and program consortiums that pool their training resources. In addition, the MA degree was accepted as the appropriate entry level for the practice of professional psychology. Vail will be best remembered as the conference at which a professional practice model was explicitly put forth. The conferees adopted the position that psychology had advanced to the point that the knowledge base was sufficient for training professional psychologists.

NATIONAL CONFERENCES ON TRAINING IN COUNSELING AND SCHOOL PSYCHOLOGY AND COMMUNITY MENTAL HEALTH

The conferences described were all convened by the APA, and the participants were broadly representative of the field of psychology. There have been four national conferences concerned with training in particular professional specialties within psychology, at which most of the participants were associated with these specialties.

A conference was convened at Northwestern University in 1952 to clarify standards for training counseling psychologists at the doctoral level (APA, 1952). The Northwestern Conference was for counseling psychology what the Boulder Conference had been for clinical psychology. It was deemed essential by the participants that psychological counseling be based firmly on psychological science, and that graduate curricula in counseling psychology encompass the basic concepts and techniques common to all psychologists. Research training was defined as a basic element in the education of counseling psychologists, and a core of specialty courses and practicum experiences was outlined.

The functions, qualifications, and training of school psychologists was the topic of the Thayer Conference held at West Point, N.Y., in 1954. Patterned after the Boulder Conference, the Thayer Conference considered a range of issues with regard to the graduate education of school psychologists at the doctoral level (Cutts, 1955). Professional issues relating to the roles and functions of school psychologists, administrative and practicum training arrangements, the accreditation of school psychology training programs, and problems associated with certification for the practice of school psychology were among the topics considered at the Thayer Conference.

In 1964, the APA Division of Counseling Psychology convened a second national conference on the "Professional Preparation of Counseling Psychologists" (Thompson & Super, 1964). At this conference, which was held at the Greystone Conference Center, Teachers College, Columbia University, there was considerable pessimism with regard to the likelihood that current counseling needs could be adequately met by traditional one-to-one counseling procedures. Discussion at the Greystone Conference also dealt with increasing social demands for a wide variety of indirect counseling services. As stated in the conference report (Thompson & Super, 1974):

Looking toward the future, counseling psychologists can anticipate more involvement with important and crucial domestic and international issues such as unemployment, education handicaps, retraining, undeveloped and under-privileged populations, and delinquency. . . . More service will have to be provided indirectly than directly, by leadership and program development . . . and through the consultative rather than direct service role. (pp. 13–14)

By the mid-1960s it was generally recognized that treatment of the mentally ill should be shifted from residential institutions to community settings. The Community Mental Health Centers Act of 1965 provided guidelines for consultation and the delivery of services within community settings as well as funds for staffing the new centers. Other factors that influenced the Zeitgeist in professional psychology in the mid-1960s included the demonstrated efficacy of psychoactive drugs, the continuing shortages of fully trained mental health personnel, the increasing acceptance of the contributions of nontraditionally trained persons to mental health programs, and growing awareness of the importance of community-based mental health programs.

The Greystone Conference on Counseling Psychology and the Chicago Conference on Clinical Psychology both recognized the increasing demands for a wide range of community services and the limitations in prevailing individual approaches to psychological treatment. These concerns were brought into sharper focus in the spring of 1965 at a national conference on the "Education of Psychologists for Community Mental Health" held in Swampscott, Mass., a suburb of Boston. At this conference, new conceptions about the nature of mental illness, the influence of environmental factors on behavior, and the importance of community involvement in treatment programs were shared concerns of the participants.

The report of the Boston Conference (Bennett, Anderson, Cooper, Hassol, Klein, & Rosenblum, 1966) emphasized the need for both study and treatment of individuals within a community context. The following specific areas in which community research was needed were identified in the final report (Bennett et al., 1966):

1. The study of man in the community, including the effects of varying physical and social environments upon his functioning both as an individual and as a member of social organization.
2. Assessment of the individual's reaction to planned change by varying methods of social intervention in a wide variety of human problems and concerns.
3. Basic research on the relationship between social-cultural conditions and personality functioning in order to add knowledge about the positive mastery of stress.
4. Examination of the effects of social organizations upon the individual, particularly those creating high-risk populations, and alternative social patterns which may serve to reduce their creation.
5. Facilitation of social-organizational change through modification of motivational and personality factors in the individual.
6. Evaluative research on consultation and other social change processes. (p. 23)

Additional recommendations at the Boston Conference stressed the need for evaluative research on consultation and for investigations of the reactions of individuals and groups to planned change. While several different training models were discussed, the conference participants recognized that it would be premature to make recommendations with regard to a specific curriculum for training programs in community psychology. It was generally agreed, however, that the medical model was no longer adequate and that interdisciplinary training experiences in psychology and other social and behavioral sciences were highly desirable. The term *community psychology* was embraced at the Boston Conference in preference to *community mental health*.[1]

[1] It seems appropriate to acknowledge at this time that the term *community psychology* was apparently first used by William Rhodes, and not "coined" at the Boston Conference, as we have previously suggested (Iscoe & Spielberger, 1970). We are grateful to Jules Seeman (1975) for calling this fact to our attention.

Boston was probably the first conference at which the participants fully recognized that the mental health needs of the lower socioeconomic classes and ethnic minority groups were not being met by traditional approaches. Substantial changes in traditional roles and functions would be required if psychologists were to play an important part in improving the mental health of citizens. For those who attended, the Boston Conference was a heady experience, but it did not provide much guidance with regard to training psychologists for expanding roles and functions in community settings. The major contribution of the Boston Conference was the impetus and the momentum that it provided for many profound changes that have subsequently contributed to the evolution and development of community psychology.

FROM BOSTON TO AUSTIN: THE EVOLUTION AND DEVELOPMENT OF COMMUNITY PSYCHOLOGY

Following the Boston Conference, the feasibility of forming a division of community psychology within the structure of the American Psychological Association was discussed at a number of informal meetings. An organizational meeting was held at the 1966 APA Convention, and Division 27 was officially approved by the APA Council of Representatives at its annual meeting in September 1967. It is of historical interest to note that the majority of the charter members of Division 27 were trained in clinical psychology, and that many of them were American Board of Professional Psychology (ABPP) diplomates with responsible positions in university clinical programs and field training settings. The Division of Community Psychology has served to focus the concerns and channel the energies of community psychologists toward constructive regional and national programs. Through its *Newsletter*, monograph series, and the *American Journal of Community Psychology*, the division has stimulated communication among its members and has served as a forum for the exchange of ideas.

During the past decade, courses and practicum experiences in community psychology have dramatically increased. In several surveys conducted by Golann (1970), identifiable course content relevant to community mental health and community psychology increased from less than 20% in 1962 to 44% by 1967. A number of departments also reported "distinguishable curriculum or specialization" in community mental health and community psychology in the 1967 survey. These trends have continued, and even accelerated, during the past decade, as may be noted by examining the chapters in part V of this volume, in which current trends in training in community psychology are reviewed.

In the spring of 1967, an informal symposium on training in community psychology was held at the University of Texas at Austin. The goals of this symposium were to provide an opportunity for the exchange of ideas among psychologists who were centrally involved in directing or developing training programs in community psychology. A volume based on the Austin Symposium, *Community Psychology: Perspectives in Training and Research* (Iscoe & Spielberger, 1970), provides information on the pressing social needs that contributed to the emergence of community psychology and clarification of conceptual issues with regard to community mental health and community psychology. An increased emphasis on training in community psychology was noted within the discipline of psychology, and the needs for research to establish a knowledge base for community psychology and for community-related field-training experience were recognized. In addition, Iscoe and Spielberger (1970) describe a number of innovative community psychology training programs within psychology departments and in multidisciplinary and field-training settings.

In 1967, the Executive Committee of Division 27 appointed a Task Force on Community Mental Health, with the mandate to develop cogent position papers on critical issues in research and practice. A series of papers was presented at Loyola University in Chicago by members of the task force, and subsequently these were published in *Issues in Community Psychology and Preventive Mental Health* (Rosenblum, 1971). The Loyola papers stress the importance of prevention and intervention strategies for dealing more effectively with mental illness and for fostering mental health, and they describe emerging roles for community psychologists as conceptualizers and planners. In the summary chapter of the Loyola volume, Glidewell (1971) discusses accountability in social interventions, the breakdown of existing boundaries between psychologists and community agents, and the special responsibilities of university training programs and community training agencies:

The community, through its agents, has begun to intervene into the special social systems in which most psychologists work—universities, clinics, hospitals, laboratories. The community agents seek a greater influence over what goes on in these special systems. The psychologists may find that they are involved in collaborative social interventions with community agents whether they want to be or not. The task is to contribute to a process of reallocation of resources and power which is self-modifying in response to the consequences of each step.

Accordingly, we propose that training agencies, especially universities, but also community training agencies, give high priority to the training of psychologists competent to design, execute, and be accountable for collaborative, experimental, social interventions to facilitate the accomplishment of developmental tasks, especially with children. (p. 151)

The growth and development of community psychology was reflected in the results of two national surveys of academic and field training opportunities in community psychology and mental health that were conducted by Bloom (1972) under the sponsorship of the Division of Community Psychology. Particuarly notable was an increase of about 50% from the first to the second survey in field settings that provided training in community psychology and mental health. Bloom summarized the results of his most recent survey as follows:

In examining the content of academically-based training settings, 80% or more of the settings report significant exposure to various elements of community mental health practice, including innovative action programs, crisis intervention and case consultation. Almost as common are discussions of mental health program planning, brief psychotherapy, administrative consultation, and preventive intervention. More than half of the academic settings report significant attention to issues in the delivery and financing of mental health services, public health concepts, program descriptions at the federal, state and local levels, after-care programs, community organization, mental health education, community social system analysis, mental health program evaluation, and the relationship of social factors to emotional disorder. . . . In field settings the same general pattern prevails, i.e., major attention is directed to the technologies of community mental health practice, while fewer than 25% of the settings devote any substantial time to examination of empirical studies. (p. 1)

THE NATIONAL CONFERENCE ON TRAINING IN COMMUNITY PSYCHOLOGY: EARLY PLANNING EFFORTS

Some veterans of the Boston Conference contend that the idea for a national conference on training in community psychology was first discussed in 1965 on the bus transporting the participants from Swampscott to Logan Airport. As previously noted, the participants at the 1967 Austin Symposium recommended that a national conference on training be convened by Division 27. Soon after the formation of Division 27, the issue of a training conference was raised by its members, and this topic subsequently entered into the deliberations of the Division Executive Committee with considerable regularity. In 1970, the Division 27 Planning Committee specifically recommended convening a national conference on training in community psychology, and this recommendation was supported with highest priority by the Division Training Committee.

In response to these widespread expressions of interest in a national conference on training in community psychology, representatives of Division 27 met with NIMH staff in the spring of 1970 to explore the possibility of obtaining federal funds to hold such a conference.[2] The NIMH staff was

[2] This meeting was attended by Donald C. Klein and James G. Kelly, who were then president and president-elect of Division 27, respectively, and by Charles D. Spielberger,

encouraging, but the APA Education and Training Board was also beginning to formulate plans for a national conference, which eventually resulted in the 1973 conference at Vail. Since the APA-sponsored national conference on "Levels and Patterns of Professional Training in Psychology" would have important implications for community psychology, the Division 27 Executive Committee postponed its planning activities and encouraged its members to support the Vail Conference.

Division 27 was well represented at Vail. Its members contributed to the formation of a special interest group, which presented a series of 12 recommendations pertaining to community psychology. These recommendations were subsequently published in the *APA Division 27 Newsletter* (1974), and have served as the stimulus for several symposia and discussions at APA regional and national meetings. The Vail recommendations that pertained to community psychology follow in abridged form:

1. We recommend that the Division of Community Psychology, in concert with [other APA state and national committees and boards] develop guidelines for the diverse roles in community psychology ... for all levels of training.
2. A realistic career-ladder structure needs to be developed for community psychology from the journeyman entry level (MA degree) to the doctorate.
3. Personal competence, skills, and related experiences should be applied ... in lieu of specific academic requirements in meeting formal training requisites ... associated with designated positions in a functional career ladder.
4. Training for careers in community psychology shall be implemented via active, continuous collaboration between multiple and diverse settings such as departments of psychology, professional schools, interdisciplinary training programs, and a variety of service settings.
5. Training in community psychology at all levels and in all settings shall require appropriate competence in the critical evaluation of programs.
6. Every university training program in community psychology shall require all staff at all levels of training to participate in appropriate continuing education for the equivalent of at least two months out of every two years.
7. Community service centers shall require all staff at all levels of training to participate in continuing education programs for the equivalent of at least two months every two years.
8. A system shall be developed for an ongoing dialogue between ... the recipients of psychological services and the professionals involved in the delivery and evaluation of such services.
9. Greater emphasis shall be placed on ... expanding the scope of services to the many in society who require help. Such changes are urgently needed

---

who was serving as chairman of the APA Committee on Accreditation and as a member of the APA Education and Training Board.

if current overwhelming imbalances between need and resources are to be reduced.

10. Psychology should place greater emphasis on, and allocate more of its resources to, the study of social institutions, how they shape behavior, and how they can be modified.

11. Community psychology should devote substantial energies to training, service, and research on topics of competence and health, in contrast to the issues of psychopathology and personal incompetence.

12. Community psychology should insure that minority persons who have been disenfranchised, and who are without the traditional access to clinical and community services, have increased opportunities to receive such services. (*Newsletter*, p. 1)

During the 1970s, undergraduate (BA) and graduate (MA, PhD, PsyD) programs in community psychology were springing up all over the country, and Division 27 was continuously bombarded with questions concerning basic curriculum and practicum experiences, internships, ethical guidelines, standards for training, certification for practice, and the like. Clearly, community psychology was rapidly gaining in acceptance within the discipline of psychology, and programs described as "clinical/community," "community/ clinical," and "community/social" were beginning to appear in academic institutions. It should be noted, however, that the term *community* in many programs, as well as in job descriptions for personnel in mental health and academic settings, was often used synonymously with *community mental health* and/or *the practice of clinical psychology in community settings.*

By January of 1974, the need for a national conference on training in community psychology was strongly evident. The Division 27 Executive Committee, at its annual midwinter meeting in Chapel Hill, N.C., with Division President J. Wilbert Edgerton presiding, unanimously approved the recommendation of the Division Training Committee to hold a national conference on training in community psychology. Ira Iscoe was appointed chairman of the Conference Planning Committee and Charles D. Spielberger, president-elect of the division, was appointed liaison between the Executive Committee and the Conference Planning Committee. The Community Psychology Training Program of The University of Texas undertook the responsibility of hosting the conference. A preliminary budget of $1,000 (later increased to $3,000) was allocated for the conference, which would be held in the spring of 1975 at the University of Texas at Austin.

The chairman of the Conference Planning Committee was urged to submit an application to NIMH by the March 1, 1974, deadline. Despite the time constraints, this application was duly prepared and submitted to the NIMH Behavioral Sciences Training Branch. If NIMH funds could be obtained, a large conference could be held with broad representations of minority groups and graduate students. If federal funds were not forthcoming, the conference would be smaller, the division would absorb the administrative costs, and participants would be asked to obtain their own travel funds. The time for a national conference on training in community psychology had come at last!

REFERENCES

American Psychological Association. Recommended standards for training counseling psychologists at the doctorate level. (Northwestern Conference) *American Psychologist*, 1952, 7, 175-188.

APA Division of Community Psychology Newsletter, February 1974, 5(2), 1.

Bennett, C. C., Anderson, L. S., Cooper, S., Hassol, L., Klein, D. C., & Rosenblum, G. *Community psychology: A report of the Boston conference on the education of psychologists for community mental health.* Boston: Boston University, 1966.

Bloom, B. L. *Training opportunities in community psychology and mental health.* Boulder: University of Colorado, 1972.

Cowen, E. L., Gardner, A., & Zax, M. *Emergent approaches to mental health problems.* New York: Appleton-Century-Crofts, 1967.

Cutts, N. E. *School psychologists at mid-century* (Thayer Conference). Washington, D.C.: American Psychological Association, 1955.

Glidewell, J. Priorities for psychologists in community mental health. In G. Rosenblum (Ed.), *Issues in community psychology and preventive mental health.* New York: Behavioral Publications, 1971.

Golann, S. E. Community psychology and mental health: An analysis of strategies and a survey of training. In I. Iscoe & C. D. Spielberger (Eds.), *Community psychology: Perspectives in training and research.* New York: Appleton-Century-Crofts, 1970.

Hoch, L., Ross, A., & Winder, C. L. *Professional preparation of clinical psychologists.* Washington, D.C.: American Psychological Asosciation, 1966.

Iscoe, I., & Spielberger, C. D. (Eds.). *Community psychology: Perspectives in training and research.* New York: Appleton-Century-Crofts, 1970.

Korman, M. National conference on levels and patterns of professional training in psychology: The major themes. *American Psychologist*, 1974, 29, 441-449.

Lloyd, D. N., & Newbrough, J. R. Previous conferences on graduate education in psychology: A summary and review. In E. L. Hoch, A. O. Ross, & C. L. Winder (Eds.), *Professional preparation of clinical psychologists.* Washington, D.C.: American Psychological Association, 1966.

Raimy, V. C. (Ed.). *Training in clinical psychology.* New York: Prentice-Hall, 1950.

Roe, A., Gustad, J. W., Moore, B. V., Ross, S., & Skodak, M. (Eds.). *Graduate education in psychology* (Miami Conference). Washington, D.C.: American Psychological Association, 1959.

Rosenblum, G. *Issues in community psychology and preventive mental health.* New York: Behavioral Publications, 1971.

Sarason, S. B., Levine, M., Goldenberg, I. I., Cherlin, D. L., & Bennett, E. M. *Psychology in community settings.* New York: John Wiley & Sons, Inc., 1966.

Seeman, J. The term community psychology. *American Psychologist*, 1975, *30*, 863.

Spielberger, C. D., & Iscoe, I. The current status of training in community psychology. In I. Iscoe & C. D. Spielberger (Eds.), *Community psychology: Perspectives in training and research*. New York: Appleton-Century-Crofts, 1970.

Strother, C. R. *Psychology and mental health* (Stanford Conference). Washington, D.C.: American Psychological Association, 1956.

Thompson, A. S., & Super, D. E. (Eds.). *The professional preparation of counseling psychologists—Report of the 1964 Greystone Conference.* New York: Teachers College, Columbia University, 1964.

Zax, M., & Specter, G. A. *An introduction to community psychology.* New York: John Wiley & Sons, Inc., 1974.

2 Planning and Monitoring the Conference

Ira Iscoe and Bernard L. Bloom

The application to NIMH for funds adequate to support a conference stressed the rapid expansion of community psychology training programs. Also stressed was the reality that 10 years after the Boston Conference, community psychology was finding itself with a proliferation of training programs at various academic levels, a growing divisional membership, and increasing demands for clarity regarding roles and functions of community psychology and community psychologists. The purpose of the proposed conference was to look at the crucial theoretical, definitional, curriculum, and training issues that had to be faced.

The proposed conference was in this sense similar to conferences that educational, clinical, and school psychology had held at certain key periods in their development, which had enabled them to define and develop training models, viable curricula, and field training experiences. The projected format emphasized the identification of the diverse models of community psychology training that had evolved in the preceding 10 years. The budget request stressed that the great bulk of the funds would be used for emerging community psychology programs, with the presumption that more established programs would be able to handle the expenses of their representatives. The application further noted that special efforts were to be employed to find support for ethnic minority group members. A portion of the funds was to be used to support the attendance of promising graduate students in a variety of programs, settings, and levels.

At the APA meeting in New Orleans in September 1974, the Executive and Training Committee met with representatives of the NIMH Training Branch in an informal site visit on the grant request. An addendum to the grant proposal was submitted later that month, and late in January 1975, the good news of funding was received. With the NIMH grant of nearly $13,000, it became possible to expand plans for the conference. Division 27 and the Hogg Foundation for Mental Health of the University of Texas made contributions; the Community Psychology Program at the University of Texas allotted funds to the conference and assumed a generous proportion of the secretarial and clerical expenses.

DEVELOPING THE CONFERENCE AGENDA

The Planning Committee wanted, at all costs, to avoid giving the impression that this was to be a meeting to settle all problems. Input from the

17

membership made it clear that the guiding principle should be the articulation of training approaches and goals. The selection of participants, therefore, was in part predicated on their ability to make substantial contributions to these issues. The main focus of this conference was to be on the PhD-level community psychologist.

The Planning Committee also was aware that since the founding of Division 27, a number of persons interested in the area had had only limited opportunities to interact with each other. A new generation had emerged since 1965, a generation that had come through a variety of training programs and experiences. It was of primary importance to get these people together and let them meet informally as well as formally. While it was important to facilitate dialogue, it was also necessary to emerge with appropriate written documents as a guide to the future of community psychology training and to make sure that the younger members were thoroughly informed of the rationale for the main recommendations of the conference.

The so-called grandfathers (there were no grandmothers at Boston) were to be prepared to pass the mantle of responsibility on to younger persons. Better representation of females and ethnic minorities was to be sought at all levels of divisional functions. The planners were acutely aware that a community psychology without adequate representation and full participation by ethnic minorities would be and should be suspect.

SELECTION OF CONFERENCE PARTICIPANTS

Too large a conference becomes difficult to keep goal directed, while too small a conference runs the danger of narrowness of input and charges of elitism and cronyism. In setting up guidelines for the selection of participants, the Executive and Planning Committees considered a number of factors, including the need to involve younger persons, graduate students, ethnic minorities, and women. The identification of training as the central issue in the grant request constituted an important determinant in the selection criteria. The general thrust was to begin a constructive consideration of salient issues related to the training of students in community psychology.

At their January 1975 meeting, the Executive and Conference Planning Committees decided to limit the number of conferees, exclusive of the University of Texas at Austin delegation and special guests, to a maximum of about 80. In a deliberate effort to democratize representation and to make sure that younger community psychologists were well represented, guidelines were developed of roughly 20% new PhDs (0-6 years after graduation), including postdoctorals; 20% intermediate level (7-15 years); 20% senior level (15 years or more); 20% graduate students; 10% observers and members of funding agencies; 5% representatives of APA and Special Boards; and 5% special categories. The committees also sought as much of a balance as possible between academic and field training situations.

PRECONFERENCE MATERIALS

In addition, the committee determined that background readings, position statements, and other materials should be assembled and made available to participants prior to the conference. This collection of preconference materials represented a concerted effort to strike a balance among: (1) the substantive areas of interest and concern of conference participants, (2) the group responsible for planning and organizing the conference, (3) the materials submitted by the members and friends of Division 27 for possible inclusion in the volume, and (4) a little reality testing about how voluminous the document ought to be.

The two most commonly expressed needs were reasonably well discussed in the preconference materials. These were issues related to academic, university-based training models in community psychology, and issues in field training and in the optimal integration of field and academic training. There was somewhat less material pertinent to the third most commonly mentioned interest—the area of the ethics of social intervention and community-based research. For another commonly expressed interest—the level-of-entry problem, that is, the issue of undergraduate, AB, MA, and PhD preparation in community psychology—there were some useful and pertinent papers.

But there were four common areas of interest expressed by potential conference participants for which little or no material was available: (1) continuing education and postdoctoral training in community psychology; (2) the role of community psychology in the formulation of social and public policy; (3) employment opportunities and the issues of reimbursement for services, and (4) applied research and program evaluation training. In addition, there were some topics that relatively few conference participants mentioned, but for which considerable material was submitted: the role of the community psychologist in the planning of human service delivery systems and in the delivery of human services; social ecology and community analysis; and primary intervention. Finally, other topics were mentioned infrequently and little material was submitted. This list included (1) the functioning of the community psychologist in specialized settings, that is, minority communities or the university community; (2) interdisciplinary functioning and territoriality; (3) licensing and certification of community psychologists; (4) accreditation of community psychology training programs; (5) sources of funding support for training programs; and (6) criteria for the selection of students for admission into community psychology training programs.

There is something to be learned from these matches and mismatches. Topics mentioned relatively infrequently may well become more salient in the coming years. Commonly mentioned issues for which little pertinent material was available may serve to identify areas for future conceptual and empirical development. And those topics for which more material was available than appeared necessary may well be on their way out as centrally important to the field of community psychology.

It is perhaps a measure of the usefulness of the preconference materials that people are still requesting copies. Unfortunately, the supply has long since been exhausted, but the table of contents of the book of preconference materials appears in appendix B. The preconference materials included descriptions of 25 community psychology training programs. Each of these programs was described along the following seven dimensions: ideology and value base, goals and objectives, units of study, knowledge and research base, technology and skills required, content area, and format for training. These seven dimensions plus others were later incorporated in a guideline for training model construction used by the conference in its discussions of training approaches.

THE CONFERENCE PARTICIPANTS

Despite the efforts to "hold the line," more people attended the conference than had originally been planned, but the number was kept within a reasonable limit so that full participation and interaction was possible. Table 1 shows the distribution of participants according to years of experience (not including University of Texas graduate students and faculty), while Table 2 gives the ethnic minority distribution of participants.

About 50% of the PhD participants had graduated within the preceding six years. There were about 20% graduate students, exclusive of those from the University of Texas. Attempts at ethnic minority representation were gratifying; attempts at balancing sex distribution were most successful at the graduate student level and less so with increasing years of experience. This is an accurate reflection of the recent increase in the number of women entering the field. About 40% of the participants were in primarily academic settings, 30% were in field settings, and another 30% were classified as academic/field. This third category was used to classify participants who were primarily involved in teaching but who also had considerable responsibilities in field activities such as directing evaluation studies, consultation, training, and program planning. The majority in this category were in the younger group, and the category as a whole indicates the linkage between academic settings and field activities. As a historical note, 11 of the participants had also attended the Boston Conference.

TABLE 1 Participants by years of experience

| | | Years past PhD | | |
	Students	0–6	7–15	15+
Male	13	35	21	23
Female	11	16	2	1
Total	24	51	23	24

TABLE 2   Ethnic minority distribution of participants

	Students[a]		0–6		7–15		15+		
	Male	Female	Male	Female	Male	Female	Male	Female	Total
Black	3	5	4	5	5		1		23
Mexican-American	6	3	1	1	1				12
Asiatic			2						2
Puerto Rican	1			1	1				3

[a]Includes University of Texas graduate students.

PRECONFERENCE ORIENTATION

The preconference materials, edited by Bernard Bloom, stressed that no single meeting could even begin to settle the many problems and issues that had emerged in community psychology in the preceding 10 years. A start had to be made somewhere, and the planners recognized the impatience expressed by some about the failure to come up with a clear definition of community psychology and its relevant parameters. They stressed that community psychology, like many other areas of psychology, was going to face some difficult times and that training programs in the future would have to take into account variables that had not been considered by other conferences. These variables included a contracting rather than an expanding economy, the rise of paraprofessionalism, and an increased questioning of the efficacy of psychological approaches to major social problems such as violence, crime, juvenile delinquency, and integration, to mention only a few of the more prominent ones. Some excerpts from one section of the preconference materials (entitled "Some Perspectives") follow:

While at the Boston Conference (in 1965) there were no directors of community psychology training programs per se, the Austin Conference will have at least seven directors of programs entitled Community Psychology, plus many from programs entitled Community Mental Health and Community-Clinical, besides specialized programs in the community area such as Social Ecology, Urban Psychology. . . . While community psychology is beginning to declare its ideological independence from community mental health, we are informed about upcoming cuts in research and training and that positions in psychology (but not necessarily in community psychology) at the PhD level will be harder to come by. The mood of the country has changed and graduate education is undergoing careful scrutiny. . . . Professional schools have emerged, and these, too, have to be considered in the training strategy. Clinical psychology training programs are undergoing painful changes, and all programs related to human services are reconsidering their thrusts, goals, and areas of functioning. Many of them are under attack for failing to deliver in the human benefit area.

FORMAL ASPECTS OF THE CONFERENCE

The Planning Committee and Executive Committee, in following the decision to focus on training, its issues and problems, used the construction of training models as a vehicle. In addition to the parameters of the models described, each participant was urged to think about the following questions, many of them related to the approach to training that they had selected and that would be considered at the conference: (1) What are the constraints to an ideal program? Given clear signs of a changing picture in terms of employment and training support, what new arrangements for support of graduate students should we be thinking about? (2) What are new sources of field training support if internship money begins to fade? (3) Where will or should community psychologists as community psychologists be employed? What are the possibilities at the local, state, and federal levels separate from mental health endeavors at these same levels? What unique skills could community psychologists bring to various positions, in contrast to those brought by people in administration or organizational development? (4) What is the relation of continuing education to field training? (5) The level of entry is a vexing question but one that community psychology has to face. What does an MA-level psychologist do, for example, in contrast to a PhD- or BA-level community psychologist? Who should be called a community psychologist?

SUMMARY

Judging from informal and formal feedback, the great majority of the participants considered the Austin Conference a significant event in which community psychology at last came of age. Morale was strengthened by the opportunity to share worries about ambiguity and complexities of varied approaches with others struggling with the same problems. The "spirit of Austin" carried beyond the meetings. A three-hour session at APA in Chicago, September 1975, was well attended, and it convinced skeptics that the enthusiasm generated at Austin had not dissipated. Some of this enthusiasm is apparent in the papers—some presented at the conference and others based on discussions that took place—that compose the rest of this volume.

II KEYNOTES: ON THE IDEOLOGY OF COMMUNITY PSYCHOLOGY

INTRODUCTION

Bernard L. Bloom

The process of selection of keynote speakers for a national conference aspiring to have a significant impact on an emerging field of endeavor is a simple one. One need merely identify speakers who are brilliant, visionary, thoughtful, provocative, inspirational, and properly hortatory—in short, the true leaders of the field.

We were enormously fortunate in securing four such persons for the National Training Conference in Community Psychology. Their presentations were scheduled at critical moments throughout the conference. The first three keynote presentations—those of Seymour B. Sarason, Robert Reiff, and James G. Kelly—are in this initial section. The fourth, by Jack Glidewell, is placed in context at the start of the next section.

Sarason, Reiff, and Kelly pointed out the limitations of our concepts and knowledge and dared us to take a breathless leap into that strange territory known as the community. To keep us from feeling lost, they provided us with valuable guideposts—important values and ideologies, a sense of direction, and the commitment of mutual support. They asked us to be Mr. Everyman and more. They asked us to try to understand the networks within which we and the other members of our communities function. They asked us to help build new networks, both in the university and in the community at large, and to help sustain those that already exist as well as those that are new. They asked us to look with our intellects, our hearts, and our fidelity at our communities and their potential for good. And they told us that it would not be easy, but that we would not be alone.

3 Community Psychology, Networks, and Mr. Everyman

Seymour B. Sarason

From the fall of 1961 when the decision was made to create the Yale Psycho-Educational Clinic, we were confronted with a question that came up repeatedly throughout the years the clinic existed: Since those of us who were starting the clinic were all traditionally trained clinical psychologists, what consequences would that have on the fact that we had no intention of remaining in traditional clinical roles or providing the usual clinical services? The question came up with regularity because it involved the relationship among our past, present, and future professional identities. It was a threatening question because one way of answering it meant severing ourselves at least partially from our professional and intellectual pasts as well as experiencing the tortures, anxieties, and excitement of starting a new life. This, undoubtedly, is an overdramatic way of putting it because the truth is that we only dimly sensed, particularly in the early years of the clinic, what was at stake. I think what really happened is that we were fully aware that we were changing fast in terms of accustomed roles and jargon, but we did not comprehend the conceptual implications of these changes.

When a marriage partner comes to the realization that he or she must get a divorce, it sometimes is experienced as a shock, but after a little reflection the person "understands" that the conscious decision had long been building up, that over the years there were symptoms that now were organized into a syndrome about which action had to be taken. I deliberately use the divorce analogy to make three points: Divorce is usually painful; its consequences are unpredictable; and once the decision for divorce is made, perception of internal and external reality undergoes radical change. Divorce can be the best thing for the parties concerned, and with the passage of years they may even be able to see this as well as to recognize that a part of each is bound to the other—and a basis for a mutually satisfying friendship emerges. So I suggest

From "Community Psychology, Networks and Mr. Everyman" by S. B. Sarason, *American Psychologist*, 1976, *13*, 317–328. Copyright 1976 by the American Psychological Association. Reprinted by permission.

This chapter was facilitated by the support and atmosphere of two sources: Yale's Institution for Social and Policy Studies, and the tri-university "network" initiated by Dr. Saul Cohen of Clark University. I am also indebted to Elizabeth Meyer Lorentz, who in different ways stimulated me to think more carefully about networks.

the divorce of community psychology from the community mental health movement because I have come to believe that it ultimately will have productive consequences for both and, more important, for our society. It is not my intention to polarize, to assert the superiority of one over the other, or, heaven forbid, to plant a flag of possession on new academic turf. If what follows is in a personal vein, it is because I think it is the best way to convey larger issues. It is apparent, I hope, that this call for a divorce is not from the vantage point of a blameless past. If you find divorce an unacceptable or precipitous action, I am willing to compromise with an interlocutory decree.

In the first year of the clinic, our building housed Murray Levine, Michael Kahn, Esther Sarason, and myself. (There was, of course, our secretary, Anita Miller, who was born to the community game.) The title *clinic* is misleading, because whatever we did or hoped to do required that we work in other people's settings. Most of the time Anita was the only person in the building. But the other four of us did meet one morning of the week to share our thoughts and plans. Those were difficult meetings. For one thing, we were not clear about what services we could provide. For another, nobody was really asking for our services. Of course, if we had said we were going to provide diagnostic and therapeutic functions, life would have been easy. But the one thing we were clear about was that we did not want to provide these services, not because such services are unimportant or unnecessary—they are vital and socially meaningful—but because they were quintessentially clinical; that is, problems had to exist and be brought somewhere for solution. What we wished to do was to figure out ways of preventing problems or, at least, to prevent them from becoming serious or insoluble ones. If we were unclear or even naive about how to think and act in regard to what we might do, we were quite clear and realistic about the manpower problem: Our society did not possess nor would it ever possess the professional resources to deal with troubled individuals. Put another way, as long as we define the problems of individuals in a way so as to require solution by highly trained professionals, the gap between "supply" and "demand" becomes scandalously greater with time. I suppose I must emphasize that I believe that any troubled individual deserves the services of a clinician who is experienced and well trained, and I would argue vehemently against any proposal to reduce the number of clinically trained professionals. At the same time, I would argue just as heatedly against anyone who maintains that we can ever train clinicians in other than miniscule numbers relative to defined needs. In fact, I consider as ignorant, socially irresponsible, and possessed of astigmatic tunnel vision anyone who says that the only way to deal with troubled individuals is through the services of highly educated professionals. In starting the clinic, we were not going to go the clinical route.

So there we were, a small group of clinical psychologists intent on not going the clinical route. As we added staff we gained, among others, more clinically trained people (e.g., Ira Goldenberg, Frances Kaplan Grossman,

Dennis Cherlin, N. Dickon Reppucci, and Edison Trickett). From what other pool of professionals could we choose? We chose from a familiar pool, but in each case the person was, in varying degrees, eager to depart from the clinical model. In the early years of the clinic I regarded myself as a clinical psychologist venturing forth into new areas, conceptual and geographical. After all, I was intent on helping, and if my goal was to help change settings in some vague way, was it not the case that I had to do this through individuals? In those days the label *community psychologist* was hardly used, and besides, how would you define it for those who asked? But I was also uncomfortable in saying I was a clinical psychologist because it would mystify people who wanted to know our patient load, where it came from, how we worked, and what our administrative structure was. When I would tell them we had no patient load, no psychiatric consultants, no social workers, but that some of us worked in schools, neighborhood employment centers, skill centers, regional centers for the mentally retarded, and day care centers, our questioners were both enlightened and mystified. They were enlightened because it sounded as if we were consultants and that is a familiar role (although when we said that that label did not cover our active participation in the affairs of these settings, we could expect a series of questions about what we "really" did and why). They were mystified because many of them knew we were trained clinical psychologists, and understandably, could not square that fact with what we said we were doing.

It is only in retrospect that I can see the earliest events that should have signaled more clearly than they did that I was headed for an identity crisis, that is, that I was beginning to separate myself, conceptually and professionally, from clinical psychology and the mental health movement. (The divorce was on its way.) The first signal came the year before the clinic formally opened, when we sought NIMH research support to allow us to study the culture of the school via different ways of being in a helping role in the schools. You well know that grant requests require, and understandably so, that you specify what you are going to do and why and the significance of the outcomes for existing knowledge. We had a variety of intensive experiences in schools, but they were not geared to the problem of understanding the culture of the schools. Essentially, what we proposed was to view the schools as a South Pacific island that we wanted to observe, become participants in its activities, and see where it all took us. This was both a congenial and an important approach for me because a decade earlier I had had the opportunity to work most intimately with an anthropologist, Dr. Thomas Gladwin, and one of the many things I learned from that collaboration (I interpreted the projective tests) was that understanding a community involved bodies of knowledge, concepts, and modes of action quite different from those on which the mental health professions were based (Gladwin & Sarason, 1953). What I contributed to that collaboration was considered valuable, and it may even be that I did illuminate some aspects of the Trukese as individuals. But if you read that monograph, I am sure you will agree that I did not illuminate very much about the Trukese community. After all, if as a clinical psychologist I was interested in what I thought was going on in their heads, it is no wonder that I could not place those heads in the larger social context. Gladwin was interested in the community, and I was interested in individuals, and we saw the world quite differently, thank God. It was not that one view was better than the other but that they had radically different consequences depending on what one wanted to understand, and increasingly but preconsciously I wanted to understand the social complexity of communities.

We wrote the grant request in an honest way, by which I mean that we recognized the ambiguities of our methodology and conceptual rationale. We wanted to understand schools in order better to see how and at what points they could be changed to prevent the myriad problems for which existing and future manpower were woefully, if not scandalously, inadequate. We were site visited by a group of mental health professionals who obviously were troubled by our request. In general they were sympathetic to us, less because they understood what we were about and more because they respected us as clinical psychologists. Try as we might, we could not convince them that we were dealing with a complexity that no one truly understood, in which the mental health professions in particular and the social sciences in general had little interest, and the nature of which would have increasing significance for our society. What we were saying, in effect, was that the mental health professions were parochial and somewhat socially irresponsible; that is, their methods, theories, and focuses were too acultural and individually oriented. Our grant request was tabled, and we were asked to rewrite and resubmit it. And so we did. And we had another site visit. And we went through the same discussion. And our grant request was denied. In my more charitable moments I could entertain the possibility that they were right for the wrong reasons. The point of all this is that we and they were thinking in radically different ways. They were thinking in the context of theories of and practices about individuals while we, superficially to be sure, were thinking in terms of intrasystem dynamics, power-political characteristics, social history, and the nature of tradition.

Another event that heightened my developing identity crisis was a growing tendency on my part to view the development of the clinic from a community-ecological perspective rather than from an individual-clinical perspective. This development was deceptively personal and initiated by this question: How would I explain that two years after the clinic started, our building housed about 20 people engaged in a variety of ways in diverse settings in our part of the state? Whereas in the first year the clinic was a lonely place populated by a handful of people worried about survival, within two years it was overpopulated with people, each of whom was dividing his or her time in at least two community settings. The question I asked myself had surprisingly little to do with value judgments. Of course, I thought this growth was a good thing, but that was a very minor stimulus for the question. (I knew that whatever we did would be in the record and that whatever judgments people would make they would make.) The major stimulus was a gnawing dissatisfaction with the answers that others spontaneously gave, that is, answers centering around my personality and ideas. It was not undue modesty on my part if I felt the answers to be typically clinical or individualistic and, therefore, misleadingly incomplete—not wrong, but incomplete in an instructive way. For example, very few people put weight in their answers on the fact that I was a full professor when the clinic started. Statistically speaking, the chances of a nontenured faculty person being "allowed" to start such a venture—at Yale or any other university—and to have it grow rather quickly are small indeed. Wrapped up in this fact are a set of considerations rooted in the traditions, history, organization, and values of the American university that are independent of individuals and personalities and that are the warp and woof in which faculty are embedded, developed, and changed. It is understandable if we put undue weight on individuals because we literally can "see" and interact with them. In that sense we cannot see the social fabric in which the individual is embedded and, therefore, we are prone to misevaluate its significance for what we are trying to explain. And the more clinical we are in our thinking and actions, the less we see the larger picture or the social fabric. The individual tends to be figure and all else ground, and we are not even aware that there is a ground. And the kind of ground I am talking about can never be seen; it has to be conceptualized, and the basis for the conceptualization is in fields other than psychology. At the very least, they are conceptualizations that can never come out of clinical psychology or the community mental health movement.

A second factor that the usual explanation ignored consists of two "variables." The first is that Connecticut is a small place; that is, one can rather easily see and know the state. It is graspable in an experiential sense. You can know it in a way that you will never know New York State if you live in New York City or Syracuse or Buffalo. The second variable that people overlooked is that I had lived and worked in Connecticut since 1942, part of the time in a state institution in a rural area and the rest of the time in and around New Haven. If you live in a small state for almost two decades—in roles requiring you to have all kinds of commerce with individuals and agencies near and far (although nothing and no one is "far" in Connecticut)—the chances are high that you are part of or know about scores of networks of people and agencies. It was this kind of knowledge that was important, if not crucial, in the creation and quick growth of the clinic.

Geographical size, work roles, status, institutions and their traditions, and age—awareness of these and similar factors increasingly forced me to see the difference between clinical-type or personality-type explanations, on the one hand, and what I will loosely call a community-ecological explanation, on the other hand. I must reiterate that these are not inherently antithetical polarities, especially in regard to the type of question I was asking. But it is unfortunately the case that in practice they emerge as polarities, and my experience has impressed upon me the limitations of the clinical mode of thinking rather than the community-ecological one.

Because the distinction I am trying to make is so crucial and can easily be misinterpreted, I ask you to consider how clinical psychology and the community mental health movement has reacted to the work of Roger Barker and his colleagues (e.g., Barker, 1963b; Barker, 1968; Barker & Gump, 1964; Barker & Wright, 1951). One way of putting it is: How can you react to what you do not know? (This point has also been made by James Kelly, 1975, in his review of a recent book by Barker & Schoggen, 1973.) If those in the movement have known about it—and examination after examination of relevant bibliographies suggests they do not—they obviously see no relevance for it in their work. This reaction is not hard to understand because the studies by Barker and his colleagues of a small midwestern community have by theory and design little or no focus on individuals, their psyches and problems. Their focus has been on collectivities, behavior settings, physical environments, ecological interrelationships, and the like. If, for example, you were to read one of their books devoted only to one boy's day (Barker & Wright, 1951), you would likely be overwhelmed by the details, all uninterpreted, and you might end up puzzled by what the point of it all is, especially if you are a clinical psychologist or even a community mental health professional. In fact, most of their reports are in the form of compendia of descriptions and analyses that are difficult for anyone to follow or to digest. But what makes it so difficult for the psychological reader is not only the form of their presentation, but the absence of what we ordinarily call psychological data. We are so used to seeing individuals and fathoming what is going on in their heads that we are unable even to conceive that there are other ways of viewing these situations. For example, in 1963 Barker delivered the Kurt Lewin Memorial Award Address in Philadelphia. Most of us have been to similar meetings, and when we have talked about them it has been in purely psychological terms: the kind of person being honored, his reaction, style and content of address, our response, audience reaction, etc. Barker (1963a) had this to say:

It is not often that a lecturer can present to his audience an example of his phenomena, whole and functioning in situ—not merely with a demonstration, a description, a preserved specimen, a picture, or a diagram of it. I am in the fortunate position of being able to give you, so to speak, a real behavior setting.

If you will change your attention from me to the next most inclusive, bounded unit, to the assembly of people, behavior episodes, and objects before you, you will see a behavior setting. It has the following structural attributes which you can observe directly:

1. It has a space-time locus: 3:00–3:50 p.m., September 2, 1963, Clover Room, Bellevue-Stratford Hotel, Philadelphia, Pennsylvania.
2. It is composed of a variety of interior entities and events: of people, objects (chairs, walls, a microphone paper), behavior (lecturing, listening, sitting), and other processes (air circulation, sound amplification).
3. Its widely different components form a bounded pattern that is easily discriminated from the pattern on the outside of the boundary.
4. Its component parts are obviously not a random arrangement of independent classes of entities; if they were, how surprising, that all the chairs are in the same position with respect to the podium, that all members of the audience happen to come to rest upon chairs, and that the lights are not helter-skelter from floor to ceiling, for example.
5. The entity before you is a part of a nesting structure; its components (e.g., the chairs and people) have parts; and the setting, itself, is contained within a more comprehensive unit, the Bellevue-Stratford Hotel.
6. This unit is objective in the sense that it exists independently of anyone's perception of it, qua unit. (pp. 26–27)

Barker was illustrating his central concept of a behavior setting: a naturally occurring unit having physical, behavioral, and temporal properties, and one revealing a variety of complex interrelationships among its parts. That is to say, there is a way of looking at a behavior setting that is illuminating, independent of individual personalities. Someone might ask: Illuminating of what? I could answer by saying that at the very least Barker's approach reminds us, and we always need this reminding, that our accustomed ways of reacting to and conceptualizing about familiar situations are no more than that: accustomed ways. There are other ways. But another part of the answer is that Barker's overarching goal is to look at and describe a total community: its parts, interrelatedness, structure, ecological balances, and processes. The community, which is amorphous ground for most of us, is figure for Barker. If he ever wanted to waste time answering the question of why our clinic grew so quickly, his answer would be radically different than the ones ordinarily given.

I have talked about Barker and his work of several decades in one American and one British town not because I am convinced that he has provided us with the most productive conceptual basis for a community psychology. I am not so convinced, although the recent papers by Price (1974) and Price and Blashfield (1975) do indicate the fruitfulness of Barker's work for community psychology. The significance of Barker's work is fourfold. He did take on the awesome task of studying a community. He has provided us with fresh insights about familiar settings, for example, schools. And, not surprisingly for someone who is in the Gestalt tradition, he has emphasized interrelatedness. Lastly, the theoretical and empirical traditions (ecology, Gestalt psychology) that are the underpinnings of his work are not those of the community mental health movement, a fact that when pursued exposes the flimsy and parochial underpinnings of the community movement. In Sarason (1974) I devote several chapters to the social-historical context that more or less guaranteed that the conceptual base for the emerging community mental health movement would be at best disastrously parochial and at worst conceptually bankrupt. Like it or not, modern clinical psychology and psychiatry—and their offspring, community mental health— arose as a rather quick response to social needs (and governmental funding), and that type of situation is rarely conducive to dispassionate reflection, planning, and decision making. But more of this later.

What I propose to do now is to elaborate on a concept I mentioned earlier and have come to see as a crucial one for a community psychology that purports either to understand or to help change aspects of community functioning. The concept is that of the network. Initially at least, it appears simple enough, and it is explicitly or implicitly used by us in our daily lives as well as formally in a variety of disciplines. If the significance of the concept of networks was forced upon me by my reflections on the growth of the clinic and its varied activities, it is another example of how we conspire with life to reinvent the wheel. Ironically, it is a concept central to the thinking and practice of clinical psychologists who always see their clients as embedded in a network of interpersonal relationships, and the overarching goal of practice as in some way or other either to use the network for therapeutic purposes or to change the quality and quantity of relationships within the network. But when mental health professionals enlarged their activities to include communities, they were utterly unprepared to deal with the fact that a community is, among other things, composed of related and unrelated networks of relationships, each of which can be ordered along a number of dimensions, for example, vocational, religious, political, recreational, neighborhood, charitable, educational. I am not restricting the concept of network to organized or formal groupings that by custom, law, or choice bring their members into relationship with each other even though that may not require or entail face-to-face contact or any contact at all. For example, as a member of the American Psychological Association I actually know a miniscule number of its thousands of members. But I know who those thousands are (there is a directory), where they live, what their proclaimed interests are, and a few of their demographic characteristics. When I get mail from the APA, I know they are getting the same mail. When I pay dues, they pay dues. I know some of the journals some of them read. I know who participates in the different activities and functions of the association. So when I say that I am a member of the APA, I am saying that I am a member of a very large network, most members of which I do not personally know but with all of whom I could be in contact if I so desired. If, for example, I were to take a 5% random sample of the APA and write each person a letter beginning with the words, "As a fellow member of the APA I am writing to seek your help in disbanding the organization," I can assume that each of the recipients would not question my right "to call upon" them, although they may have doubts about my personal stability. Ordinarily, neither I nor they would think about ourselves as part of a network—one thinks of oneself as a member of a large, impersonal collectivity that can do things for us as individuals—but it takes the kind of letter I would write to remind us that we can do things for each other, at the very least we can "call upon" each other. The truth is that if I wanted to achieve my goal I would never write to a random sample of the APA. Some people in the network are more influential than others in the sense that if they take a stance they can garner more support than others who may hold the same position. My task is to find out who these people are and which of them may respond congenially to my plea for support. The point is that however I proceed, I am assuming that I feel I have a right to proceed and that those whom I will contact will perceive this contact as right and proper; that is, I can call on them for knowledge and support as they can call on me.

But now imagine that I have chosen a 5% random sample of the American Psychiatric Association and I write to them saying, "I am a member of the American Psychological Association and I am writing to secure your support for the disbanding of the American Psychiatric Association." The prepotent response would be "Who the hell are you to contact me about such an outrageous suggestion?" I am not in their network, and I have no warrant to call upon them for help. I am an outsider. But am I an outsider? I do know a number of psychiatrists. We are part of a network independent of all other networks in which we are embedded.[1] How do I use that network to find out how I should go about locating people in "the other APA" who may be congenial to my purposes? The psychologist-psychiatrist network of which I am a part extends over a wide geographical area, but relatively speaking it is very small. Are there other networks of which I am a part or to which I can potentially relate that can provide me with more knowledge and potential support? The answer, of course, is yes. If it were my major passion in life, I could tap scores of, if not countless, existing networks in order to gain knowledge and support from within and without the American Psychiatric Association. All of this, I presume, is obvious enough. *What is not so obvious, however, is that in the process of pursuing my goal, I very likely will have become part of new and existing networks.*

But why use the term *network*? Would not *relations* or *interrelationships* serve as well? Or *contacts*? The difficulty with these terms is that in ordinary

---

[1] There is a real question about whether *any* network is independent of all other networks. That is to say, however stringently one defines a network, I think it is possible to show that each person in that network is part of another network, and in that sense one network is not independent of all others. When I have taken pencil to paper to map out the networks of actual people of widely different statuses in the community, I could in each case demonstrate that each person could, if she or he wanted, relate to any other network I could dream up.

parlance they refer to an actual connection among two or more people, whereas the term *network* includes such connections and in addition emphasizes that they are an extremely small sample of connections potentially available to us. The different visual pictures that our minds conjure up when we use the terms *network* and *relationships* reflect the kind of differences I am trying to convey. A further advantage of the term *network*, as I used it in regard to my membership in "our" APA, is that it forces on us the awareness that we are part of many networks, in each of which we have call upon others whether or not we know them in the sense of actually having had some sort of commerce with them. In any one network a wide discrepancy usually exists between the number of people potentially available to us and the number we actually know.

Just as I was writing the above paragraph a student came into my office. He is in a seminar that Dick Reppucci and I are teaching entitled "Policy and Management Issues in Human Services Institutions." The students have been divided into four groups, each of which is devoted to a different problem they are to investigate. Each group must write a sizeable report. This student is part of the group working on deinstitutionalization.

Him: Our group wants to interview state senator _____. Do you know her?

Me: No.

Him: Do you know anybody at Yale who knows her?

Me: I assume, knowing where she lives, that there are a number of Yale people who know her. But at the moment I can't think of anyone who knows her and would be willing to run interference for you. I could call her up, but God knows how many days it would take for us to connect. And even if we connected I am not sure she would go out of her way to make herself available to your group in the next few days.

As he left the office and I began again to think about networks, it suddenly hit me that sitting in my outer office was, of course, Anita Miller, whose father is very much a part of a state political network of which state senator _____ is a member. Anita and I are "related," but if I had not at that moment been thinking about differentiating between a network and a relationship, I would not have "seen" Anita as having easy access to a network by no means easily available to me. And that is the point: It is natural to think of people with whom we interact in terms of relationship. It is not natural to see them as part of numerous networks. You can see people. You cannot see networks.

If you begin to apply the concept of the network to a community, it becomes immediately apparent that a community is composed of networks countless in number and probably countless in degree of interconnectedness.

The traditional bases for describing and understanding a community—social class, economic, legal, religious, political, governmental, etc.—have obviously been productive, and it is not my intention in any way to underplay their importance. Indeed, it is my opinion that we have not used such variables in the most productive ways precisely because we tend not to view or understand them in their interrelatedness. I venture the hypothesis that if we were to begin to view the community in terms of networks we would begin to get a better picture of this interrelatedness. At the very least, we would have to confront more realistically than we have that a community is impressively, if not overwhelmingly, complex and that our traditional ways of thinking about and dealing with it have not taken this complexity into account. It would also become apparent that the view of the community that has powered the community mental health movement is parochial, distorted, and mischievous. Fairness requires that I say that this is only somewhat less true for other psychologists who proclaim a community orientation.

I did not introduce the concept of networks for theoretical or propagandistic purposes. I have no desire to push or sell the concept, and I would be the first to confess to bewilderment at how systematically to apply it to better understand a contemporary community. Certainly, one of my purposes was to make the point that if we arrogate to ourselves the title *community psychologist* or the characteristic of a "community orientation," we should at least have the humility to confess that we hardly understand how the inhabitants of a community are actually or potentially interrelated. When I see clinical psychologists and others in the community mental health movement smugly proud of their community orientation and unbothered by the superficiality of their knowledge of what that community consists of, how it is organized, its truly dynamic processes, its interrelatedness—utterly unaware that their presumed focus (the community) cannot be comprehended in terms of the theories and practices of the movement, and their minds uncluttered by the knowledge that when they center their attention on this or that group or this or that setting they are confusing the part with the whole to which the adjective *community* gives priority—I react not with anger or criticism, but with sympathy, because I made most of the mistakes they are making. Some of us at the Psycho-Educational Clinic focused on schools, and because schools were in the community, that, we thought, made us community psychologists. Some devoted a major part of their time to starting programs for and with the community action agency. And there were others who literally created new community agencies on a scale or degree of community involvement that was, relatively speaking, galactic. But, queried a small voice, are there not a lot of people who are not psychologists who do what you do? Are they community psychologists? To which the big voice replied: These other people, like us, are trying to better understand or to conceptualize more fruitfully how things are. Do you mean, said the small voice, that doing what you are doing in these different places is furthering your understanding of a community? It seems to me that it furthers your understanding of these different places, but it is not clear how it furthers your understanding of the community in which they exist. Is it possible, continued the voice, that you use the word *community* the way people use the word *personality*; that is, that it stands for something important and complicated, but you don't deal with it in its complexity, you deal with its parts and wrongly assume that you understand the relationship between whole and part. I cornered my critic with the crusher: It is literally impossible to deal with this complexity; you can only deal with parts, on the basis of which you get better glimpses of what the whole is like. And the appropriate retort was: But how you actually approach and deal with the part must be influenced mightily by where you see it in relationship to the whole; that is, what you hope to do and the ways in which you go about it are consequences of how you think it is embedded in the larger picture.

What the years at the Psycho-Educational Clinic taught me was that the small voice should have shouted earlier in my stay there, because as time went on I realized that if I had forced myself to confront what I did know about the community and whom I knew in it, I definitely would have proceeded in different ways with different groups and different focuses. More important, such a confrontation would have told me what I did not know about the community and whom I did not know, and how both types of ignorance would inevitably affect what I proposed to do. The fact is that I was using the term *community* without bothering to examine what its references were for me.

If I finally learned something, it is primarily because the clinic was created to deal with, among other important considerations, the myth of unlimited resources (Sarason, 1972). In his own way, George Albee (1954, 1968) had been yelling, with data no less, at the mental health movement to face up to the scandalous and socially irresponsible discrepancy between supply and demand. I was sympathetic to his message because I had come to see that what professionals characteristically do, with the best (or, at least, not with the worst) of intentions, is to define a problem so that its solution requires *only* professionals, thus rendering the problem unsolvable (Sarason, 1971, 1972). As soon as you take this indisputable conclusion seriously, one of the questions you have to deal with is, How do I locate people who have the requisite skills but are not employing them, or who have the potential to acquire quickly some or all of the needed skills? How do you think about this question (assuming your professional preciousness permits you seriously to pursue the question, if only for kicks) and the numbers you come up with will be determined by the scope of your concept of a community and the number of networks you can tap into. More correctly, the number of networks you can tap into is a criterion of the scope of your concept of a community. If you play with this way of thinking, you may find, as I did from experience, that the numbers you come up with are surprisingly large and that you are thinking about parts of the community ordinarily outside your interests and ken.

A concrete example follows. We were helping to create a new state facility for handicapped children (Sarason, Grossman, & Zitnay, 1972). If you know anything about how such facilities are planned and created, you know why they become the graveyard for high hopes and for fantasies of innovative practice. The reasons are many, as I have pointed out elsewhere (Sarason, 1972), but high on that list is limited manpower. Our task was to locate people who had skills we needed and who would seriously consider giving them to us for free. We were not only looking for the volunteer who could answer telephones or put stamps on envelopes or help in the kitchen; we also needed people with special knowledge and skills. Where were they and in what numbers? For the sake of brevity I shall start with the fact that we found ourselves in the office of the society editor of the local newspaper. We came away with a list of over 100 organizations, facts about the relatedness or overlapping among them, and some sound advice about how to go about our task. The important point in all this is that we learned a great deal about aspects of the community we never dreamed of as being either interesting or important for us. In practice, the scope of our networks was small, but potentially it was and did become vast, and our conception of the community broadened.

It could be argued that the concept of networks may be of some value for the purpose of understanding and broadening our conception of a community and conceivably would be productive in dealing with the resource issue if one were so inclined. But was it not more than a little silly and wasteful to go the route we did rather than advertise? It would take me too far afield to justify (as I could) our approach in the specific case, but I wish to use the question to discuss the larger and crucial issue it raises: How does one get community support for what one is trying to do? How can one get support for what others in the community want to do and with which you are in sympathy?

My last three books (Sarason, 1971, 1972, 1974) have been concerned with the basis for and the processes of institutional and community change. In writing each of these books I had the unsettling problem of how many instances of failed and catastrophic attempts by mental health professionals to implement their community orientation or program I should describe. I say unsettling because I felt uneasy about being perceived as a cataloguer of unwitting disasters or as a dyspeptic observer of the current scene, especially because I did not feel that I was *that* much wiser than they. I do not think it was a wise decision to limit the number of cases because I have met a number of people who have reacted approvingly to what I have written but who go on to describe their activities in a way to suggest that my generalizations were not well comprehended. For example, one of the most frequent mistakes that is made is to neglect or vastly underestimate the importance of answering these questions: What individuals or groups will be directly affected by the proposed program? What issues of territoriality will it raise for which agencies, professions, and other interest groups? Who can be counted on to put obstacles in the way of the proposed program? Who has the power, actual or potential, to prematurely terminate the program? When you try systematically to answer these and related questions—and these questions refer to one's own organization as well as to external ones—you will find that what you propose to do impinges on networks radiating far into the community, that is, that what you propose to do will become related to quite an array of existing relationships. Indeed, performing this exercise is instructive in giving one a healthy appreciation of the myriads of interlocking networks that exist in a community. Unfortunately, an appreciation of this has always come after the program has failed, or has been aborted, or has fallen far short of the mark, or has been so transformed that its original goals are no longer in the picture. But even that is too charitable an assessment because in many instances the major "lesson" articulated is that there are a lot of stupid, selfish, power-hungry people in the community who feed on well-intentioned, health-giving professionals.

There is a problem in dealing with these questions that can easily be overlooked (it almost always is), and once stated, it is obvious. Those who conceive the program, passionate and committed to a set of substantive ideas they consider innovative and needed, are not in the best psychological set to deal ahead of time with the radiating community consequences of their program. They are psychologically in a set in which optimism and hope and possession of their version of the truth obliterate a systematic approach to the question. In my experience, even when there is a sensitive awareness to these questions, one can predict that they will encounter in themselves two sources of resistance. The first is that it will take time, more time than they are willing or prepared to give. The second is that as they tap into existing networks to get soundings, they are likely to find—they will always find—nodes of opposition. They are, in fact, likely to find that their ideas can be expected to galvanize existing networks, near and far, in opposition to their program. Even if their proposal is to give away large sums of money to afflicted individuals or community agencies—to ask nothing of the community but to accept the money—they will encounter all sorts of opposition and criticism.

It is apparent, I hope, that in raising questions about consequences I have been leading up to the crucial point that a community venture requires support, the kind of support that one can count on to surmount the numerous obstacles that the answers to the questions indicated. And that is the point; the process of tapping into networks to obtain information and soundings is the first stage of the process of answering the question, How much support will we require from what networks to provide us with a fighting chance? And the chances are always fighting ones. It is beyond the scope of this chapter to pursue the processes of gaining support and the dilemmas of compromise.[2] I wish to conclude this part of my presentation by emphasizing that the root cause of the failures I have observed inheres in a conception of a community that ill prepared us for understanding its complexity and our actual and potential relationships to it, as well as for harnessing its resources behind our efforts.

What are the distinguishing characteristics of a community psychologist? In stating characteristics, I make no pretense at inclusiveness. He or she is a person who stands in awe of the discrepancy between firsthand experience of the community and the knowledge needed to comprehend its complexity. She or he is also a person who has made it a point to become familiar with that part of the social science literature that deals with the history and organization of communities, particularly as that literature bears on the ways in which communities are changing. It is this kind of knowledge that allows one to tolerate the discrepancy I described earlier because it provides a kind of compass directing one's efforts to enlarge this firsthand experience. But the community psychologist is one who also knows that the picture of a community to be gained from reading in the social sciences is painted in broad strokes and usually from a standpoint that does not in any direct way point to action for change. The community psychologist, precisely because he or she is involved in understanding *and* change, is one who learns that these broad strokes, while illuminating, are not sufficient for explaining myriads of interrelationships among networks in the community. It is like the situation of the clinician who knows from theory that the behavior and personality of members of a family are a function of various, specifiable factors in familial interactions, but who also has learned from practice how these factors can be differently manifested and patterned in different families. Community psychologists are pursuers of new knowledge and new networks in the community, not only because of immediate or long-term purposes but also because they see themselves as helping unrelated networks come into relationship with each other in light of their mutual needs. Community psychologists seek for themselves and others a sense of community (Sarason, 1974), and acceptance of this value requires them to play the "good broker" role. They are not neutral about values, if for no other reason than that nobody is. But because they take on the label of community psychologist, they have come to grips with the shoulds and oughts of community functioning. Community psychologists lack the grandiosity that alone can permit individuals to believe that they (or their groups) can change a community, but they possess the certainty that their efforts to understand and change a part of a community are doomed if they do not in some way conceptualize these efforts in terms of the larger picture.

---

[2] I will have little to say here about how community psychology has come to grips with issues of values, that is, how one justifies one's actions and programs in relation to community involvement. This problem I have discussed in some detail in Sarason (1974).

Community psychologists are not clinical psychologists or mental health professionals. They are not superior to them, just different. They do not start with theories of the individual, and they are not absorbed by intrapsychic complexities. Pathological behavior is of interest to them primarily in the context of how resources are defined and used so as to maximize the psychological sense of community. They are wary of professional imperialism and preciousness because guildism, however well intentioned in its origins, resists community scrutiny and influence. Conflict is no stranger to them, but it is not the kind of conflict contained in traditional psychological theory in which the individual is usually figure and all else is ground. For the community psychologist, conflict stems from the different traditions, interests, and statuses and other characteristics of different groups, differences producing more or less impermeable boundaries among them—leading to a degree of ignorance of each other not explainable on or even very productively in purely psychological terms. The economics of the mind are one thing; the economics of a community are another. The politics of a family are important and fascinating, but so are the politics of a community to the community psychologist. Sibling rivalry is a valid and productive construct for the clinician; conflict among community groups for limited resources is a stock-in-trade concept for community psychologist. The clinician seeks to use an individual's strengths to combat his weaknesses; the community psychologist is no less sensitive to a community's strengths as weapons against its weaknesses. The clinician seeks allies, internal or external, to the individual. Building alliances is also second nature to the community psychologist.

The truth is that the community psychologist I have described does not exist, or hardly exists. Certainly, our training programs do not produce such a person. When World War II gave rise to modern clinical psychology it was assumed—the way we assume that the sun will rise—that its viability required an alliance with psychiatry and the medical setting. For those of you who doubt this or were in elementary school at the time of 1948 Boulder Conference, I suggest you read those proceedings. (I confess to some satisfaction in being part of a small minority at that conference who considered such an exclusive alliance as equivalent to aborting the potentialities of a differentiated and innovatice social-clinical psychology.) As someone once said: It hasn't been all bad. I quite agree. Therefore, when I suggest that a viable community psychology needs allies, I should not be interpreted as recommending other than a loose confederation among community psychology, ecological psychology, and the social sciences.[3]

---

[3] I have elsewhere (Sarason, 1974) made the point that the characteristics of American social psychology—in its own ways an individualistic, experiment-worshiping fugitive from the social world in which we live our lives—provided no conceptual framework for either modern clinical psychology or the community mental health field. The absence of social psychology from the confederation is not an act of exclusion on

When modern clinical psychology was born, it had to contend with psychiatry, a professional war not yet over. (Why is it that, to my knowledge, there has been no doctoral dissertation on this professional fight? The ahistorical stance of clinical psychology and psychiatry is but one indication of why neither field could give birth to a productive community orientation.) Community psychology will not have to contend with such opposition. Indeed, my experience suggests that there are individuals in these allied fields who would be warmly supportive of attempts to forge new relationships. Note that I said individuals, not departments, because the modern university has many of the characteristics of a community, and the person who seeks to forge a new set of relationships to implement a new kind of program is faced with all the issues I have already discussed. One must use one's existing networks, tap into new ones, and develop a basis of support. Before we venture into *the* real world, we have to solve the same problems in *our* real world, and from the standpoint of action and change the two worlds are similar. Before we save other people's worlds, we should first be able to demonstrate that we can save our own.

In conclusion, I would like to deal with a criticism directed at my position by a student. Paraphrasing his remarks:

The way you describe community psychologists, they are remarkably similar to a lot of people in the community. Police, organized criminal syndicates, politicians, business people, fund raisers, and Mr. Joe Blow himself—all of them would say that what you are describing are people with common sense who have lived in the real world and have tried to get something done. They will all tell you that you have to get to the right people, you have to learn who the right people are, and that you have to know the territory like the guy in "The Music Man" said. They would also agree with your criticism of professionals who screw things up when they want to do good in the community. What, they would say, do these professional do-gooders and bleeding hearts know about life in the real world? I would not be surprised if they looked on what you have said as another glimpse of the obvious described by another academic who does not know the difference between common and uncommon sense.

These remarks bothered me because there was a part of me that was ready to agree with my critic, and yet, if I agreed, if only in part, I felt that the strength of my position would be considerably weakened. Besides, even if I were convinced he was wrong, I was not convinced by my reply to him, and,

---

my part but simply the belief that it has little to offer. Again, this is not intended as a way of manifesting any superiority on my part or that of the fields upon which I would base a community psychology. The fact is that when all of us entered the post-World War II era, we were conceptually bankrupt before we began. Please remember that bankruptcy does not mean one is without assets, just that one does not have enough assets to carry on one's business. I am petitioning for a reorganization.

of course, neither was he. Reflection, if not candor, forced me later to realize that what bothered me was the illness of professional preciousness. I wanted a community psychologist to be a distinctive and, perhaps, unique kind of person and, therefore, I was not going to look kindly at a criticism that said that far from being distinctive, the community psychologist was like a lot of other people. That thought forced me to go back and read Carl Becker's 1931 presidential address to the American Historical Association (Becker, 1935). In this address, entitled "Every Man His Own Historian"—which I would make mandatory reading for anyone pretending to seek a liberal (liberating) education—Becker shows the communalities between Mr. Everyman (today it would be Everyperson) and the professional historian. I cannot present here Becker's arguments—they defy brief summary. But this quotation will give you the aroma if not the taste of the intellectual dish he serves:

If the essence of history is the memory of things said and done, then it is obvious that every normal person, Mr. Everyman, knows some history. Of course we do what we can to conceal this invidious truth. Assuming a professional manner, we say that so and so knows no history, when we mean no more than that he failed to pass the examinations set for a higher degree; and simple-minded persons, undergraduates and others, taken in by academic classifications of knowledge, think they know no history because they have never taken a course in history in college, or have never read Gibbon's *Decline and Fall of the Roman Empire*. No doubt the academic convention has its uses, but it is one of the superficial accretions that must be stripped off if we would understand history reduced to its lowest terms. Mr. Everyman, as well as you and I, remembers things said and done, and must do so at every waking moment. (pp. 235–236)

Toward the end of his address, Becker reassures the professional historian that he has both a common and uncommon role to play:

The historian, like Mr. Everyman, like the bards and storytellers of an earlier time, will be conditioned by the specious present in which alone he can be aware of his world. Being neither omniscient nor omnipresent, the historian is not the same person always and everywhere; and for him, as for Mr. Everyman, the form and significance of remembered events, like the extension and velocity of physical objects, will vary with the time and place of the observer. After fifty years we can clearly see that it was not history which spoke through Fustel, but Fustel who spoke through history. We see less clearly perhaps that the voice of Fustel was the voice, amplified and freed from static as one may say, of Mr. Everyman; what the admiring students applauded on that famous occasion was neither history nor Fustel, but a deftly colored pattern of selected events which Fustel fashioned, all the more skillfully for not being aware of doing so, in the service of Mr. Everyman's emotional needs—the emotional satisfaction, so essential to Frenchmen at that time, of perceiving that French institutions were not of German origin. And so it must always be. Played upon by all the diverse, unnoted influence of his own time, the historian will elicit history out of documents by the same principle, however more consciously and expertly applied, that Mr. Everyman employs to breed legends out of remembered episodes and oral tradition. (pp. 251–252)

"More consciously and expertly applied"—that is the kernal of the answer I wish I had given my student critic. We are similar to and different from Mr. Everyman, and that should be a powerful reassurance for the community psychologist. And if we forget that bond, we have lost our roots and, as Becker says, "our proper function."

REFERENCES

Albee, G. *Mental health manpower trends.* New York: Basic Books, 1954.

Albee, G. Models, myths, and manpower. *Mental Hygiene,* 1968, *52,* 168–180.

Barker, R. G. On the nature of the environment. *Journal of Social Issues,* 1963, *19*(4), 17–38. (a)

Barker, R. G. *The stream of behavior.* New York: Appleton-Century-Crofts, 1963. (b)

Barker, R. G. *Ecological psychology. The stream of behavior.* Stanford, Calif.: Stanford University Press, 1968.

Barker, R. G., & Gump, P. V. *Big school, small school.* Stanford, Calif.: Stanford University Press, 1964.

Barker, R. G., & Schoggen, P. *Qualities of community life.* San Francisco: Jossey-Bass, 1973.

Barker, R. G., & Wright, H. F. *One boy's day.* New York: Harper & Row, 1951.

Becker, C. Every man his own historian. In *Essays on history and politics.* New York: Crofts, 1935.

Gladwin, T., & Sarason, S. B. *Truk: Man in paradise.* New York: Wenner-Gren Foundation for Anthropological Research, 1953.

Kelly, J. G. (Review of *Qualities of community life* by R. G. Barker & P. Schoggen). *Contemporary Psychology,* 1975, *20*(3), 193–195.

Price, R. H. The taxonomic classification of behaviors and situations and the problem of behavior-environment congruence. *Human Relations,* 1974, *27,* 567–585.

Price, R. H., & Blashfield, R. K. Explorations in the taxonomy of behavior settings: Analysis of dimensions and classifications of settings. *American Journal of Community Psychology,* 1975, *20,* 335–351.

Sarason, S. B. *The culture of the school and the problem of change.* Boston: Allyn & Bacon, 1971.

Sarason, S. B. *The creation of settings and the future societies.* San Francisco: Jossey-Bass, 1972.

Sarason, S. B. *The psychological sense of community. Prospects for a community psychology.* San Francisco: Jossey-Bass, 1974.

Sarason, S. B., Grossman, F. K., & Zitnay, G. *The creation of a community setting.* Syracuse, N.Y.: Syracuse University Press, 1972.

4 Ya Gotta Believe

Robert Reiff

The future of community psychology is related to its past history, to the history of psychology as a whole, and to the growth and development of professionalism during the last two decades. The future of community psychology is a vacuum that is going to be filled by the biographies of those who have contributed to it during the past 10 years and of those who are here today. Note that I said that history is to be *filled* by these biographies; I did not say it was to be made. That remains to be seen. And that is why this conference is so crucial. Whether the future of community psychology is going to be made behind our backs, as it has been thus far, or whether we are going to make it is a moot question. The results of this conference will in part determine that. I would like, therefore, to talk for a few minutes about the history of community psychology in the past 10 years so that we may get some perspective on the future.

First, as a community psychologist I would like to ask two simple questions: How has community psychology been affected by the historical period in which it has grown? What are the social conditions under which community psychology was developed? Community psychology was born in a social context in which there was a great deal of interest and investment in social reform. It took place in an era of great social mobility. The professions experienced an unprecedented increase in numbers. As people with low incomes moved up the social scale, the professions themselves changed in nature from organizations of elite, upper-middle-class people to a mix of upper-middle-, lower-middle-, and upper-working-class people.

There was at the same time an air of dissatisfaction throughout academic institutions, with widespread accusation that they were irrelevant and were not doing anything about social problems. In general there was an abundance of funding for reform programs and, in spite of the criticisms, there was also an unprecedented growth and expansion in academic institutions.

A very important professional condition was the growth of the community mental health movement, which in theory moved away from one-to-one individual remedial healing to a more conscious effort to develop healing processes as a social experience rather than an individual intrapsychic, interpersonal experience. Some psychologists, primarily clinicians, reacted to these social and professional conditions by proclaiming that psychologists should be social interventionists. There was an emphasis on social system intervention, but it did not necessarily reflect any knowledge about social systems. Rather, it more than likely reflected the belief that there was some kind of cultural lag in psychology, that psychology was behind technology and science because it didn't know anything about social systems and, therefore, ought to catch up. Because the people who were responsible for developing community psychology were clinicians, there was a great deal of emphasis on primary prevention, and there was also an emphasis on the professional as an activist. All of these ideas were ambiguous. They were like emotional statements without conceptual clarity. And while these ideas were couched in the language of a proactive program, they were, in fact, a reaction to the social conditions of the time, a much more reactive than proactive program.

After 10 years community psychology still does not have a conceptual framework, a value base, or an organizing concept. As a result of these lacks, it has become mostly a job opportunities movement. As soon as the jobs in community mental health dry up, community psychology is likely to become something else. That may be good or it may be bad, depending on what we accomplish at this conference. Unfortunately, community psychology at the present time is an association similar to the Association for the Advancement of Psychologists in Private Practice. It is an Association for the Advancement of Psychologists in Community Mental Health. I think if it remains that it is going to die a horrible death.

At this 10th anniversary what we have on hand is a 10-year-old creature who doesn't know where its mouth is, who can't comprehend what its eyes see, who spends its time working with skills it acquired before it was born, and who on anniversary occasions looks down at its navel trying to decide to what species it belongs. I think if you had a 10-year-old child like that it would worry you, and I wonder how you would judge its future in the absence of some very drastic intervention.

That is the past. Let us turn to the future. What are the social conditions likely to be in the next 10 years? Certainly there is going to be an atmosphere of social regression, social conservation. The social reforms of the past decade or two are going to be eroded. There will be an air of economic stringency, perhaps even economic crisis, if it isn't true that we are already in one. There will be continuing attempts at contraction of human services. The political climate will be one of tightening our belts, rolling up our sleeves, and biting bullets. These are likely to be the social conditions with which we will have to contend.

What are the professional conditions that might prevail under these social conditions? There will be an atmosphere of retrenchment in the universities. There will be further retreat from relevance to academic neutrality and conservatism. There will be further attempts to incorporate the community mental health establishment completely into the medical establishment and the further erosion of the concept of social causation in mental illness. And there will be the further incorporation of professionals into civil service or bureaucratic agencies, with the concomitant result that professionals will lose control of their knowledge. Already more than 50% of the psychologists in the U.S. are either in civil service or employed by bureaucratic agencies of one kind or another. Those are likely to be the conditions under which we will be trying to develop community psychology. We can remain reactive and allow these conditions to shape our future, or we can become proactive and make some conscious attempts to change them.

The future of community psychology is inextricably linked to the welfare of the people in our society. Unless we understand that, we are likely to become what C. Wright Mills calls "cheerful robots" who dissociate what is going on in society from their own professional status and privileges. How do we become proactive? I think there are three important dimensions to the task we have to accomplish in the future. Seymour Sarason made a marvelous argument in his presentation at this conference (see chapter 3). He pointed out, as the first dimension, that we have to shift our perspective away from the individual to the social structure. The second dimension is our value system. We have to shift from individual values to social values; that is, define problems not in terms of achievement, competition, and success, but in terms of freedom, distributive justice, and other such values. Closely linked to the problem of values is the third problem of social ideology; that is, what is our ideological position with regard to our professional body of knowledge? How do we define problems? It is easy to talk about internal conflict, conflict between ego and id, conflict between ego and superego, people exploiting themselves, etc. But rarely do we hear anybody in a psychology meeting say that this is a class society where people exploit each other on a class basis as well as on a psychological basis. We cannot deal with the problem as a psychological problem only, for it is not just a psychological problem. I reveal to you my social ideology. I believe this is a class society, that we exploit each other, and that exploitation produces human misery. As a psychologist I have something to contribute to alleviate such human misery. For me that is an organizing principle. I am willing to declare it and ask you to join me.

I see three important professional ideologies in community psychology. There is the *healing* ideology, espoused primarily by clinical psychologists, with its emphasis in restoring the sick individual. All problems—social, political, and economical—are interpreted in terms of that healing ideology. I would place most of the clinical theories about social change under the healing ideology. Then there is the *developmental* ideology, with programs whose emphasis is on the realization of full potential of individuals. Many of the ecologically based programs fall in this category. Finally, there is the *social problems* or *social change* ideology, with its emphasis on changing the social structure. Persons who advocate the healing ideology see all problems as primarily needing healing skills. Developmentalists look at problems and say they require the skills of the developmentalist. The social structure people say problems require primarily the skills of a social change agent. It seems to me that the lesson to be drawn from this is that people in each ideology tend to define problems in terms of their own skills. Clinicians look at a social problem and define it in terms of one or more of the different therapies.

Developmentalists define the problem as requiring the skills of environmental manipulation. However, there is one difference between these three ideologies that I think is crucial. If you maintain the healing ideology, all the dependent variables in the study of a problem can be psychological ones. If you are a developmentalist, dependent variables will also be psychological. But you cannot be a social change agent and insist that all dependent variables be psychological. That is an important difference, and it has many implications for the definition of problems.

We all talk about social systems and about tackling problems from the social systems point of view. But few of us know very much about social systems. Behind our difficulties there is an assumption that leads to confusion and superficiality in our social system approach. That assumption is that if one works in a social system, one is producing social system change. That is an absolutely false assumption, and I am going to show you why. Let us first differentiate the various levels of social organization at which one might work. The least complex is the *individual*. Some people say we can look at an individual as a system. The second, and more complex, level or organization would be *group or family*. The third and even more complex level would be *organizations or institutions*. Above that would be the fourth level, the *community*, and above that the most complex level, the *society*.

The assumption is that if you work in a school system you are changing that community. The fact of the matter is that working in a system does not automatically guarantee that you are working toward system change. There are three kinds of changes one can possibly make: (1) One can work in an organization to change individuals, that is, to *change the dispositional factors* in the individual, the intrapsychic or intrapersonal behavior. (2) One can work at any level to produce *situational changes*, or changes in the immediate milieu. And (3) one can work at any level to produce what can be called *social structure changes*. For the most part the clinician works at the individual and group level and less frequently at the organizational or community level. The clinician produces dispositional and situational changes but rarely gets to social structure change. Using this taxonomy to define community psychologists, I would say that the community psychologist ought to be working at any of the system levels with the primary aim of producing social structure changes. That is where we have to go to meet the social problems of the next 10 years. And we had better move fast.

I would like to introduce another concept. C. Wright Mills makes a distinction between what he calls "personal troubles" and "social issues." I think that is an important distinction to keep in mind. Let me give you an example. A marriage might be threatened by the fact that there is an intrapsychic or interpersonal difficulty with one or the other of the partners. This is a "personal trouble." It may also be threatened by something within the situation, such as an economic problem. This is a "personal trouble" related to situational factors. But when 50% percent of the people in the U.S.

get divorced, then there is something beyond the intrapsychic and inter-personal, something beyond the situational, and something in the social structure that accounts for these personal troubles; and that something is what community psychologists ought to seek. That would open up a whole new world for us. It also is a tremendous problem to acquire the skills to do it. A lot of us are going to be scared and say that is too heavy a load to carry, that they are getting out. But some of us may not. When one begins to think in those terms, some new problems arise. Nothing is ever easy.

There are certain tensions already existing that are going to be increased if we take the social problems approach. One existing tension is between disciplines and the social problem approach. This approach requires inter-disciplinary knowledge and cooperation. There is tension in the university today between maintaining individual disciplines and moving in an interdisci-plinary direction. I defy anyone to tell me what the basic core of courses for a PhD in community psychology would be to prepare a student to work on social problems. Until we decide whether we are going to operate on the basis of a healing ideology, an environmental and developmental ideology, or a social structure ideology, it is premature to talk about a PhD in community psychology. I think that if you take the social problems approach, then you have to study social problems as they are and not as a discipline defines them.

At this conference we deal intellectually with the problems of where community psychology should go. The nonintellective work, the real work, begins when this conference is over. The question is, what should that work be? What have been the mechanisms by which community psychology has changed? The usual mechanisms have been the traditional meetings and conferences among ourselves. I think we have to develop a number of new mechanisms to change community psychology, including one that provides us with the conceptual knowledge and viewpoints that we need in order to attack social problems. We need allies, and we need them badly. We can find allies among individuals in the social sciences in the university, if not in departments. We should begin to develop joint liaison programs, joint seminars around social problems, with other social scientists. We need that conceptual, nutritional mix. It will be good for us organizationally, as well, because we won't be able to do it without some informal or formal organization. We need some kind of organizing principle if we want to become a substantial and recognized group of people with a function and an ideology.

There is another tension—the tension between the university and social change. Can one engage in social change and be part of the university? Is the university necessarily the best place to engage in social change? Frankly, it is not the best place. That doesn't mean we shouldn't try to do it there if that is where we are. How can we create social change in the universities, recognizing the tensions? One way is to begin to develop students whose careers are in research, teaching, and other roles in which there is an opportunity to influence and participate in policy decisions that contribute to the promotion of human welfare. Let me explain further. There are two kinds of knowledge: knowledge to know and knowledge to change. These are not necessarily the same thing. If you do research to develop knowledge to change, more often than not you are going to be involved in some change process—that is where activism comes. If you do research to develop knowledge to know, there may not be an activist component to it, but it can still be an important contribution to social change. Social policy research, for example, can be of either kind or a combination of both. I think it is important for every community psychologist to learn social policy analysis and research. That means changing a number of things about the university. For example, learning to use history as a tool in social policy analysis and research is essential. But the colleges have been turning out a generation of students who are ahistorical in their thinking, who hardly ever think in terms of history. You cannot engage in social policy analysis and research without consciously and deliberately taking into account the history of the policy or problem.

Aside from changing the attitudes of the university, is there anything we can do organizationally to resolve the tensions between disciplines and the social problem approach? I think there is. I would say that the best strategy would probably be to work toward setting up a program in social policy research as a minor for all social science students and give up the idea, at least for the time being, of a PhD in community psychology. Students can get their PhD in any of the social sciences, and together with all the other social sciences we can offer a minor in social policy, research, and analysis.

Another possible route would be to develop interdisciplinary centers that give certificates or even masters' degrees in social policy. We have to be creative in developing organizational forms that promote an interdisciplinary effort in the approach to social problems.

Someone recently asked me why the nonprofessional citizen can't do what I am proposing the community psychologist do. There is an important difference between the professional's and the citizen's effort to bring about social change: The professional tries to bring some methodological order into social change efforts. As far as I am concerned that is the only distinction, but it is an extremely important one. I think that is where the future of community psychology lies.

5 Varied Educational Settings for Community Psychology

James G. Kelly

Community psychology has attained a valid place within the profession of psychology. The variety of training programs, the number of books and articles published, and the growth of the Division of Community Psychology in the APA are testimony to this observation. For example, there are at least 18 doctoral training programs in community psychology; 30 universities report community psychology as an area of concentration for the master's degree (APA, 1974); two professional schools are providing a focus for community psychology; and there are schools where education of the community psychologist is going on in a multidisciplinary setting (Binder, 1972; Vallance, 1976). The content of community psychology is also taught at the undergraduate level. In addition, a number of associate in arts degree programs in mental health work emphasize content within the boundaries of community psychology. In terms of scope and levels of training, the field is active.

Viewing the field in terms of published articles and publication outlets, community psychology is visible. In addition to articles contributed by psychologists to the *Community Mental Health Journal*, the number of community-oriented citations appearing in the *Journal of Clinical and Consulting Psychology, Journal of Abnormal Psychology, Psychological Bulletin,* and *Professional Psychologist* is increasing. There are now two important journals solely for the field, the *Journal of Community Psychology* and the *American Journal of Community Psychology*. The *Annual Review of Psychology* has featured chapters on significant community material, such as the Design of Social and Community Interventions, Primary Prevention, Social and Cultural Influences on Psychopathology, Psychology and Culture, and Program Evaluation, with more to come. And let's not forget the publication of books. The publication of the *Handbook of Community Mental Health* is an important

This is an expanded statement of ideas expressed at the evening session of the National Conference on Community Psychology in Austin, Tex., April 28, 1975. Prompted by the mood of the conference, the author offered personal recollections of his experiences as a graduate student at the University of Texas and his career as a community psychologist. The ideas that were briefly stated on that occasion are now amplified in these comments.

These ideas were emended by the critical review of Ricardo Muñoz, Ben Gottlieb, Mary Harvey, Mele Koneya, Ed Lichtenstein, John Monahan, Lonnie Snowden, Norm Sundberg, Dave Todd and Ted Vallance. I appreciate their investment.

historical moment. The number of books primarily related to the topics of community psychology published between the time of the Swampscott Conference on Community Psychology in 1965 and the Austin Conference in 1975 is conservatively estimated at about 500! We are present and visible in our trade.

Now that community psychology is a distinct field, my hope is that we will seize the opportunity to complete the "rite of passage" and consciously work to create the conditions for doing our intellectual work with a collective sense of optimism and good will. Now that we have arrived, I hope our profession, which has as one of its aims the creation of emotional and social support systems, will develop personal and social support systems for the individual community psychologist and the profession of community psychology.

COPING WITH THE TENSIONS OF OUR WORK

The tensions in carrying out the work of community psychology are many and expected. Such tensions are common when doing something new and different. I suggest that the tensions will be managed differently, depending on the type of educational setting where we work. The first point I want to stress is that education in community psychology should take place in different settings. My premise is that varied settings will assist the creative evolution of the field. Second, I ask for the development of supportive social systems within these educational settings. My premise here is that the profession will be renewed if we all can benefit from our varied educational settings, and if we can design social settings that are supportive to the creative management of tensions in the field. Seymour Sarason, as I read him, has suggested a similar need in his appraisal of the constraints on community psychology in higher education and in his appeal for the psychological sense of community (Sarason, 1974).

A way to aid both ourselves and the field of community psychology is to consciously design and create ways to share and try out ideas, to give and receive feedback for our efforts in research and practice. Can each of us relate to each other as a respected and valued kin, rather than as someone to impress, exploit, manipulate, compete against, and be "one up" on? I really believe that our survival as individual community psychologists depends very much on our creative ability to adapt to our varied settings. Our survival also depends on our personal commitment to help each other manage the tensions of doing work while we are engaged in marginal roles.

In the spring of 1969, in a survey-and-interview study of the role strain, marginality, and communication patterns of academic community psychologists, Maher (1970), found that 15 community psychologists reputed by peers to be leaders in the field did not communicate with each other about substantive topics and did not cite each other in their publications. He found that 15 leaders in the field were doing their own thing! During the past six years there have been indications that there is more sharing, with a sense of common mission emerging. If there is a perceptible change in our behavior, we can be explicit about the potential benefits of varied educational settings and interrelated supportive behaviors. Several years ago, I suggested that we need an analogue to the Woods Hole Experiment Station in biology where we could work informally for the good of ourselves and our chosen field (Kelly, 1970). This idea is still in my head. It seems appropriate to repeat it for review and reflection at this time, now that the field is established and congealing.

I have been struck by the historical accounts of the role that the Marine Biological Laboratories at Woods Hole, Massachusetts, has played in the development in biology (Conklin, 1968a, 1968b). For many years, Woods Hole served as a social setting with a mixture of functions. It was a place where biologists could come to work; it was a place where the leadership attracted the stimulating and provocative minds. It was a place where faculty came with their students and, under very informal and casual conditions, worked, talked, and shared their ideas and hopes that so frequently do not appear in the final publication of scientific reports. Biologists with whom I have spoken are unanimous in their praise for this institution and for the major influence that the setting has had in the development of their own work.

The picture of Woods Hole, as sketched by those who have been associated with it, can take on the properties of a romantic south sea island. Putting aside such reveries, the creation of an analogue to Woods Hole for the training of community psychologists seems to me to be an idea worth pursuing on its own merit. An idea that, if implemented, could play a critical role in the updating of the faculty and the generation of students who can become the eminent and accomplished innovators.

When I begin to consider the means by which a Woods Hole laboratory can be created for the training of community psychology, some features occur to me that are different than those of a research laboratory located in a scenic marshland along the Massachusetts coastline. Such a facility would not be in one place, but would be scattered in different parts of the country and would be located in geographical areas where there are varying political conditions, different opportunities for the delivery of community services, and where each of the laboratories would have contrasting styles of working with citizens. Such facilities could provide a node for regenerating community psychologists rather than creating totally new communities. (p. 530)

In his closing to *The Structure of Scientific Revolutions*, Thomas Kuhn (1970) says:

Scientific knowledge, like language, is intrinsically the common property of a group or else nothing at all. To understand it we shall need to know the special characteristics of the groups that create and use it. (p. 210)

Here are some personal views about the roles of community psychologists working in varied educational environments and how we can self-consciously develop our identity as a profession.

Community psychology is a strange field. The two words, *community* and *psychology*, do not easily go together. The qualities and characteristics of individuals are not quite the same as the qualities and characteristics of social issues and events. In addition, there are several natural and expected tensions in working out the mission of community psychology. An *intellectual* tension exists in understanding and clarifying relationships between persons and large social organizations. There is a *methodological* tension in adapting the procedures and paradigms of laboratory work within psychology to the topics of community psychology, which often demand different strategies. There is a tension within the *ideology* of the university faculty for the preservation of autonomy and freedom versus the expectations of many psychologists, particularly community psychologists, for the university to respond to and cope with social issues. There is as well the tension of *cultural* heritages between the goals of the professor, often white and male, and the aspirations of minority faculty and citizens who wish to see psychology directly useful to minority people. Lonnie Snowden (1976)[1] has reminded me of another major tension—the tension between security and adventuresome behavior, which contributes to the everyday conflict and dilemma of doing something new and different versus doing business as usual—a particularly pertinent and real-life dilemma for all nontenured assistant professors.

Many of us have experienced some of these tensions as we have tried to do our work. I hope that we can self-consciously build the personal, social, and supportive relationships for our field so that the resolution of these tensions has a direct consequence for our work (Glidewell, 1975).[2] Varied settings for the education of community psychologists can offer extended opportunities to cope with the tensions derived from the traditions, the values, and the social norms of each setting. While these tensions are present and are being coped with, there is a simultaneous and, we hope, long-term benefit in the creation of occasions for new traditions to enhance our personal development. The question is, can we create preventive interventions to help ourselves cope with the crises latent in our own work? The paradox for us in community psychology is that we will have to know much about ourselves as people and our ability to be resources for each other if we are to contribute something to the "psychology" of community psychology. The quality of the profession that emerges in community psychology, I believe, will depend on the creative resolution of these tensions. We, ourselves, are involved in social change when we create new ways of doing our own business. This is a truism that often we prefer to put out of our minds.

[1] Snowden, L. Personal communication, February 20, 1976.
[2] Glidewell, J. G. Personal communications on many occasions when talking about the educational enterprise for community work and community psychology, 1972-1975.

Developing educational programs characterized by their multiple tensions is a difficult task. Creating a sense of community for the community psychologist as we do it is even more difficult. We will be pushed and pulled by the traditions of professional work in ways that are antagonistic to building personal and social supports. As we try, we will be asked to be autonomous, reflective, and private, if not solitary; to be self-serving; and to be a member of our own preferred social clique rather than a resource in a social network. The distinction between a clique and a network is important: a clique focuses on social status, prestige, and exclusiveness; a social network aspires after mutual help, respect, and admiration derived from shared goals and reciprocal appeals for genuineness.

We will be asked to behave in nonpersonal ways in our different educational settings, not as an explicit assignment but because such ways are the dominant life styles of faculty in higher education. In essence, I'm offering suggestions for putting collegiality back in the educational enterprise.

THREE VIEWS OF THE UNIVERSITY

J. Mitchell Morse (1975), a professor of English at Temple University, cited a pertinent comment by Charles Sanders Pierce, who had remarked in 1896 that it was morally impossible for a gentleman to have an original idea of any consequence. Morse builds on this appraisal by adding that Thorstein Veblen three years later observed that most of the great consequential ideas in science at the time had arisen outside universities because university faculties consisted largely of gentlemen, to whom unorthodox thoughts could not occur.

The field of community psychology is probably at a similar place in our history. As we engage in the pursuit of unorthodox ideas, we are not sure of our status as "gentlemen," and we are definitely ambivalent about losing our identification as gentlemen, even if it is thrilling to test the limits of our colleagues' tolerance for gentlemanly work when doing community psychology.

Until 1960 many of the ideas, service programs, and preventive interventions in community mental health and in community psychology occurred outside the university. Even today, the work of community psychology produces conflict and challenges the daily life and values of higher education. To cope, we will still need to produce our own sense of purpose and our own sense of history.

There have been at least three points of view on the role of the university and social issues. One view, expressed by the late Jacques Barzun (1968), is that the university should be above, beyond, and separate from the surrounding dilemmas of social consequence:

The university must make up its mind and choose between two attitudes which go with two messages incessantly heard. One is: "Behold our eminence—it deserves your support and affectionate regard after you have attended and shared our greatness." The other is: "We are a public utility like any other–drop in any time." Both messages are spoken by the same voice and both, perhaps, should remain unspoken, but the first should secretly inspire the "university conceived." Let it be clear: the choice is not between being high-hat and being just folks. It is not a question of hospitableness–a university should be hospitable; it is a question of style, reflecting the fundamental choice as to what the university thinks it is. . . .

It can, from generous but misguided motives, yield to the assimilating effect of cooperation with the world. Then a big grant for a noneducational purpose brings out scholars in a goldrush, though they do their best to keep the rest of the show going not too badly. This defection has occurred before. "In my time and my country," says Montaigne, "learning has a salutary effect on the pocket, rarely on the mind." (p. 285)

Barzun favored the university as an honored, protected, and safe haven for ideas. But the 1960s put aside the fantasy that universities are safe and protected. The 1970s, with a sanguine and intrusive public asking for evidence of what we do, further belies that fantasy. Universities are vulnerable, fragile, open systems.

John Maher of the Delancey Street Foundation, in Sales (1975), offers a contrasting point of view.

To academics and intellectuals in the U.S., what you *say* is far more important than what you *do*. If you cured fifty lepers, but spoke like a hard-hat, a Southerner or a black–the three maligned elements in the culture–you would receive no more. But if you can express humanistic drivel in a language acceptable to the ideology of that vast band who confuse impotence with morality, they call it "openmindedness" and cheer, whether you do anything or not. . . .

Talk is cheap. If you're in the Women's Movement and did nothing but picket McSorley's Ale House because it's for men only, or if you're in the Black Movement and all you've done is scream "white motherfucker"–haven't helped educate any kids–or if you were against the War and only gave a cocktail party so you could meet more playmates, then kindly take your place among the followers and stop blocking the leadership. Either you struggle in your own lifetime for a better world–or you become part of the problem. (p. 28)

Barzun appeals to the great and noble traditions and ideals of a university. Maher taunts and kicks us to really worry about societies beyond our own, and suggests direct and immediate ways to help. Behind the contrasting dictums of Barzun and Maher are the political forces that we as community psychologists must reckon with: how to contribute knowledge, to be personally useful, and to solve *real* problems (Sundberg, 1970). This brings us to a third point of view.

Roger Heyns has expanded the domain of university activities to contemporary problems (Heyns, 1968). He starts by asking three questions:

1. Can anyone else do it better?
2. Is there a body of content, a discipline to be learned?
3. Does the proposed [community] program draw on, as well as enrich, other [university] programs? (p. 35)

These are educational questions. In answering them, Heyns believes that the university must have a great deal of control over the field situation to obtain optimum results. He then offers four criteria in defining how a university can relate to the community. First, "the students must be geared into the [community] to be sure that they aren't just additional manpower, or given routine assignments; *real* opportunities for learning must be provided" (p. 35). Second, it is not worthwhile for the university to operate the field agency themselves:

One little noticed but very real objection to university-operated and university-run social agencies [is that] the autonomy of the community itself may be compromised. We should be just as sensitive to the ability of the community to determine the kind of services it wants as we are to protecting our own freedom. (p. 35)

Heyns' third point is that the practical learning experience must be related to the on-campus learning. "The classroom learning must inform practice and vice versa. Mere uninterrupted experience is not enough" (p. 36). Fourth, Heyns affirms: "The guiding concept for student behavior and experience is that he is a student—not a general citizen, not another member of the troops, and not an employee" (p. 36).

Barzun suggests that we can remove ourselves from the external world. Maher advocates that we plunge directly into it. Heyns offers us a chance to adapt the university in order to participate in new work while meeting the needs of persons outside the university and preserving the historical mission of the university.

To uphold Barzun's thesis as a reference point creates problems because it prevents us from sanctioning applied and useful work. I listen to Maher, but I reject a wholesale embracing of society's problems by the university, even though I advocate university and professional work on controversial issues defined by citizens as problems. Heyns suggests criteria by which we can resolve the tensions between reflection and action, between being useful and being thoughtful, and between contributing to the profession and contributing to a community. I believe that the field of community psychology should be measured by the varied ways in which we cope with the resolution of these universal tensions when creating our educational programs.

As a start, I will present three examples of how the training and education of community psychologists can be diverse: (1) graduate education within a department of psychology, (2) graduate education within a multidisciplinary program, and (3) undergraduate education. I have selected these examples because I personally have been a part of these settings and have observed some good effect, along with some definite stress on my energy level and strain, in realizing my aspirations for these settings. All three can help the field of community psychology grow, and each can make contributions to the other two. Most of all, all these settings can be interrelated, supportive, educational settings. We may still argue and fret about some issues, such as who has primacy rights, who is better trained, and who has more power within the profession, but what I'd really like is to reduce the fatiguing and destructive features of the universal tensions I named. By valuing diversity we can celebrate our complementary educational missions and appreciate the field as a whole. Some professions have trouble with pluralism. We in community psychology can be different.

THE DEPARTMENT OF PSYCHOLOGY AS HOST AND GREENHOUSE

The commitment to analysis, reverence for conceptual and integrative abilities, and deep involvement in methodological innovation are mainstreams of psychology. In my personal experience these qualities are not only useful but essential for the design and analysis of social and community interventions. I believe one must know *something* to solve a problem. We can take pride in the fact that there *is* something intrinsically good about the explanatory power of ideas, systematic inquiry, and revering a conceptual ability and empirical data. Ideas such as role conflict and role ambiguity, cognitive dissonance, the Hawthorne effect, and conflict resolution, and knowledge about concepts such as dogmatism and trust are very helpful for a community psychologist. Many important ideas for community work, such as reference group, reinforcement, conformity, and that old idea, the Zeigarnik effect, have come from academic psychology. The academically-oriented community psychologist has the satisfaction of seeing research influence the actions of others, even if the impact is indirect and includes not only lags in publication but lags while practitioners read, absorb ideas, and then make them work.

The scientific features of community psychology can be developed if the department of psychology can encourage the display of explicit criteria for community work and if Heyns' principles can be tested. Within different departments of psychology, a variety of approaches to the academic development of community psychology will occur with the variation related to the unique interests of individual faculty members. Provisions for faculty development programs can be a reservoir for retesting ideas and integrating concepts, methods, and styles of work from other areas within psychology. The written qualifying examination, the oral examination, the internship, the preparation of reviews of literature, and the doctoral dissertation are all occasions for expressing and improving conceptual and integrative abilities as well as for thinking analytically and clearly. Doing community work and unraveling the direction and impact of organizational and social forces requires an ability to scan, to digest, and to pull together the bits and pieces of personalities, settings, social events, and political underbrush. Learning community psychology in a department of psychology is valid because there is something needed and useful to be learned there. The role identity of psychologists in a department of psychology is explicit, and the organizational values are very well expressed. Several generations of psychologists are available within a departmental structure to pass on the benefits of the psychological perspective to the next generation.

What are the limitations of the department as host? Perhaps within a department of psychology there is a tendency to anoint and encourage research fads rather than initiate a genuinely new direction. Since it takes time to develop a new method, it is understandable that once it is born, the psychologist is interested in having others test and replicate. There is also a palpable, even coercive, pressure to complete doctoral work and publish something. There is the convenience of the college student (the universal subject), who is relatively easy to control and who has short periods of time to contribute to research data. This convenience is sought perhaps too often in order to publish and in order to be revered.

Because of the need within community psychology to deal with multi-variate topics over time, there is tension regarding how long university faculty can wait to see if and what the community psychologist produces. Interim criteria are needed for promotion and tenure appraisal until the "real" data comes in. There is a compelling need when criteria for promotion and tenure are being considered for the community psychologist to include a review of work in progress.

Departments of psychology generally do not seek to receive influence from professionals and citizens outside the departmental structure. The inevitable isolation and perhaps resulting narrowness of the department can be troublesome to the community psychologist. However, there are at least two ways of reducing the pain of such dilemmas. One is to seek out those faculty members in other universities who are working on similar topics and involve them as consultants and resources for departmental colleagues. This helps to collectively share tensions and reduces the problem of one faculty member managing the unresolved tensions generated from role strain and marginality. The other way is to create formal and informal occasions where influential citizens, clients, and professionals can publicly express their views about social issues and how the work of the community psychologist can be helpful. While such occasions may produce unrealistic expectations for both the citizen and the psychologist, such occasions can be the beginning of the next insight. The adaptive requirement for the department of psychology is: to self-consciously create opportunities for nonpsychologists to express views on new topics of study and new ways to study them.

The department of psychology can be a valid host for community psychology if it is an "open system," if it welcomes and nurtures the planned intrusion into the university of debate about topics of intervention and social policy. In this way, the worries of outsiders can appeal to the theoretical queries of the psychologist as problems for psychological work. Education for community psychology in a department of psychology can be good and useful if there are planned occasions for renewal and update that include the nonpsychologist.

MULTIDISCIPLINARY EDUCATION AS A CATALYTIC SATELLITE

There are several situations within higher education where it is possible for doctoral students in psychology to expand their graduate study by being a part of an explicit and intact multidisciplinary program or by having access to faculty from different parts of the university. Psychology students and faculty are just one discipline represented in these programs. At first glance such education seems a very attractive aid in understanding the complexity of social forces acting on national and community life and efforts to evaluate or create public policy. In this educational option, there is in one setting a variety of professional resources for shared problem solving—an intriguing possibility indeed! While the department of psychology offers clarity of traditions and bounded knowledge, the multidisciplinary program produces some definite ambiguity in that there are few traditions and unbounded opportunities for creating knowledge. My guess is that the optimum beneficiaries of multidisciplinary training are people who have had extensive and diverse professional experience, are emotionally and professionally mature, have a clear personal identity, and really love tackling new and unfamiliar topics and making sense out of them. I also believe it is important for the academic background to be sufficiently broad to allow one to move easily into quantitative methods in such fields as geography, urban planning, etc., and to appreciate the benefits of topics like gaming simulations and econometrics. This setting is a real opportunity for adapting the psychological perspective, but the setting is also a test of personal adaptability.

For the spirited generalist moving toward a career in public policy, the multidisciplinary educational program offers a setting in which to learn new methods and become acquainted with ideas that go beyond the inevitable constraints developed within a single professional boundary. For the psychologist, being immersed in methods and content that have implications about new dependent variables, fresh topics, and alternative points of view provides new opportunities.

A recent study by Bloom and Parad (1976) offers a cautionary note on the interest of psychologists in multidisciplinary work. They received reports from 55 of the 87 federally-assisted community mental health centers and 67 of the 77 professional training programs in psychiatry, clinical psychology, social work, and psychiatric nursing in 13 western states. Psychologists expressed the least interest in interdisciplinary training of the four professions in both center and training samples. This finding suggests that we in psychology, at least in these settings, are balking in working with nonpsychologists.

One of the consequences for the graduate student in psychology is that the investment in the profession of psychology may be lessened. The impact of a saturated experience in this kind of multidisciplinary environment may be that the person will not develop his or her identity as a psychologist. Still, the psychologist could very well stay and become an ambassador for the psychological perspective.

Multidisciplinary training programs present the profession of psychology with a catalytic challenge to learn from the outside world. In terms of Pierce's thesis about gentlemen not having innovative ideas (Morse, 1975), the psychology profession can benefit from its mavericks in such settings. If you believe, as I do, that much of the generative spirit in creating new knowledge does occur at the margin of organizations, then we do want to follow up the experiences of psychologists who have been working in multidisciplinary settings. If we systematically move beyond our own traditions and develop communicative channels with these psychologists, we will have created our own adaptive options for organizational renewal, our "outreach" resources for our planned change.

The impact of being a psychologist in a multidisciplinary program will be stressful. Language, values, and goals for education will likely differ between participants and differ from the goals articulated in a department of psychology. On many occasions the psychologist may not know what the other persons are talking about, and the psychologist will have to cope with the feeling of being "the odd one out." There may be no available reference groups and no peer groups to share opinions, doubts, and aspirations. The psychologist in a multidisciplinary group could, however, emerge as a local psychotherapist. It is human nature, particularly for nonpsychologists, to want to know more about what is going on within ourselves and others. The risk under these conditions is that the psychologist will be seen as a "token shrink" and be applauded without any reference to substantive issues.

A particularly vulnerable role strain for the psychologist in a multidisciplinary setting is the tension between doing a time-limited, cross-sectional study, using conventional methods, in essence a safe study, and working with nonpsychologists on a promising, long-term, but vaguely defined expedition with a very uncertain outcome. That choice is there quite often; certainly it is an occasion to call upon that personal support network for reasoned reality testing.

Membership in a problem-solving group with a variety of people from different disciplines suggests that the psychologist (if not all members of the group) will require a well defined personal identity, a strong sense of self-assurance, purpose, and self-realization. One cost of being a member of a multidisciplinary enterprise is the fatigue that sets in when trying to cope with uncertainties of group goals, ambiguities of crossing over disciplinary boundaries and topics, and anxieties over achieving a common purpose. Here is where access to psychologists with similar interests is helpful and where psychologists who are in similar settings can clarify and integrate with us and coach us.

If these stresses and strains can be overcome, there is something valuable to be learned. A multidisciplinary environment sharpens the thinking about solving practical problems. There is less opportunity to hide behind the canons of tradition. There is an intrusive and compelling excitement in extracting an idea from wherever it is found and bringing it to the solution of a problem. The spirit of intellectual pragmatism takes hold in a setting where a variety of research paradigms and theories is close at hand. This setting gets close to realizing the benefits when intellectual wisdom pops up in an active social network of diverse persons.

The field of community psychology can learn something about the role of stress in group problem-solving when the community psychologist is among persons with differing values, experiences, and points of view. The ingredients of social development and social change exist on a smaller scale within the experiences of the community psychologist being a stranger in a strange land.

UNDERGRADUATE EDUCATION AS A REHEARSAL FOR REAL LIFE

Undergraduate education for professional roles has been expanding, yet the major emphasis has been on identifying the BA-level person as a preprofessional who performs a variety of professional roles on a smaller scale. If the dominant ethos of undergraduate education is designed to prepare students for a future career in psychology, then it is possible that community psychology education at the undergraduate level will be brief, serving as just another orientation to another field of psychology. However, if the functional roles of community psychology can be identified, there is a chance for undergraduate education in community psychology to be distinct from other undergraduate education.

Whether the PhD-trained psychologist likes it or not, many public community services in the U.S. are provided by BA- or AA-degree persons. The undergraduate college has the opportunity to design a curriculum that provides both a liberal education and the technical competences to perform service roles. This point of view has been the orientation of the New Careers movement, stimulated by Art Pearl and Frank Reissman many years ago (Pearl & Reissman, 1965).

The operation of such educational programs provides a chance for working professionals with less than BA degrees to obtain the education that will help them perform valid roles and sometimes new roles in community service. To achieve this logical goal, university-based education must change. It must become field oriented, worry more directly about the skills and competences to be learned, and involve the professional community in the educational program. The Lila Acheson Wallace School of Community Service and Public Affairs at the University of Oregon is an example of one effort to achieve such goals (Kelly, 1973, 1974, 1975; Sundberg, 1970, 1972). When the Wallace School began in 1967, participating faculty members encouraged the recruitment of faculty from a variety of academic disciplines and authorized students to have a full academic term in supervised field work. Consistent with Heyns' criteria for university leadership, the students are required to participate in a theory–practice integration seminar with a member of the school's faculty.

The benefits of operating the New Careers program at the Wallace School were foreshadowed by positive experiences of the faculty with undergraduate field-based education. The Wallace School's commitment to undergraduate education has achieved sufficient permanence so that the New Careers program can now have an experienced host for experimentation (Wallace School, 1975). On the basis of experiences so far, the working professional in the New Careers program who receives release time from his or her work setting to attend the local community college or the university has more significantly improved job status and income than working new professionals not in such a program. Whether it is a "Hawthorne Effect" or not, it works. What is not clear is how many of the New Careerists continue on in *new* careers with a community orientation and how many maintain a clinical role identity.

A subtle, often invisible and unmentioned, benefit of this type of undergraduate education is seeing students adopt a professional identity that is not doctrinaire or self-centered in a specific profession. Students can develop a comfort and ease in participating with topics, problems, and issues that are beyond any one discipline. It's a pleasure for me to see students develop a professional identity without the trappings, trinkets, and tokens of professionalism. I am itching to understand and document this apparent effort.

There is satisfaction in seeing this type of professional identity emerge. There is satisfaction in seeing the impact of the integration of ideas, skills, practice, and theory on occupational choice. Shaping and reinforcing a career does occur! If we put a little extra effort into the educational adventure, we can keep up, find out how students' future professional identity develops, and sense that our early educational efforts have helped.

The negative features of operating an undergraduate professional school are visible in ways different than in the other two educational programs. It is unclear how the educational experience contributes to a professional identification for the hundreds of graduates each year. There are too many graduates to know personally. It is also not always possible to know about the quality of the service being provided by the graduates who are employed in a variety of public and private agencies, or to know first-hand the impact the graduate has upon her or his agency in working to improve the quality of service with a BA degree. The student may enjoy the *doing* so much that faculty wonder if the total educational program is challenging the students to consider a broad array of choices for their future career roles. Both the constraints and the opportunities are present to design education without the traditions, the long time-period, and the theroretical and methodological format of graduate education.

There are costs for the faculty. The visible day-in, day-out incentives to participate in intellectual discussions are lacking. Faculty focus is on how to teach, how to integrate classwork with field instruction, and how to design an education that is experientially appealing. There is also a nagging, ever-present sense that the faculty are not really viewed as equals in the university. There is an annual epidemic of stress when promotion and tenure decisions are made by the school's personnel committee, the dean, and the university personnel committee.

In spite of these constraints, I believe that more emphasis within psychology should be given to undergraduate professional education, for it offers the opportunity for experienced persons without degrees and inexperienced persons aspiring for careers to receive an education that begins to cement a professional role identity. Time and again, the graduates of the Wallace School now in graduate work say that their undergraduate education was not only superior to that of their peers, but that it was superior to the education they are receiving in graduate schools of social work, urban planning, or psychology. The graduates also report that they are able to obtain positions with new responsibilities when they seek employment in careers in community and public affairs after the BA degree. While the faculty don't experience it, the students seem to be able to extract and integrate the diverse experiences of undergraduate education.

There is no reason to wait for graduate study to design analogues for community work. If field experiences are available and the university faculty believe in generic education, the university can make useful contributions to the declaration of undergraduate professional roles. The faculty will want to be alert to the developmental capabilities of the students and be prepared to cope constructively and creatively with the marginality of being a professional in a university. The satisfaction is genuine when the BA-trained person performs quality work and maintains an optimistic commitment for professional growth.

CONCLUSION

The field of community psychology has arrived. Tangible signs illustrate growth and success. I believe the goal for community psychology is to create and sustain a conception of the profession that includes diverse educational settings. The personal and social supports generate innovative thinking, not the number of training programs, textbooks, and journal articles alone. Three examples of varied settings—graduate education in psychology, multidisciplinary graduate education, and undergraduate education—have been presented. Each has unique contributions for the profession, and each is expected to serve as part of the larger support system for the culture of community psychology.

Satisfactions derived from each of the three settings are somewhat different. The appeal for rigor, set in traditional paradigms for empirical research in the department of psychology, is complemented by the enterprising focus of the multidisciplinary setting, where there are plentiful opportunities to adapt ideas and a clear incentive to go in new directions. Both of these graduate educational settings offer something different, yet powerful, for the field. Each setting, with its press of being disciplined or adventuresome, will require personal supportive means for the work to be done. The psychologist in one place can help the psychologist in the other. The field needs the interchange of both experiences as well as the undergraduate setting.

The undergraduate setting in turn needs both graduate settings, where ideas and issues are proclaimed. The undergraduate setting can be the place where the values, the frame of reference for community work, are established, where the career is defined and set in motion, and where the role of the person with a BA degree in service and policy making can be appraised. All three educational settings offer clear and valid roles. Each setting, paired with each other setting, can radiate ideas to resolve the tensions of community psychology work. In combination, they each assert a shared involvement in the diversity of the field.

The thesis is that we as community psychologists, in order to be true to ourselves and to be meaningful participants in the profession, should work toward the creation of personal and social support systems for each other. It's essential for every community psychologist to do this. In doing so, each community psychologist will become even more useful, contributing as a valued individual to a social network of community psychologists and to a unique profession.

REFERENCES

American Psychological Association. *Graduate study in psychology for 1975–76*. Washington, D.C.: Author, 1974.

Barzun, J. *The American university: How it runs, where it is going.* New York: Harper & Row, 1968.

Binder, A. A new context for psychology: Social ecology. *American Psychologist*, 1972, *27*, 903–908.

Bloom, B. L., & Parad, H. J. *Interdisciplinary training and interdisciplinary functioning: A survey of attitudes and practices in community mental health.* Unpublished manuscript, 1976. (Available from Department of Psychology, Muenzinger Building, University of Colorado, Boulder, Colo. 30309).

66   J. G. KELLY

Conklin, E. G. Early days at Woods Hole. *American Scientist*, 1968, *56*, 112-120.

Conklin, E. G. M. B. L. stories. *American Scientist*, 1968, *56*, 121-129.

Glidewell, J. G. Personal communications on many occasions when talking about the educational enterprise for community work and community psychology, 1972-1975.

Heyns, R. W. The university as an instrument of social action. In W. J. Minter & I. M. Thompson (Eds.), *Colleges and universities as agents of social change*. Berkeley, Calif.: Center for Research and Development in Higher Education, 1968.

Kelly, J. G. Antidotes for arrogance: Training for community psychology. *American Psychologist*, 1970, *25*, 524-531.

Kelly, J. G. *Careers in community service and public affairs at the B.A. level: The University of Oregon experience*. Paper presented at the meeting of the American Psychological Association, Montreal, August 28, 1973.

Kelly, J. G. *The hallmarks of CSPA: Criteria for work and fun*. Paper presented at the faculty meeting of Lila Acheson Wallace School of Community Service and Public Affairs, University of Oregon, Eugene, September 18, 1974.

Kelly, J. G. *CSPA as a resourceful organization*. Paper presented at the faculty meeting of Lila Acheson Wallace School of Community Service and Public Affairs, University of Oregon, Eugene, September 18, 1975.

Kuhn, T. S. *The structure of scientific revolutions* (2nd enlarged ed.). Chicago: University of Chicago Press, 1970.

Maher, T. H. *Differentiation within university departments: A case study of emerging forms of community psychology*. Unpublished doctoral dissertation, University of Michigan, 1970.

Morse, J. M. The retreat from articulacy. *The Chronicle of Higher Education*, 1975, *10* (April 21), 24.

Pearl, A., & Reissman, F. *New careers for the poor*. New York: Free Press, 1965.

Sales, G. The gospel according to John Maher. *San Francisco*, 1975, *17* (April), 24-28.

Sarason, S. *The psychological sense of community: Prospects for a community psychologist*. San Francisco: Joseey-Bass, 1974.

Sundberg, N. D. The community concern of the university. In F. Robert Paulsen (Ed.), *Higher education dimensions and directions*. Tucson: University of Arizona Press, 1970.

Sundberg, N. D. *The Lila Acheson Wallace School of Community Service and Public Affairs, Five-year Progress Report 1967-1972*. Eugene: University of Oregon, 1972.

Vallance, T. R. The professional non-psychology graduate program for psychologists. *American Psychologist*, 1976, *31*, 193-199.

Wallace School of Community Service and Public Affairs. *Undergraduate education for professional careers: An Oregon story*. Symposium presented at the annual convention of the American Psychological Association, Chicago, September 1975.

III TRAINING MODELS AND APPROACHES IN COMMUNITY PSYCHOLOGY

INTRODUCTION

Ira Iscoe

One of the main tasks of the participants at the Austin Conference was to work on an approach to training in community psychology. An analysis of the 25 training program descriptions, or models, submitted as part of the preconference materials led to the selection of 7 such approaches for deliberation and study:

1. *Clinical Community* An extension of the clinical model. Trainees receive basic clinical training, work with individuals or groups, but may also work in community mental health centers at individual or group levels. Focus is on the amelioration of symptoms, although there is some intervention and consultation.

2. *Community Clinical and Community Mental Health* Less emphasis on clinical but still a strong clinical flavor. Aim may be the improved mental health of the community. Psychologists may do more administrative and planning work. There is responsibility to a more or less defined community.

3. *Community Development and Systems* Aim is a better quality of life for the community. Activities include conceptualizing and planning, managing, evaluation. Main emphasis is still on mental health, although there is a strong interdisciplinary flavor.

4. *Interventive Preventive Systems* Stress is on fostering competence. Frequently involves utilization of non–traditionally trained personnel. Psychologists work in community and organizational settings, including schools, departments of public health, etc. Clinical knowledge is minimized, evaluation and consultation strongly stressed.

5. *Social Change Models* Emphasis is on changing of institutions and society. Interdisciplinary flavor; sophistication in politics and influence of legislation important.
6. *Social Ecology and Environmental Models Systems* Systematic assessment of community forces and the planning of multilevel interventions. Interrelationships of various environmental forces and the consequences and constraints are considered, including the relationship of housing, population density, and other physical factors.
7. *Applied Social Psychology and Urban Psychology Systems* Emphasis is on the external factors acting on persons. The intrapsychic receives little stress. Activities are directed toward achieving social change designed to promote human well-being. Emphasis is on urban problems; evaluation and consultation are stressed; field research is stressed.

In making its classifications, the planning committee was aware that the approaches could not be completely separated from one another but instead tended to overlap. Further, the committee recognized that the approaches selected were neither exhaustive nor mutually exclusive. They do, however, constitute a continuum of training, from a traditional clinical approach through an applied social approach to an ecological approach. Thus, they recognize the great diversity in community psychology and at the same time provide the participants with specific areas of concentration for the duration of the conference.

Several weeks prior to the conference the participants received a description of the seven models along with other preconference materials. Included was a request to submit the approach they wished to pursue in depth. Expressed interest in the clinical community model was so sparse that the model was combined with the community clinical/community mental health model, thus reducing the number of approaches from seven to six. On the other hand, interest in the interventive and preventive approach was so great that this model was split into three sections, while interest in the social change model led to the addition of one extra section.

Each group consisted of 9 to 14 persons. During the three days of the conference a total of about seven hours was allocated for formal discussion, with an additional three hours scheduled for a plenary session in which all of the approaches were discussed. The challenge facing each group was a formidable one, and conference planners recognized at the beginning that it was unlikely that the groups could complete these tasks by the end of the sessions. Therefore, on the final day group chairmen and recorders met to formulate plans for continuing their work after the conference, to set up communication details, and to establish completion deadlines. The diligence of the chairmen in carrying out the follow-up activities and editing the final reports resulted in the material in this section.

It should be noted that the groups accomplished more than developing a training approach. They also served an important and previously neglected informal function, providing an opportunity for community psychologists to get to know one another and to work together toward conceptualizing a particular approach to training in a direction of mutual interest.

To provide some cohesiveness to the diverse approaches as well as to allow for comparisons across models, each group was given a Guideline for Training Model Construction. Flexibility and creativity were emphasized, and the participants were urged to avoid minutiae—no small request of academes. The guidelines incorporated the seven areas used in the preconference materials to describe the programs: (1) ideology and value base of the training approach, (2) goals, (3) level of operation, (4) research and knowledge base, (5) technology and skills required for graduates to function effectively, (6) content area, and (7) training format. Additional areas included financial support; locus of employment; provisions for continuing education; level of entry; career ladder and lattice opportunities; essential and recommended courses; and type of field training settings, including recommendations about practicum and internships.

Not all of the areas were addressed by each group, and the reports vary in degree of comprehensiveness and completion. All, however, represent a distinct contribution to community psychology within the broad areas of the approach selected. Questions not answered usually resulted from the participant's concern that the particular approach or the field itself was not sufficiently involved or clarified for answers to be more specific at this time. Thus, the reports in some ways reflect the degree of evolution of the particular approach espoused.

Readers can judge for themselves how well each group succeeded in meeting its goals. An analysis of the models en toto is provided at the end of this section.

6 Competence and Conflict in Community Psychology

John C. Glidewell

Having read and reread the accounts of the 25 models prepared for the Austin Conference, my impression is that there is one theme: complexity. The complexity is manifested in the remarkable variety of roles for which community psychologists are trained; in the complex weaving of social problems into client concerns; in the crosshatched psychosocial phenomena into which a community psychologist is expected to intervene; and, more fundamentally, in the cultural preoccupation surrounding the roles, the client concerns, and the phenomena to be modified.

Before I explain my analysis of the training models, let me call your attention to a bit of life in the city. I think it lends some concreteness and specificity to what follows. You may know that in Chicago there is a special "El" train that doesn't go anywhere—it just goes round and round the loop in the center of the city. The train is used for making some of the complex connections available in the loop and for local traffic. It is called the shuttle train. I ride it a lot. I keep looking for Bob Newhart, but I have never seen him on the El.

Behavior on the El is quite regular. It makes me think about the incredible regularity of the general behavior of people and the general preoccupations of our time and civilization. People get on and they sit down—usually—and they try as well as they can to act as if there is nobody else on the train. There is a sort of bubble of privacy around each person. If someone accidentally touches another person, she breaks the bubble. He quickly draws back. She apologizes. In a crowded train in a crowded city, privacy is dear and treasured.

People usually carry something: a lunch box, a shopping bag, a briefcase, or just a plain brown bag. One fellow got on with a long telephoto lens, about 200 millimeters. He held it very gently and kept examining it. Now and then he would hold it up to his eye and look through it. You could tell his new telephoto 200 mm lens was his key to the good life. That was really pride.

A lot of people carry newspapers. I like to read over their shoulders. (Yes, I am farsighted.) One lady was reading a feature on department store charge accounts being closed to women after their husbands died. Now and then she'd say to herself, "Bastards, dirty bastards!" That was really outrage.

One man in a worn suit, about 80 I'd say, sat in the back with a bag of dog food between his knees. When he thought no one was looking, he would sneak a pellet of dog food into his mouth. And he would grin to himself.

Once I saw an old woman, so feeble she could hardly take the step at the entrance. She was in pain and so cold she was shaking. Everyone pretended not to notice her, but you could feel the surge of tension in the car. People watched out of the corners of their eyes. We thought she was going to fall, but she didn't. When she finally dropped into a seat, you could feel the relief, the unexpressed sigh. She made it!

The El is a speck of life in the city and maybe, thereby, in the urban civilization. There are efforts to enhance life with special lenses; to solve social problems, human problems; to find justice in the distribution of food, people food; and to relieve pain and distress in the bones of people, old and young.

In the curricula of 25 training programs there are efforts as diverse, as ambitious, as complex as life in the city. I am reminded of the fact that, as knowledge grows more complex, it is distributed in smaller and smaller fractions. As the practitioners specialize their practices in order to conform to their particular fractions of the available knowledge, they often need perspective, and they turn to their colleagues to try to find it. I think the trainers of community psychologists are now seeking perspective. Let me make a provisional try at drawing some perspectives out of the accounts of the 25 training programs.

The theme, I have said, is complexity: complexity of role, complexity of client concerns, complexity of psychosocial phenomena, and complexity of cultural preoccupations. Within these complexities are deep and abiding conflicts: conflicts of values on cooperation and values on contention, conflicts between quick emergency relief from distress and gradual growing enhancement of life, conflicts between direct paths to goal attainment and roundabout struggles toward justice, conflicts between changing individual behavior to fit social systems and changing social systems to accommodate individual behavior. Let me try to put the complexity into a manageable structure. My review of the programs led me to believe that each reflected four dimensions: (1) the varying cultural preoccupation of the times, (2) the varying conceptions of the phenomena to be changed, (3) the varying roles of the clients, and (4) the varying roles of the practitioners (see Table 1).

I'd like to analyze the broadest first: the varying cultural preoccupations of the times. I maintain that such cultural preoccupations are constantly shifting from fierce competitive goal attainment to fine cooperative coordination, from distributive justice to life enhancement—and that people tend to be preoccupied about just one at a time. We neglect conflict as we focus on cooperation. We neglect long-term qualities of life as we concentrate on short-term goal attainment. In this country we have shifted from the cooperative 1950s to the battling 1960s, from long-term enhancement of our environment to frantic production of energy. The cycles will always be with

TABLE 1 The matrix of professional practice

Cultural preoccupation	Psychosocial phenomenon	Client	Practitioner	Point of intervention
Life enhancement	Dreaming, planning, inventing, affluence	Participant-developer	Planner, designer, evaluator	Policy-making
Social conflict	Resolute contention, struggle, deviation	Misfit, deviate, subordinate culture	Consultant, negotiator, conciliator	Conflict arena (on-site–off-site)
Distributive justice	Poverty, discrimination, neglect	Have-not, discriminated against, neglected	Advocate, organizer, agent	Local exchange point–mass media
Pain-distress	Illness, injury	Sufferer, patient	Healer, therapist, counselor	Private life-institution

us and always affect the practices of community psychologists. We seem to move in cycles through four preoccupations: life enhancement, social conflict, distributive justice, pain and distress.

My time on the El reflected in miniature the inherent conflicts and preoccupations about life enhancement, social conflict, distributive justice, and pain and distress. In the training models I studied, I counted 15 programs preoccupied with two goals: social problem-solving and distributive justice. Social problem-solving was most often to be accomplished by conflict resolution and coordination. The linked distributive justice was to be accomplished by organized community action and advocacy. Another 16 programs addressed both life enhancement through planning and distributive justice through advocacy. It is important that only four models expressed an explicit preoccupation with relief from distress.

Consider whether these preoccupations are not mutually exclusive. Can any professional practitioner really address more than one at a time? It would seem that community psychologists and their trainers may be trying to do the impossible.

Let me take the analysis one step further. Leaving the cultural preoccupations, there are four classes of phenomena in which community psychologists are meant to intervene: (1) development, social and individual, (2) social conflict and deviancy, (3) discrimination and neglect, and (4) pain and distress.

Consider the prime values of intervention into each of these phenomena. In development the prime value is life enhancement, in social conflict the value is resolute contention, in discrimination the value is distributive justice, in pain the value is relief. I am pretty sure that I cannot pursue all those values at the same time.

Consider the primary processes involved in the four phenomena. Development involves leaving familiar supports and taking unclear risks. Conflict involves mobilization of resources and unwavering loyalty. Discrimination involves intergroup suspicions and strongly defended boundaries. Pain involves the most intense need and the most ready dependency. One simply cannot facilitate all at once: risky shifts, unwavering loyalty, defended boundaries, and ready dependency.

Community psychologists should have a ready knowledge in depth of the psychosocial phenomena in which they intervene, and they must have an effective technology for this intervention. Is it better to know one of these phenomena well and thoroughly, or is it possible to know all of them well enough? We must face this question here and now.

But let me change focus again, from the phenomena to the client in whose interests the psychologist intervenes. There is an intricacy about helping relationships that almost defies analysis. What indeed is help? What are the spontaneous social supports, the degrees of autonomy, the speed of the outcomes, the enabling initiative?

Once when I made the mistake of telling my younger daughter that she was too little to carry my suitcase, she said, "I bet you a hundred dollars that I can push something in the wheelbarrow from here to the street—and you can't push it back." Yes, I lost. What you are thinking is exactly correct. When I took the bet she said simply, "OK, hop in." Some things I can do for myself. Some things I can't.

The programs are oriented to a remarkably wide variety of clients: (1) the developer-inventor-dreamer (I'll call her the inventor); (2) the social antagonist, the misfit; (3) the chronic have-not, the poor; and (4) the acute sufferer.

Consider first the autonomy expected by each. The inventor expects enormous autonomy. She must have room to experiment. The antagonist expects loyal support but no constraints. He is overly resistant to constraints. The poor person may expect much or little. If militant, she tolerates no interference. If apathetic, she expects others to act for her. The sufferer quickly surrenders autonomy in exchange for relief.

Consider the spontaneous social supports of each client. The inventor seeks support from the affluent who have discretionary funds: foundations, corporations, governments. It may turn out that she makes the rich richer. The antagonist or the misfit seeks support from his fellow antagonists, and they take over his usual duties when he is protesting, negotiating, or waiting and waiting in court. The poor person must try to find support in collective action and solidarity. Embargo, boycott, and strike depend on collective action, witholding those resources that the poor may collectively command.

The sufferer is relieved of his usual social duties until his distress is over and he is offered sympathy and expressive support to supplement or compensate for submission to the healer's instrumental intervention. The client roles are so different that to serve more than one at a time is to tear oneself apart.

Without leaving the client, let me turn to the complementary practitioner. He can be the planner-designer, she can be the consultant-negotiator, she can be the advocate-organizer, he can be the healer-therapist. Many program accounts reported that they were training the participant-conceptualizer, only a few the scientist-professional. None really were. Let me be more specific.

We are much influenced by the image of healers. They relieve suffering. They have arcane and dependable knowledge not available to the laymen. They are constrained by ethics to act in the best interests of their clients. Indeed, they know better—because of their arcane knowledge—what is good for their clients than the clients do themselves. The healer's is a prestigious role with enormous social power and, often enough, deeply dedicated to relief of distress.

Advocate-organizers, on the other hand, have no arcane knowledge. They substitute a special charisma. Consultant-negotiators, still different, act jointly with or through their clients, with a combination of personal style and professional skill. Planner-designers are technician-visionaries. They accept joint accountability to produce a plausible invention.

In the descriptions of the training models, take note of the frequent specification of planning skills. I counted six such programs. Look then at the social problem-solvers. I called them consultant-negotiators, but only the consultation was in focus; the negotiation was implied. I counted ten such programs. Now turn to the advocate-organizers. I found five such roles specified. There were many mixtures—most were mixtures—and few full houses.

As I have proposed, if the cultural preoccupations are mutually exclusive, if the phenomena involve conflicting processes, if the clients have conflicting expectations, consider the conflicts among the four practitioner roles.

The prime value of the planner is the long-term enhancement of life. The prime value of the healer is immediate relief from pain. The prime value of the consultant-negotiator is conflict resolution and synthesis. The prime value of the advocate-organizer is distributive justice. Is it possible to pursue any two of these values at once? Can I both cooperate and contend? Can I both plan and relieve? Can I both confront and give quick relief? Can I both plan and contend? Possibly I could—sometimes—but rarely, I think, very rarely.

For what, then, shall we train? How shall we cope with the inevitable role conflicts, the inevitable conflicts between practice and cultural preoccupations? Can I be a planner in a time of crisis? Can I be a healer in the context of neglect? Can I be an advocate in a time of cooperative social problem-solving?

The combinations of cultural preoccupations, psychosocial phenomena, client needs, and practitioner skills are just too many. Some go together well, very well indeed; some don't go together at all. All community psychologists must get together and decide upon our kind of clients, our role repertoire, the psychosocial phenomena we really must know about in great depth, and especially the cultural preoccupations we shall address. And we must—I am certain we really must—fit the role to the client, the phenomena, and the preoccupation as carefully and as deliberately as we can.

I think we must do even more. I think community psychologists are going to find themselves specializing even when they didn't intend to. As a practitioner, once one grasps the excitement and the confidence of really knowing what one is doing and really producing visible improvements for clients, one will stay with that phenomenon, that role, and that kind of client. Think what it means to a person to understand really, deeply, and comprehensively one cultural preoccupation, such as social conflict. Think what it yields to know thoroughly all the ins and outs of one psychosocial phenomenon, such as deviancy. Think of the fulfillment gained from the confident mastery of one professional practice, such as consultation. Think of the self-authentication of competently, calmly, and carefully serving the acute interest of one client, such as the neglected. One could take a justifiable pride in professional accomplishment subject to a professional discipline created in the joint interests of a diminished client and of a concerned community.

Then, and maybe only then, a person can take up a secondary role, a secondary preoccupation, a secondary psychosocial phenomenon. But if so a person must, as always, take on another primary client.

Given such commitments, a community psychologist could go home after one of those miserable days of failure and frustration and reflect upon the experience with confidence and challenge. One could systematically consult one's knowledge, analyze one's day, and after a time say, "Now I know what I did wrong and why. Now I know what I should try tomorrow." That is the prime test of competence: to make mistakes, to analyze them clearly, and to know how to correct them—to know what to do in trouble. Such competence, I am sure, requires that one understand thoroughly the cultural preoccupations, the psychosocial phenomena, and the client role in response to which one conducts one's professional practice.

7 Clinical Community and Community Mental Health Models

Joseph F. Aponte

IDEOLOGY, VALUE BASE, AND SOCIAL ETHICS

The main focus of a community psychology program should be on the well-being, enhancement, and betterment of all persons, rather than exclusively on the mentally ill. There must be a sensitivity to well-defined community needs, as determined by analyses that reflect a wide range of perspectives and sources of information including surveys of citizens and citizen participation in the determination of priorities among identified needs.

Community psychology must have a broader base than solely a clinical program, with a greater emphasis on the social structure, organization, and processes of the community itself. Community psychology, still recognizing the importance of intrapersonal and interpersonal experiences, can be viewed on a continuum with clinical psychology and need not be conceptualized as a separate entity.

Thus, the clinical community and community mental health group recognized the legitimacy of a plurality of models, namely, the scientist and practitioner models. They considered it important to acknowledge the necessity of research for the sake of knowledge and social understanding as well as research for the sake of social change. The greater emphasis in community psychology should be on social change. (See Table 1 for examples of potential content areas.)

GOALS AND OBJECTIVES

The student of community psychology must have a broad based training program. This would involve changing the structure and curriculum of preexisting psychology departments. The student must receive both the support and the encouragement of the department to seek interdisciplinary training when necessary, as well as to maintain some, but not all, of the preexisting clinical-interpersonal skills.

Participants in this model: Clifford Attkisson, Keith Barton, Bernard Bloom, Robert Callahan, Louis Cohen, Aubrey Escoffrey, Ricardo Esparza, Charles Haywood, Swen Helge, Bernard Lubin, Sherman Nelson, Rodney Nurse, Louis Ramey, Gwendolyn J. Roquemore, Lynette Smith, Charles Spielberger, Stanley Sue, Henry Tomes, Forrest Tyler, Tom Van Hoose, Edward Zolik.

TABLE 1 Clinical community model

	Psychology	Nonpsychology
General	Developmental—life cycle Personality Social Sensation—perception Motivation and emotion Learning Multiethnic psychology Ethics and human rights	General systems theory Public administration Economics Political science Social policy and planning Epidemiology Ethnology (anthropology) Literature History Philosophy of science

Clinical	Individual behavior in groups
	    and organizations
	Psychological assessment
	Growth facilitation
	Individual, group, and
	    organizational intervention
	Psychopathology	

Community	Consultation Organizational psychology Environmental psychology Systems intervention Community psychology Program evaluation Community assessment	Urban planning Criminal justice Community organization

Research Methods	Measurement (field, naturalis-
	    tic, demographic, and
	    social area analyses)
	Program evaluation	

Field Training	Practicum Internship Special experiences	

LEVEL OF OPERATION

The community psychology student should work on multilevels, with bimodal points being: (1) individuals, groups, and families; and (2) communities and society as social entities as well as institutions and other social systems. It should be emphasized that inherent in the individual, group, and family level is the recognition that this model is a very real part of the broader-based community model, but it retains its intra- and interpersonal base.

RESEARCH AND KNOWLEDGE BASES

The knowledge and research base needs to move beyond traditional laboratory models to incorporate the interfacing and impact of organizations, communities, and society on individuals, groups, and families. Action research, program evaluation, and epidemiological studies, for example, should be the proper domain of the community psychology student.

TECHNOLOGY AND SKILLS REQUIRED

Each trainee should have an array of assessment and intervention skills across multiple levels, including: (1) individuals, (2) groups, (3) families, (4) organizations, (5) communities, and (6) society. It would be unrealistic to expect each person to be expert at each of these levels. Rather, the student would be expected to have a general knowledge of all of these areas and to be expert in a few. Skills in individual, group, and family assessment, organizational assessment, community needs assessment, and social indicator construction and usage are of paramount importance. Interventions at these multiple levels of case, organization, and system consultation also are important. In addition, program evaluation skills to measure the impact of these interventions are needed.

CONTENT AREAS

The content areas of the training program should build on existing knowledge bases in the areas of general psychology, clinical psychology, and community psychology. It should also include nonpsychology content courses that cut across the general, clinical, and community areas. Flexibility that allows responsiveness to changing problems and needs in the community and larger society must be built into the training programs.

In the general psychological domain, courses such as developmental, personality, social, learning, ethics and human rights, and multiethnic psychology are important. General systems theory, public administration, social policy and planning, epidemiology, anthropology, and philosophy of science should be interfaced with the training program.

Individual behavior in groups and organizations, psychological assessment (at individual, group, and family levels), growth facilitation, individual and group intervention, organizational intervention, and psychopathology are courses that have importance in the clinical psychology domain. Nonpsychology courses could be drawn from other disciplines such as sociology, medicine, and education.

In the community psychology domain consultation, organizational psychology, environmental psychology, systems intervention, community assessment, and program evaluation are important. Nonpsychology community courses include urban planning, criminal justice, and community organization. A number of other courses can of course be added to this list.

Research methods would cut across the psychology and nonpsychology content areas. Measurement in field and naturalistic settings would be the focus. Demographic and social area analysis are examples of needed skills. Social action research and program evaluation in a number of settings with a variety of problems would be stressed.

FORMAT

Training can and should take place in a number of settings (academic departments, medical settings, community mental health centers, school systems, etc.), but the program should be based and principally supported in a university setting and allow for experimental programs within newly developing schools of professional psychology. Relationships should exist with these other settings in the form of joint appointments, sharing resources, and sharing of faculty and staffs.

Course content and experiences would be sequenced so that core general and clinical courses would be taken in the beginning of the student's career. Community courses should also be built into the beginning years, with the bulk of the courses and experiences coming later. Placement in the field at an early stage is essential.

Practicum, job placements, internships, and special experiences should be designed to interface with the didactic courses and to maximize the learnings of the community psychology student. Theses and dissertations should also be relevant to the area of community psychology, with university settings accepting field and naturalistic research and not just laboratory studies.

FINANCIAL SUPPORT

Faculty, student, and program support should come primarily from institutional committed funds and secondarily from outside sources. Examples of such outside support might include federal stipends, work study programs, and local or state agency stipends. The essential components of the underlying ideology are that community psychology program support should be stable, yet of multiple origin, and should be guided by a sense of responsibility and accountability.

In addition, there should be encouragement of potential new sources of funds from federal, state, and local categories such as juvenile justice and manpower areas. Student stipend support should be encouraged through local/ state psychological associations and successful local groups of practitioners such as family and group therapy centers and private practice groups that contract to provide services for local mental health agencies.

LOCUS OF EMPLOYMENT

Community psychology program graduates entering the employment market can work in positions already legitimized for psychologists; create new jobs; or earn the opportunity to work in positions ordinarily occupied by persons with other kinds of training.

Some graduates will work in traditional settings—teaching, mental health service, and research. Others will move into broader arenas such as human service delivery systems focusing on the integration of human service networks, community consultation, or social structure analysis and modification. All of these activities can take place in both the public and the private sector.

CONTINUING EDUCATION AND RELATIONSHIP TO TRAINING

Adequate attention has not been given to community psychology continuing education and to the related area of recertification and relicensure. Perhaps the first step should be to identify the continuing education needs of professional psychologists, then to identify the areas in which community psychology can contribute to meeting these continuing education needs. It is also imperative to begin including community psychology in those growing state programs (e.g., California) where psychology continuing education is being built into the ongoing structure of psychology.

LEVEL OF ENTRY

The MA is recognized as the present level of entry for a community psychologist. In principle, entry may be possible at other levels (BA and AA), but no adequate pre-MA designation of skills particular to specific roles, functions, and responsibilities is clearly articulated at these levels. Further clarification is needed in this area.

With regard to MA and PhD training, individuals with either degree are recognized as capable of providing services, but the individual with the PhD is viewed as having more in-depth and conceptual skills. The person with the MA is considered competent but narrower, while the person with the PhD is viewed as competent but broader. Each can fit within a practitioner, scientist, or scientist-practitioner model.

CAREER LADDER AND CAREER LATTICE OPPORTUNITIES

Both career ladders and career lattices are strongly supported. Development within levels and movement into other levels are essential for the vitality of community psychology. Upgrading of skills should be a responsibility of the training program and of the profession. Ideally, each should work closely together.

ESSENTIAL COURSES

The type and number of essential, desirable, and ideal courses has not been explicated. This would depend on a detailed specification of basic skills that community psychologists should have in their armamentarium. It would, however, be essential that courses and experiences of a general, clinical, and community nature within and outside of psychology be incorporated in the training program.

FIELD WORK EXPERIENCES

Job placements, practicum, and special experiences in the field are crucial to the training of community psychologists. Appropriate role models in which people are providing service and conducting research in the field need to be established. Interdisciplinary exposure and the utilization of nontraditional as well as traditional settings are also important.

Placement in the field needs to begin early in the career of the student, preferably in the first year. Flexibility is essential in the training program so that arrangements can be made to have students in the field for varying lengths of time. Programs should move away from the semester or quarter concept with regard to field placements. The task should determine the length of time in the field.

Close coordination of field work experiences is necessary. This would include on-site supervision, reciprocal funding and service arrangements, and cooperative agency and university ties. Joint appointments and exchanges of staffs would facilitate this type of coordination.

8 Community Development and Systems Approaches

Raymond P. Lorion

Given the focuses of the training models, the unique component of the community development and systems model is its emphasis on the conceptual and empirical delineations of the dimensions of communities and their social systems, which are relevant to the personal-emotional adaptation of their members. The development of this body of information should enable the social scientist to implement systematic changes in communities and their institutions in a responsible fashion. The direct and indirect, positive and negative, and intentional and unintentional consequences of proposed interventions can then begin to be identified and anticipated prior to the implementation of changes.

IDEOLOGY

Professionals operating within this model

1. assume that the community as environment, sense of belongingness, or however defined shapes an individual's behavior in both positive and negative ways, providing resources for adequate coping as well as imposing forms of stress and restricting the range of alternative solutions.
2. assume that within a community there exists an identifiable set of systems (i.e., educational, social services, legal, judicial, political, recreational) affecting positively and negatively the psychological status of its members.
3. assume that communities and their relevant systems proceed through identifiable stages and transitory forms, which can be considered systematically in the design and implementation of interventions.
4. assume that involvement in communities and their systems requires a synergistic exchange between conceptualization and program implementation such that each develops through the efforts of the other.

VALUE AND ETHICAL BASE

Professionals operating within this model should

1. recognize and constantly attempt to clarify their personal values and goals

Participants in this model: Bruce Bailey, Tom Cripps, Meg Gerrard, Judy Kramer, Meg Meyer, Francis Miller, Chris Padesky, Henry Pitts, Margaret Rust, Brian Sarata, Wade Silverman, Karl Slaikeu, Edison Trickett, Neomia Turner, Christine McLean.

in order to minimize ethnocentric conflicts with target communities and enhance the culture of the community.
2. recognize that at times their goals (e.g., the elimination or reduction of racism) may be directly antagonistic to those of the target population (e.g., "antibusing" parents).
3. appreciate the ethical implications of assuming the role of social activist or social respondent. This implies genuinely confronting the pros and cons of our assumptions (e.g., "prevention is good") and models of health and dysfunction.
4. direct their efforts toward reinforcing community autonomy and independence and modifying their input as members of the community expand their options.

GOALS AND OBJECTIVES

The professional trained within such a model should be able to

1. identify and modify the dimensions of communities and their systems relevant to psychological adaptation.
2. maximize the impact of community resources.
3. work collaboratively with members of a community across social, economic, and ethnic groupings.
4. utilize existing systems within a community's structure to "improve the quality of life" for its members.
5. evaluate the needs of a community and the impact (positive and negative) of interventions to meet these needs, and communicate this information in such a way that the process of development can be enhanced.
6. facilitate the implementation of community and system changes through consultation efforts.

LEVELS OF OPERATION

Although professionals operating within this model would occasionally intervene with the entire community, the primary target of their efforts would be systems functioning within the community. Among the likely targets are: preschool services; established health service facilities; social welfare services; and legal, judicial, and recreational services. Professionals may also intervene in organizations less traditionally associated with mental health services, such as churches, civic groups, labor unions, etc. An important focus of professional activities would be the identification and resolution of conflicts between and within human service systems.

RESEARCH AND KNOWLEDGE BASE

In view of the focuses of the other training models, it seems appropriate to expect that professionals trained with a community development and systems model would generate much of the conceptual and empirical material necessary for direct program implementation and social change. The program should emphasize research into community and system needs and resources; analyses of organizational functioning; and estimates of the mental health "ripple" effects of social, economic, and political changes on a community. Not only is much new knowledge needed in the general area of community and systems analysis but, more essentially, existing knowledge and research methods from other social disciplines (e.g., urban planning, public health, economics, political science, etc.) must become available to the area of community psychology. Techniques such as survey strategies, systems analysis, and epidemiology should be included within the empirical armamentarium of the community psychologist.

TECHNOLOGY AND SKILLS REQUIRED

A person emerging from a training program in community and systems development should be able to

1. conceptualize communities and their systems within an ecological perspective and recognize their relevant structural components.
2. interact with individuals and organizations across the social and economic levels within the community.
3. evaluate communities, systems, and programs, using the research and conceptual skills described.
4. assess and maximize linkage across relevant human service agencies.
5. describe the mental health needs and resources of a community or a subgroup within the community.
6. facilitate the development and implementation of programs by "on-line" staff.
7. possess specific skills ranging from program evaluation to community organization, consultation, and development.

CONTENT AREAS

A training program in this area should provide the knowledge base needed to identify and ameliorate the human dysfunctions that arise from social-community conditions. This would seem to require an understanding of normal and pathological human growth and behavior through studies of traditional psychological areas such as personality, development, and psychopathology, and appreciation of less traditional perspectives such as systems analysis, community organization, and public health. In many ways the complexity of working with communities and systems may require specialized attention to a limited range of such institutions. Overall, training should provide an understanding of person-system interdependence as an essential base for the development of strategies for community development and/or remediation.

FORMAT

Little attention was given to this question. Given the focus of the training program, it is clear that didactic material must be balanced with direct, intense experience in the community. At present, continuing contact with the core knowledge base of psychology as a science of human behavior should be maintained.

FINANCIAL SUPPORT

Training programs may find it necessary and, ultimately, preferable to negotiate part of their support through direct contract for program evaluation and community consultation. Other support may be pursued through traditional federal channels, the U.S. Justice Department, and university, etc.

LOCUS OF EMPLOYMENT

Ideally, the products of this program should be able to fill planning and evaluation slots in community mental health centers, positions in city planning offices, and positions in county, state, and federal mental health/mental retardation bureaus. The broad-based interdisciplinary knowledge of the product of this type of training should be able to contribute to almost any system affecting the "quality of life."

CONTINUING EDUCATION

This is certainly necessary, although it was not discussed. Among the potential options should be included exchange sabbaticals between academicians and agency staff.

LEVEL OF ENTRY

As defined in this discussion, the conceptualizer-empiricist-program planner would be a doctoral-level professional.

Career Ladder, Essential Courses, and *Field Work Experiences* were not dealt with by this committee. The committee believed that these were matters for further discussion and that it had gone about as far as it could go dealing with the areas cited.

9 Intervention and Prevention

I. Preventive Intervention

Darwin Dorr

The members of this group came together because of an expressed interest in an interventive preventive model. The general mandate was to construct a training program consistent with the focus expressed in this model. A "Guideline for Training Model Construction" was provided to help organize the final product. While the group recognized some urgency about completing this guideline, it was agreed that a careful look at and understanding of the specified model would help organize and focus the ultimate report.

Therefore, discussions began with a close look at the meanings and implications of prevention and intervention, together with a look at how this focus overlapped with, or was different from, the focuses in the other training models. As a guide in this effort, the group took a second look at the description of the cited model together with the other six models, and noted three things.

First, the seven possible models tend, in a very rough way, to fall on a continuum ranging from a primarily clinical emphasis to a socio-environmental emphasis. For example, the description of the first model notes that it is "an extension of the clinical model. . . . Focus is on the amelioration of symptoms, although there is some intervention and consultation." On the other hand, the seventh model notes "The intra-psychic receives little stress. The activities are directed at achieving social change designed to promote human well-being." Each model involves a balance between concern for individual and concern for environmental factors, but the proportion of each of these two factors differs. For example, the first model is about 95% clinical-psychological and 5% socio-environmental, while the last model reverses this proportion. Being in the middle of this rough continuum, the interventive and preventive model represents an approximate balance between individual and group focuses.

Second, this model focuses on fostering competencies in individuals and communities. As the group perceived it, *competence* refers to any given strength, skill, resiliency, etc., necessary to deal effectively with a given task or a situation. There are at least two arenas in which a person can be

Participants in this model: George T. Brennan, Larry Bugen, Rosalie Cripps, Ralph Culler, Steven Danish, Ben Dean, Darwin Dorr, Dee Fruchter, Len James, John Kalafat, Karen Kamerschen, Steve Larcen, Ricardo Muñoz, Mary Teague.

competent: the impersonal, or cognitive, arena and the interpersonal, or social, arena. Further, competency of the individual may differ somewhat from the competency of the group.

Third, the title of the model includes the word *prevention*, a rather vague term, since it does not make clear precisely what is to be prevented. On the gut level it could be said that a major goal is to prevent human affective misery and behavioral inefficiency. While no one wished to dispense with the concept of prevention, it was agreed that a focus on the positive alternatives to misery and inefficiency is desirable; that is, enhancement is the thing to stress. The group discussed the concept of *enhancement* at length and concluded that the term does not necessarily imply either enrichment or the lofty goal of self-actualization. Rather, it emphasizes the development of positive capabilities that are inconsistent with maladaptation.

FOCUS

With these factors in mind, the participants renamed the model *preventive and enhancing interventions*. The training program was seen as representing a balance between exclusive concern for individual factors and exclusive concern for group factors. Hence, it seemed that this training program would involve (1) a basic foundation in those aspects of psychology that relate to the understanding of and development of human competencies and (2) sufficient familiarity with social-political variables that the interventionist will be able to contribute positively to the development of competencies of groups. While the target of intervention is an entire system, the interface might be with an individual member or group that is a part of the system.

With this general focus, the group addressed the questions raised in the training model guideline.

IDEOLOGY, VALUE BASE, AND SOCIAL ETHICS

The goal of the model is to promote or strengthen the variety of competencies necessary to deal with the demands of the environment. This could be accomplished by helping the individual or the community to cope with tasks or demands of the environment. The aim is prevention, but the hope is to prevent problems by enhancing individual and group functioning.

Values were discussed intensively. The complexity of value issues became increasingly clear. On the one hand, it was argued that it is wrong to impose one's values on other individuals and/or groups (e.g., insisting that poor people adopt middle-class mores). On the other hand, it was argued that any intervention will by its nature involve a certain value judgment, and that it is next to impossible to avoid imposing certain values on target populations (e.g., the belief that slum children will get along better if they can read). It was recognized that everyone has values, and that these play a role in determining the nature of interventions. Since one cannot really avoid the matter of values, it is best to be intent on becoming aware of values and to share these values in open discussion with others.

GOALS AND OBJECTIVES

It was agreed that the primary mode of functioning would be indirect service. Such activities as program planning, program development, and evaluation would be desirable. Teaching and consultation would take priority over direct clinical service.

LEVEL OF OPERATION

The level of intervention theoretically can range from the individual to the broadest reaches of society itself. It was realized that the closer an intervention can come to the social end of this continuum, the more highly an effective intervention will be rated on indices of social effectiveness. However, it was also realized that the radical modification of the very fabric of society is a futuristic goal, and that intervention at lower levels is also necessary. The aim is always to intervene at the highest feasible level, and it has been suggested that one way to achieve this goal is to identify and intervene at the level of the epiphenomenal community.

As conceptualized by Panzetta (1971), *epiphenomenal community* refers to a sense of community experienced by a group of individuals who share a common oppressor or stressor and who are unified by leadership. The boundaries of the epiphenomenal community may be characterized either by shared external characteristics or by factors that are less obvious at first glance. Racial and ethnic minorities may share a sense of community, although they do not necessarily do so (e.g., poor blacks vs. wealthy blacks in urban Chicago). However, other groups may also experience a sense of community that transcends ethnic or racial characteristics or even social class. For example, the parents of retarded children share a mutual stressor and, with leadership, have developed into a powerful community in the United States. They have worked long and hard to develop legislation aimed at providing better facilities for retarded citizens. According to Panzetta (1971), the psychologist who is aware of this sense of community is more likely to be successful at the point of intervention than is the psychologist who perceives community solely as a physical area (i.e., the population of individuals residing in a particular community mental health center "catchment area" may not sense any feeling of community with each other and hence will not respond as a community to issues critical to their problems).

RESEARCH AND KNOWLEDGE BASES, TECHNOLOGY AND SKILLS REQUIRED, AND CONTENT AREAS

Since these questions overlap considerably, the issues and questions raised are addressed here in a single section. A potential training program might consist of three tracks of courses and experiences looking something like this:

Individual Factors	Social Factors	Integrative Experiences
Human development	Epidemiology	General systems theory
Personality	Social psychology	Philosophy of science
Motivation	Organizational psychology	Epistemology
Social deviancy	Sociology of organization	Social welfare
Experimental analysis	Anthropology	Planning philosophy
of behavior	Organizational assessment	Man–environment relations
Biological health	Behavioral ecology	
	Community development	

The first track would give the student foundations in basic individual psychology; the second series, intermingled with the first, would provide greater sensitivity to those social, environmental, and organizational factors that affect the individual. The third track consists of experiences that would help the student integrate the material from the first two tracks.

Additionally, the student would be exposed to methodological approaches ranging from basic experimental design to quasi-experimental designs to naturalistic research, applied research, and action research. The list of possible courses could be infinite. Each student would have to plan out a sequence commensurate with his or her particular goals. For example, interventionists interested in children should seek experiences in developmental psychology, education, reading, etc. Those interested in particular minorities, such as blacks, should seek courses pertaining to the problems of those minorities.

Technology and skills should build on the knowledge base, though skills are more often acquired via guided practice in the field. Hence, field experiences should be woven in with the academic experience from the earliest days of training (much as is done in the more effective clinical training programs). Of the many desirable skills, communications skills are close to the top. Others include program planning, professional writing abilities, consultation, evaluation, the ability to communicate easily in the public arena, and lobbying. Administrative skills also are extremely useful. These include both the ability to assess the strengths and weaknesses of an organization and the tenacity to administer the goals of the organization through to completion.

Choosing one or two content areas to emphasize is indeed a difficult matter. However, since the initial focus was on promoting the development and competence in individuals or groups, the training program should emphasize those factors that are the most relevant to these goals. Hence, human and organizational development would seem to be paramount.

FORMAT

The consensus was that the ideal base would be a multidisciplinary consortium or institute. Departments of psychology may not be the ideal location for training in community psychology, but it is conceivable that a model on preventing and enhancing interventions could issue from an academic department with proper administration.

FINANCIAL SUPPORT

If anyone should be sensitive to the practical issues of source of dollars, it should be the community psychologist. Several alternatives were suggested. First, the general tone of clinical psychology is moving in the community direction, and it is not unreasonable to expect that some NIMH clinical training programs would tolerate the general thrust outlined. Additionally, it would be possible to finance students on other types of training grants. For example, gerontology programs are beginning to take on a more applied, clinical-community look, and a community approach to the problems of the aging would seem to be a major priority. A portion of the students' support could be generated by actual community services. Contracts with community agencies could be written and the students, working under the supervision of their professors, could "work their way through" their training. It may be possible to press for additional university funding for the support of community oriented programs. These programs are likely to be attractive to students, and the tuition monies yielded by students of all levels could be returned to the training program in the form of salaries, etc.

Finally, money from the private sector should not be ruled out. Charities, private foundations, and even private industry might be willing to help. For example, alcoholism in industry is a massive problem. Many industries might be willing to support the training of students who would learn to deal with this problem on a broader scope and who would be willing to serve the particular industry for a period of time after graduation.

LOCUS OF EMPLOYMENT

The list of potential employment possibilities is endless. In addition to the traditional jobs found in academia, hospitals and community mental health centers offer what might be called "entrepreneurial" positions funded by private and public funds. For example, one may wish to set up a drug abuse program and make oneself the head of the program. Other employment possibilities are schools and industrial settings that might permit community psychologists to do their "thing." Political and civil jobs would be ideal. One example is being commissioner for mental health in a city or county, a position that carries with it tremendous power; and although this type of position is usually held by a physician-psychiatrist, some psychologists have been appointed to and succeeded in this capacity.

Finally, if psychologists are willing to give up their identification as psychologists, there are an infinite number of human service positions that community training would prepare them for (i.e., law enforcement, social work, education, etc.).

CONTINUING EDUCATION AND RELATIONSHIP TO TRAINING

The group was enthusiastic about continuing education. It was viewed as important both for the product of the program and for psychologists already in the field who are in need of further training.

At the Vail Conference the suggestion was made to set aside two months every two years for continuing education. This group thought that was a rather unrealistic idea, especially for those working outside academic settings. An alternative model would be a system of modules designed to provide training in specialized areas of interest in compact form. Training modules could be offered at national conventions, regional conventions, state conventions, or even in local organizations. Wherever they are offered, the group concurred that the leadership of Division 27 should exercise an aggressive role in implementing such training.

Regarding format, it was suggested that since skill training is usually of greater interest than academic or cognitive training, procedures should be used that tend to foster skill acquisition. For example, management games and laboratory exercises have been found to be extremely helpful ways to teach management skills. The same procedures could be used in helping psychologists acquire skills in analyzing and dealing with complex organizational processes germane to community problems. While area and regional conferences may be good places in which to organize convention or preconvention workshops, it is sometimes difficult to get away from one's own project. Hence, it was suggested that Division 27 might help organize mobile consultation services; for example, the consultant could visit the actual performance site to provide analysis and support. Additionally, it was suggested that a telephone consultation service could be established, using WATS lines, in which various major leaders in psychology and experts from related fields, such as management, might be paid to be available for phone consultation on various problems.

While workshops and consultation services would be helpful, there is a major resource for continuing training that is often overlooked—the civic leaders and influential persons in one's own community. Every community has a group of individuals who have an enormous "seat of the pants" knowledge of how their community works (e.g., when to bring a program before the voters), and these people can be valuable sources of training for young and experienced psychologists.

Also discussed was the possibility of organizing a system for documenting and recording continuing education credit. Peer review and/or program accreditation are possible related functions.

The last matter discussed was the need to educate the public, as well as psychologists, about emotional-behavioral problems. Tasteful "PR blurbs" could be developed and aired over prime time television. The Church of the Latter Day Saints is one group that has done this successfully through a series of TV vignettes. One shows a little girl being ignored by her family, the way in which this hurts her, and the need for the other family members to care for her. The piece is presented in a straight-forward, tasteful manner. Division 27 might consider a similar approach for such topics as prevention, early identification, resource utilization, etc.

LEVEL OF ENTRY

This issue met vigorous discussion. Suggestions for entry level ranged from AA or below to a postdoctoral master's degree similar to the master's degree in public health. No consensus was reached on this matter, though the group generally acknowledged the value of people trained at the AA and BA level. The group worked hard on the issue of role and function. There was basic agreement that individuals at the lower levels (e.g., AA) would be specially trained in a limited number of specific functions; that is, they would be specialists. As these workers acquired additional competencies regarding additional kinds of tasks, their "rank" would increase. Workers at the highest levels would be generalists in that they would develop competencies in a large number of areas in which they could then supervise.

No consensus was reached regarding a name for the persons at the lower levels, but the suggestion that they need not be called psychologists did not meet with great opposition. "Human development specialist" was one possible alternative job title.

REFERENCE

Panzetta, A. F. The concept of community: The short circuit of the mental health movement. *Archives of General Psychiatry*, 1971, *25*, 291–297.

10 Intervention and Prevention

II. Systems Analysis and Organizational Dynamics

Meg Gerrard

IDEOLOGY, VALUE BASE, AND SOCIAL ETHICS

One purpose of community psychology is to maximize the quality of life. Thus, community psychologists should be concerned with enhancing the functioning of individuals, organizations, and society through competency-based programs designed to maximize coping skills and access to resources. They might accomplish this by working with individuals, but they can be more effective on the organizational or systems level, working for changes in organizational structure that will allow for better client functioning or working for changes in laws that will affect large numbers of individuals.

While community psychologists do not operate in a value-free framework (they are committed to maximizing individual potential, for example), they must be careful not to impose a particular set of values that might be foreign or constraining to given clients. It is up to the clients to determine how to maximize their potential. Community psychologists can be facilitative, but they should not determine the clients' courses for them; their role is to help the clients better determine their own courses.

Community psychologists should be honest and nonmanipulative in their dealings with clients. They should make it known in advance how they expect to benefit from interaction with their clients. It is also important for community psychologists to evaluate the effectiveness of their services to determine what factors account for the success or failure of the service, as well as to show that they value the scientific model of investigation as a tool for improving these services.

GOALS AND OBJECTIVES

To develop individuals with political savvy who are able to look at problems from a systems point of view, with a knowledge of networks, communications, and power structures.

Participants in this model: Celia Cintron, Jerry Goodman, Len Haas, Steve Hobfoll, Bill Rooney, Bill Sirbu, Kemba Young, Nancy Jo Derby, Martha K. Key, Carol Roehl, and David Hoffman.

To resolve issues:

1. What kind of people want to hire community psychologists? A constituency should be built of future employers of community psychologists; they could provide input into program goals.
2. What are the criteria by which a community psychologist decides whether or not to respond to a request for help?

To create roles for community psychologists, such as: organization and systems change agent (including the judicial and legislative processes); systems analyst; community quarterback; assessor (group, organization, community); intervenor (group, organization, community); organizer, grant writer; educator; evaluator.

LEVEL OF OPERATION

The levels at which students would operate would depend to a large extent on the opportunities open to them in their department and community, as it is important that students and faculty work together to maximize the supervision provided. Probably the most common base of operation for the community psychologist will be at the organizational level (schools, police departments, etc.). There students can acquire skills in assessing, intervening, and evaluating. Some students may get involved at other levels, such as in communitywide (e.g., epidemiological) studies, policy analysis, or legal consultation. Students should have the opportunity to gain extensive experience in a minimum of one area and should obtain at least a working knowledge of intervention in other content areas such as mental health, education systems, and law enforcement agencies.

RESEARCH AND KNOWLEDGE BASES

A new knowledge base and research methodology are urgently needed in community psychology. Students should be trained in the traditional research methods of psychology as well as in field research techniques. In this way the next generation of community psychologists will be able to establish themselves as both pure and applied researchers and to develop the necessary knowledge base.

TECHNOLOGY AND SKILLS REQUIRED

Community psychologists basically will be involved in problem solving. The fundamental steps in this process are (1) assessing the problem, (2) designing and implementing an intervention, (3) evaluating the intervention. The students should be skilled in all of these areas, at either the organizational or the societal level.

In addition, students should be prepared in the basic reading, writing, and speaking skills necessary for gathering and disseminating information; the administrative skills required in program planning and implementation, including budgeting and supervision; group process and leadership skills; and applied research skills.

CONTENT AREAS

The specific content areas to be offered in a community psychology program will depend on

1. the setting available,
2. the interests of the faculty, and
3. the social and political concerns of the time (the individual can take either a reactive or a proactive stance).

FORMAT

A community psychology program ideally might be based in an interdisciplinary program, for example in a school of human relations. There is concern, however, that direct relations be maintained with psychology departments.

FINANCIAL SUPPORT

Basic support must come from psychology departments. Supplements should come from training sites that support students in advanced stages of training, for these students have more to offer the training site in the way of services.

CONTINUING EDUCATION AND RELATIONSHIP TO TRAINING

Continuing education can only be offered on an elective basis, with some incentive offered through continuing education credit units for workshops and training sessions.

ESSENTIAL COURSES

These would include systems analysis, consultation, and organizational dynamics.

FIELD EXPERIENCE

There is a concern about the isolated practicum experience in which students are sent out to agencies for four to eight hours a week, often with inadequate supervision. Therefore, the proposed model incorporates team apprenticeship, in which a team of faculty and graduate students (and perhaps undergraduates) is involved in an intervention project in an agency or in the community.

This model would allow for maximum learning by the students, since they would have extensive contact with the faculty/supervisor through all phases of the project. The faculty member could serve as a direct model for the students, as well as provide them with immediate feedback on their professional skills. A pyramid model of supervision might be adopted, with faculty supervising graduate students and the latter supervising undergraduates.

11 Intervention and Prevention

III. The Enhancement of Competency

William F. Hodges

The characteristics of the group formed to discuss interventive and preventive models of training in community psychology were mixed, and the problems that arose in trying to agree on a model were many. Several persons who chose to work on this model were actively involved in preventive programs or training; others joined the group to learn something about the area. And several members noted that this model was only one of several areas of interest.

The group had extreme difficulty trying to obtain consensus in answers to the questions. There was a strong concern for semantics. Many participants objected to the structure given the group in terms of how to go about its task. There was a question raised about the model as a "pure" type. Most programs familiar to the participants were mixtures of several of the models being discussed at the conference; no single program that the group knew about followed strictly an interventive and preventive model. The group bogged down quickly and experienced a great deal of frustration in trying to come up with necessary and sufficient aspects of an interventive and preventive model. On the second day of meetings the attrition rate for the group was large, dropping from 15 to 8 or 10 members. At the Swampscott Conference, participants had reported that they considered it premature and perhaps unwise in principle to formulate a specific curriculum, which might inhibit growth and exploration. The remaining participants in this Austin group agreed that community psychology is to some extent still in this embryonic stage where premature closure in terms of what are the essential aspects of a training program would have unfortunate repercussions in terms of the growth of the profession.

Once the group agreed that the task presented was impossible, it had no problem following the instructions. The participants, however, were only able

Participants in this model: Cary Cherniss, James K. Cohen, Anthony R. D'Augelli, Kristine Fleischer, William F. Hodges, David B. Hoffman, Edward Katkin, Maurice Korman, Jack Nottingham, Manuel Ramirez, Dick Reppucci, Maxin Reiss, Sherry Payne, James Smith, Linda Davis, Ira Semler.

to proceed by listing potential components of such a training program, rather than its necessary and sufficient conditions. After getting into the task, there was surprising unanimity of opinion on several central issues. It should be noted, however, that the ideas and opinions listed are all collections of comments by the group members and should not be viewed as agreement on the appropriate components of an interventive and preventive model. The only sufficient condition agreed to by all members of the committee was that research and evaluation is a basic component for developing a knowledge basis for intervention and program evaluation. The interaction of social change and research was viewed as absolutely essential in a training program and in intervention in the community.

Trying to separate training issues for graduate students in community psychology from the necessary skills for a community psychologist operating in the community was another difficulty. Thus, it was not unusual for the discussion to focus on what community psychologists should be doing and what skills they would need to do what was specified, rather than specifically on what a training model would look like.

Answers to the first five questions were developed at the conference. The other answers are based on comments provided by participants who had time to respond after the conference had ended. Since these were not reviewed by the group as a whole, that part of the report should be viewed as tentative and not as group consensus.

IDEOLOGY, VALUE BASE, AND SOCIAL ETHICS

The group proposed a move away from the prevention of specific psychopathologies and toward an increased emphasis on enhancement of competencies. Thus, perhaps this model should be named *Interventive and Social Enhancement Training*. The model's ideology is based on a number of needs and perceptions:

1. To foster competence at the individual and community level; to increase options and develop freedom of choice for individuals by enhancing skills
2. To foster participation in the decision-making process, identify and develop latent or potential skills in the community, and foster a psychological sense of community
3. To recognize that resources exist within the social system that the system can use for solving its own problems; to understand that it is better to intervene at the social environment level than at the individual level; and to intervene with antecedents rather than consequences
4. To reduce stress or maladaptive stress responses within the community; to perceive the social system as one with far-reaching reverberations that are both interrelated and interdependent
5. To have concern for powerless victims and those who are neglected within

our society; to develop environmental supports for change within the community and maximize the benefits for all

6. To develop a value base on the part of the professional that is explicit to the consumers
7. To recognize the importance of political, economic, social, and historical as well as psychological factors in developing social and individual behaviors
8. To realize that the abnormal/normal continuum is socially defined and not inherent in the system
9. To enhance freedom for the individual and social groups, weighing one against the other to provide stability and an opportunity to change for both

GOALS AND OBJECTIVES

The group had difficulty responding to this question. Some believed that goals could not be determined before a data base was established. It was agreed, however, that programs are needed to train all types of professionals, with strategies selected for evaluating their relative effectiveness. Specifically, community psychologists should be trained to serve as:

1. Community assessors, social change agents, evaluators
2. Linking agents between programs and needs
3. Advocates, leaders, administrators, and conceptualizers

Further goals include acquainting the student with as many roles as possible regarding values and behaviors, and making research and intervention complementary.

LEVEL OF OPERATION

Levels of operation begin at the level of social settings, not of individuals. The higher the order of abstraction from situations to social systems, the greater the potential impact, the greater the ethical problems (such as legitimacy), and the greater the impact of failure. Intervention at any level is legitimate, but the level should be the highest feasible, given the knowledge base, legitimacy, and resources for the behavior or problem being addressed.

Research and Knowledge Bases

The group had no difficulty in generating a rather long list of potential areas of important knowledge bases for the community intervenor and enhancer. Although none of the areas was seen as absolutely essential, there was rather broad agreement that the more areas in which people are knowledgeable, the better able they would be to deal with a community change. The areas include:

1. Crosscultural studies to explore opportunities for change
2. Open systems theory
3. Organizational behavior and applied behavioral analysis
4. Ethnic studies and ethnomethodology
5. Small group dynamics and person-settings interventions
6. Action research and survey research
7. Naturalistic field studies and community organization
8. Social history
9. Program planning and development, including computer-based models and experimental design
10. Consultation research
11. Epidemiological findings
12. Social learning and imitation
13. Program evaluation techniques and needs assessment techniques

TECHNOLOGY AND SKILLS REQUIRED

Group response to this question was limited, partly because of time considerations. While some of the technology and skills required are implied by comments made in response to previous questions, others specifically mentioned include:

1. Interpersonal sensitivity and skills. Training in individual therapy and diagnosis is one way to develop these skills. The need for interpersonal sensitivity, and the fact that clinical training may actually enhance such skills, may be one reason why community psychology has been reluctant to divorce itself from community mental health and clinical psychology. It was agreed, however, that there may be alternative models for training individuals in interpersonal sensitivity. Individual diagnostic and individual psychotherapy skills were seen as irrelevant.
2. Systems analysis and consultation
3. Field research skills
4. Ability to implement the knowledge base, including the language and dialect needed for working in certain settings
5. Grant writing
6. Community diagnosis and intervention planning

CONTENT AREAS

1. Organizational theory, including psychopathology of social systems
2. Criminal justice, schools, mental health
3. Specialized research methodology
4. Program evaluation and needs assessment of human services
5. Personality development and small- and large-group processes

6. Urban planning, political science, and public relations
7. Focus on enhancement and on alternative models of organization and change

   Most of the content areas that have become associated with programs in community psychology (e.g., community organization and development, social learning theory and application, systems analysis, criminal justice, public and alternative education, etc.) are appropriate for a training model in community psychology that focuses on prevention and intervention.

   Public and private sectors in international, national, state, local, and neighborhood communities intersect in broad areas such as government-administration, legal-judicial, legislative-political, defense-military, education, health, welfare, and economics-business; and they involve potential content areas with implications for historical data, conceptualization, and short- and long-term planning. Each intersect provides a valid position from which a community psychologist can work.

FORMAT

There was no concensus on this issue, with views ranging from housing a community psychology program within a department of psychology to total divorce from a university setting. Individual comments reflected the diverse views:

   "Not in any setting more concerning with social action than evaluation of community needs, the processes of change and effectiveness, and the development of concepts, ethics, and evaluation. Not in any setting where community psychologists are not working in the field getting their hands dirty. However, community psychology must not lose its identity with psychology as a science and as a profession. The processes of conceptualization, research, and intervention must not be separated."

   "The department of psychology can serve as a coordinator, with courses in many other departments."

   "A consortium of academic and training resources, with a strong emphasis on field training and dual supervision by faculty and field placement representatives."

   "Not in a department of psychology. An interdisciplinary professional college that explicitly fosters working relationships between various areas on social problems seems appropriate. A content explicitly dedicated to applied work seems necessary to avoid the endless issues of professional identity many community psychologists experience in traditional departments. A broad academic and administrative structure that validates the basic notion of community intervention is necessary."

   "Not in a department of psychology. Within a distinct school or department (such as a school of human ecology or a school of public health) that identifies its focus as a study of human behavior in its relationship to systems and their consequent interrelationships. The observed incompatibility between community psychology and traditional departments of psychology cannot be resolved. Traditional departments remain unable and/or unwilling to recognize and reinforce emerging and admittedly different behavioral repertoires of community psychologists."

"Because of the incredibly time-consuming demands of field supervision, programs should be encouraged to subscribe to a pyramid structure of supervision, in which more advanced students play active roles."

"Supervisors should have prolonged and sustained relationships with a community system."

FINANCIAL SUPPORT

Few of the participants contributed to this question. It was generally agreed that a definition of the package had to be determined before one could sell the package to the public. One participant noted that there is a need to develop specific products and skills that can be sold to both the public and private sectors. When the roles of trainer of paraprofessionals and program developer-evaluator become more legitimate, agencies will seek students with such skills.

The need to find sources for support of graduate students and professionals potentially can undermine values. Students and professionals have a tendency to go where the money is rather than where the needs are (and the two are not always synonymous). Needs for service and for training may not overlap. The source of funding may play a fundamental and defining role in determining whose needs are being met—the university, the student, the community agency, or the government.

Additional suggestions for financial support include obtaining revenue-sharing monies controlled by city, county, and state sources; intern programs sponsored by numerous state agencies; and training grants from social service agencies, day-care facilities, etc. One participant noted that it is sometimes easier to get funds at the federal or state level. Communities frequently have short-term perspectives and will not tolerate long-term solutions unless they are not directly paying for it.

LOCUS OF EMPLOYMENT

Once again, the question produced little concensus. Areas and positions suggested include:

1. State and federal administrative and legislative staff
2. Architectural and environmental agencies and firms; area planning and development commissions

3. School principals; lobbyists
4. Local government policy-makers—county commissioners, school board members, etc.
5. Universities and community colleges—academic positions and staffing training programs
6. Nonprofit corporations seeking federal grants and contract funds; research and development centers
7. Federal justice system
8. Welfare systems and area network offices—delivery of services and development of programs
9. Volunteer organizations
10. Traditional settings—program designers and evaluators
11. Community mental health centers—developing ways of disseminating psychologically useful information to agencies and the public
12. Human services agencies
13. Departments of agriculture in the U.S. and abroad—problem solving directed toward nutrition and energy needs

CONTINUING EDUCATION IN RELATIONSHIP TO TRAINING

1. Summer workshops for both short (one to two weeks) and extended (six to eight weeks) periods—the evaluation program held at Amherst each summer could offer an appropriate model.
2. Intensive workshops and seminars offered at regional and national meetings
3. A communication system established among departments and campuses to provide information for potential faculty exchange programs, vis-a-vis leave of absence, senior stipends
4. Skill training workshops
5. A clearinghouse for information on programs and for continuing education
6. Interdisciplinary conferences, with critiques by peers

LEVEL OF ENTRY

Once again, there were strong differences of opinion among committee participants. Some supported only PhD-level community psychologists, some supported PhD level until the field becomes more delineated, and some advocated participation of the paraprofessional through the PhD in the profession. One problem not yet resolved in the profession is whether the MA is a specialist and the PhD a generalist, or vice versa. Many programs begin with broad, general conceptualizations in psychology and at the PhD level allow a person to specialize in one particular area. This seems an expensive way of developing master's-level people who may not have the specific skills to handle any one problem. A more appropriate model would be to allow the master's-level person to specialize in one field and the PhD to generalize across fields.

Other comments included:

"The entry level involves not who is more competent but how many competencies we have."

"Three (BA, MA, PhD) levels should be integrated within one program. In this way the different levels of expertise and sophistication can dovetail. From a preventive-educational model, titles like *community, individual, family,* and *developmental specialist* are useful as generic terms."

"At the BA level, skills involve casework, and terms like *family specialist* or *interventual development specialist* are appropriate. At the master's level, *program development specialist* or *paraprofessional specialist* are appropriate terms. PhD level seems to involve research and conceptualization."

"If any distinction must be made, perhaps we are enriching the PhD level in areas related to theory and research while emphasizing competent service action at the MA level." (The person suggesting this, however, was not completely comfortable with these distinctions, either. Historically, PhDs have often remained in academic settings, but the community psychologist PhD is needed in the field as well.)

CAREER LADDER AND CAREER LATTICE OPPORTUNITIES

There was little postconference response to this question. One person commented on a general preference for a specification of skills needed in behavioral-competency terms, so that a ladder-lattice can be built; another noted that knowledge can be expanded at any level by anyone. Appropriate skill training, so that the knowledge can be secured (at whatever level), reported, and validated, would be the responsibility of professionals in both the career ladder and the career lattice program.

ESSENTIAL COURSES

In many ways the essential courses have been covered under the previous topics. The following additional courses were considered essential:

1. Action research methodologies
2. Ethics and responsibilities of social interventions
3. Systems consultation
4. The nature of social change from historical, sociological, anthropoligical, and psychological perspective

In addition, some political science, sociology, and economics courses that would present an overview of interactions between these areas and traditional psychological areas would enhance a training program.

FIELD WORK EXPERIENCES

On the whole, participants favored field work experiences that go beyond what most programs presently provide. Suggestions ranged from a half-day per week for two years of field work experience to ten hours per week for four years. It was also suggested that there be a balance between in-depth experience with one agency or setting and exposure to a variety of settings.

Individual comments included reference to one BA program in which there is one term of full exposure to human service setting, casework and other typical service, and research in some kind of agency. At the graduate level the program includes at least one year's experience in developing, running, and evaluating development-enhancement-type programs for the community, family, group, or individuals in a human service agency. Training of paraprofessionals and their supervisors is essential in both. Another commented on the need to have a flexible internship program that may overlap for several years with the field placement training. Others noted that the field placement program should have a built-in feedback system requiring continuous review and revision.

Pointing out that distinctions should not be exaggerated between essential and desirable placements, participants suggested that strong attempts be made to increase the range of placement areas. For example, one program gets placements with the state legislature. Openness in terms of possible placements was strongly encouraged.

12 Social Change

I. Guidelines for Social Intervention

Leonard Hassol

The social change task force consisted of four young faculty members, five graduate students, and three aging veterans of the Swampscott Conference who wanted to persuade the young folks that the world was still worth saving if only *they* could figure out how to do it. But the ambience had changed in 10 years; the crisp, bright light of 1965, reflecting the optimistic and venturesome spirit of those times, had been replaced by a somber illumination through which support for social change could be seen only with effort. Nevertheless, we decided to look because, as Alfred North Whitehead suggested some time ago, societies never think their way through social problems, they need to see possible solutions acted out. Working alternatives to present social arrangements are clearly needed, but is the Zeitgeist right, can we discern trends in the society that are responsive to efforts at social change?

The task force began with the observation that while America is a class society in which people exploit each other as often and as casually as they breath, psychologists, even community psychologists, make poor revolutionaries, and, in any event, a heavily ideological approach to social problems has never flourished in American soil. The closest this country has come to accepting a class conflict viewpoint has been that folksy, down home, largely agrarian brand of reform known as *Populism*. Populist movements have always appeared when groups with clearly convergent interests have perceived themselves to be exploited beyond tolerable limits. If such groups exist in significant numbers today, they could become the future employers of community psychologists trained in social change methods and values. There are signs that a neopopulist tide, with urban as well as rural elements, is beginning to run.

- Economists, such as J. K. Galbraith, are saying that, with the recent appearance of very sharp limits on continued economic growth, the era when at least those within the system can advance and can prosper is

Participants in this model: Sally Andrade, Rima Blair, Louis Cohen, Robert Reiff, Israel Cuellar, Sue Doty, Gayle Hill, Ernest Myers, Humberto Gonzales, Jeff Whitely, Brian Wilcox.

over. From now on, for some to win others must lose, and the ranks of those with much to lose are growing.

- There is considerable polling data indicating that for the last several years a variety of groups—urban workers, farmers, consumers of all sorts, many women, many minorities, to name a few—have been feeling increasingly angry and "ripped-off."
- There are many specific issues that focus the discontent and sense of rip-off. Some major examples:
  a. Growing inequities in both the distribution of wealth and the distribution of burdens during adverse economic times
  b. Growing discontent with the cost, quality, and availability of health services
  c. Growing pressure behind the demand for a system of child care services that would meet the needs of both children and their parents
  d. Minority rights movements facing extensive, incomplete realization of their agendas
  e. Consumerism, broadly defined to include concern for the rights of consumers in relation to products and services as well as the full environmental costs of both

IDEOLOGY, VALUE BASE, AND SOCIAL ETHICS

Underlying these specifics is a set of social values that could be useful to community psychologists trying to decide where and how to engage themselves with such issues and movements. These are values that, in their general form, seem to be widely accepted in the American culture; making them operational in American life is an attractive way of defining the principle task facing community psychology.

- *The Value of Sustaining Life.* All objects and activities that help satisfy people's basic requirements for food, shelter, healing, survival, and personal meaning are life-sustaining goods that society ought to nurture and protect. To the extent that the pursuit of other objects and activities threatens these goods, society ought to be in a posture of resistance and change.
- *The Value of Esteem.* This refers to everyman's sense that people are beings of worth, that they deserve a fundamental respect, and that, therefore, they are not being used as an object or tool by others for the attainment of purposes and goals to which they have not given their informed consent.
- *The Value of Freedom.* A most vexing but eternally beckoning ideal which probably can never be fully reached but which, at the very least, implies an expanded range of choice for societies and their members.

Such choice must take place against a background of awareness—awareness of the nature and range of the real options, of the unavoidable constraints, and of the consequences, as best they can be foreseen, flowing from each choice. In short, rational selection must be free of deception, coercion, or manipulation by the state, corporations, or individuals.

Whether or not this particular set of social values wins the concurrence of community psychologists, the group agreed with Robert Reiff's idea that the field must develop some consensus on social values before it can decide on the social goals it wishes to support and the constituencies in whose interest it will work.

The task force also agreed that a fundamental concern for the social context in which the work is used ought to inform whatever actions are undertaken. Community psychologists should regularly ask and find working answers to such ethical questions as:

• How, by whom, and to what ends are my findings or my work likely to be used?
• Are my efforts genuinely directed toward increasing not only the clients' range of choices but also their ability to choose?
• Are forces operating that will yield short-run gains to the client system while leaving it vulnerable to greater domination in the future?
• Am I guarding against the subtle imposition of values by teaching the client system how to resist my own or anyone else's manipulation?

In a social change model social policy is clearly the main target of change. However, the experience of trying to influence social policy over the last 10 years suggests that such efforts do not have to be national in scope; indeed, there is good evidence that policy can best be influenced by numerous demonstrations of alternative options at the local level. The health care system, for example, has seen the development of community-generated methods of service delivery that, for the first time, have demonstrated viable alternatives to the traditional fee-for-service model of health care. The student-run free clinics that began in the 1960's, the community-run neighborhood health centers associated with the Model Cities program, and the gynecological and abortion clinics developed by women's liberation groups made possible a change in the belief structure about medical care. Community psychologists could play an important role in the very large task remaining of expanding the constituencies for visible alternatives in other areas of health care, and then helping such enlarged constituencies move toward changes in social policy, such as rewritten medical practices acts and well-conceived national health service legislation.

GUIDELINES AND GRAND ILLUSIONS

Careful consideration of the opportunities for social change activity available at the local level suggested several guidelines that should help community psychology to develop both significant community leverage and genuine change-oriented settings in which to train its students.

Someone must identify a problem and set action processes in motion. Community psychology has not been noted as a proactive field; with a few exceptions it has accepted definitions of social problems developed by others—usually those who could pay the freight for research and demonstration projects—and contented itself with the technical functions of getting the job done. Much as clinical psychology for so long accepted the medical definition of what was appropriate for the psychological agenda, community psychology has accepted the political, or bureaucratic, or corporate rules of where and how and for whose benefit the game was to be played. It is time we started initiating social change efforts shaped by our own social values. In a word, what community psychology needs to provide in order to gain control of its professional identity is leadership.

Community psychology programs tend to exist and function in isolation from one another, each training setting and each program trying to "brighten the corner where we are" but rarely coordinated with other community psychology programs working the same corner. A half-dozen university programs agreeing, say, to work cooperatively on a system of child advocacy could, out of their different but coordinated local efforts, develop both the kind of clout and the knowledge (unified evaluation instruments, common definitions, enlarged data bases, etc.) that would lead to much more rapid and basic change in social policy toward children. The economies of scale and division of labor available from such collaboration recommend themselves with special urgency in these undernourished times.

Not all social issues are amenable to intervention by community psychologists. As Peter Edelman (1973) puts it:

The problem has to be small enough so that efforts for its solution do not turn into naive pursuits of some all-encompassing agenda. . . . It must be manageable . . . and it must have specific remedies: there are many reasons why the Kerner Commission produced little change, but one, surely, is that there are no specific remedies for racism. (p. 639)

Nor are there, as we now know to our chagrin, any specific ways for community psychology to crusade against such globally perceived evils as poverty or mental illness. In making strategic choices as to what approaches to take to local manifestations of such general problems, a weather eye must always be kept on questions of how a given tactic, as popular as it may be with a given constituency, contributes to the elimination of underlying causes. From that perspective, mental illness might be better tackled in programs aimed at eliminating slumlords than in community mental health center efforts to help public school teachers understand the emotional problems of children living in slums.

In recognizing a fundamental social problem from which many others flow, the task group took note of a nearly universal tendency toward the unrestrained growth of symbiotic governmental-corporate relationships, whose mission is clearly not the serving of human needs but simply the aggrandizement and the power of those who manage them. The specific, local manifestations of what J. K. Galbraith (1973) calls "the planning system and the techno-structure" are everywhere. They range, for example, from the ability of the high-technology weapons manufacturers to preempt the lion's share of the national budget by making their products appear to constitute national security, to the effort at co-opting and defusing the women's movement via the deceptive use of women's liberation ideas in advertising ("today's independent woman makes up her own mind about which brand of hair spray is best for her"). While community psychology cannot, by itself, go charging out after the multinationals, it should make a self-conscious effort to ally itself with the many groups who are trying to educate the country to the realities of the late-20th-century economic system. In order to bring the community psychology point of view and knowledge into useful connection with others who share these values, community psychologists and their students need some training in modern economics, a social science area almost totally missing from the psychology curriculum of the past and present. Without such training many of the most controlling influences on the community will seem remote and "obviously" subject to impersonal and inevitable market forces about which nothing can, or for that matter should, be done.

An important aspect of any model for change is the encouragement and room it provides for wild ideas, the sudden visions, the grand illusions that lead who knows where. In that spirit of adventure the task group indulged in a brief fantasy about what community psychology might best be doing.

While government can have a massive influence on the success or failure of social change efforts, almost nothing has been done to study the interaction between government and social change efforts. At the national level, the government has initiated many social change programs (witness the War On Poverty as a major example), but the same government has also killed, or at least neutralized, its own creations (again witness the War On Poverty). Between the birth and death of such efforts is a large and unexplored field of forces that determine governmental shifts in policy and support. At the local level, where much social change effort will be focused in the future, there is also intensive terra incognita between program proposals at City Hall and final outcome in the neighborhoods. For example, the Community Action Programs of the middle 1960s were welcomed by mayors in some cities and excommunicated in others. Simple explanations pointing to good guys and bad guys miss the complex community interactions influencing those differing responses; we clearly need to know a great deal more about how the process works, and community psychologists ought to be leading the needed action research. In the absence of such knowledge it will be very difficult to mount new change efforts that require long-term governmental sanction or support; no one wants to be burned twice by the same flame.

The past 15 years have seen a good deal of idealistic, often haphazard, sometimes planned, and sometimes crazy experimentation with alternative life-styles and intentional communities. Groups based on nontraditional notions of land tenure, family and sexual arrangements, reduced reliance on ecologically damaging technology, etc., have bloomed and, for the most part, died off. But clearly new forms of community life will be needed to adapt to the new conditions of life coming at us with "future shock" speed. Just as a group of natural scientists on Cape Cod—calling themselves the New Alchemists—are trying to develop, in a professional and scientific way, "soft technologies for living in balance with the environment," so community psychologists ought to be applying professional and scientific thought and effort to developing pilot demonstrations of new structures for community life. A new breed of community psychologist will be needed to meet this challenge. They will have to take the participant role just as seriously as the conceptualizer role, something that the Swampscott generation did only rarely. But then, we are now in the Austin generation, and community psychologists have some distinctly new outlines and coloration.

LOCUS OF EFFORT

Group thinking concerning how a social change model for community psychology could develop moved to the notion that certain of the broad-based coalitions of consumer groups and minority groups now forming might provide excellent starting points. Such coalitions must have local, grass-roots groupings of citizens equipped to take on complicated tasks of organization and persuasion, tasks in which the skills of community psychologists and their students could be useful. One instructive example was mentioned in which a community psychologist and two graduate students taught a group of women on welfare how to constitute a community action agency and how to apply for, win, and keep control over an OEO Community Action Program grant.

There are also advocacy groups of many kinds that might welcome the participation of community psychologists. At the national level, for example, there is the Children's Defense Fund, an organization seeking to create a new climate of understanding, policy, and law concerning children's rights. At the state level there is a counterpart organization, The Massachusetts Advocacy Center, trying to do similar things. Community psychology students from The University of Texas and from Wheaton College will shortly be working in that organization. In a similar manner, certain labor unions, some governmental agencies and departments (more often at the municipal and state than at the federal level), certain foundations, some mental health agencies, and the staffs of some selected officials could all be promising and receptive points of effort for community psychology. Extended activity in such settings would certainly help to build the knowledge base for community psychology.

There is also need to restudy the settings in which psychologists have traditionally worked to see if, with a change of ideology and emphasis, new social policy initiatives might evolve. Again, by way of illuminating example, a participant told of a very large, very chaotic public high school in which undergraduate community psychology majors were able to gather, via survey and interview methods, the perceptions of students, teachers, and administrators concerning the quality of life in the school, and each group's view of the actions of the others. These data were then used to motivate the three constituencies to start the difficult process of generating new social policy for the school. Clearly, traditional psychology skills—in this instance interviewing and survey research—can be used in the service of new social goals, and this can take place within very traditional service settings. In most rural areas the community mental health center ought to be able to function as a kind of mini-university in the sense that the center will usually contain the only available manpower trained to think systematically and methodologically about assisting communities to define social problems and to experiment with new solutions. If the staff of the center can accept such a role redefinition, they will find many possibilities to participate in social change efforts.

The task force wrestled with the many obvious questions concerning how to train students and faculty for the partially new role implied by the goals and values of a social change model. Various groupings of courses at undergraduate and graduate levels were considered, new forms of curriculum and fieldwork organization were mulled over. There was agreement that students engaged in social change activity need to be particularly sharp in written and spoken communication since much of the community effort swirling around them will be relatively imprecise and easily misunderstood by both friends and adversaries. Mass media utilization is another necessary skill, and one not usually attended to in graduate school. The ability to read and interpret research reports accurately and quickly, along with a basic familiarity with knowledge retrieval methods, was seen as another foundation or core skill.

At the Bachelor of Arts level enduring needs could be seen in such areas as social system intervention in communities and organizations, investigative reporting and the use of social statistics, survey research and evaluation skills, group process and consultation abilities. Master's-level people would add training in budgeting, administration, grantsmanship, and social and political analysis, while the PhD would need all of the above plus sophisticated ability to plan programs of social policy change, to supervise their execution, and to evaluate them in the light of best available research techniques.

But in the end the group decided that such musings were idle; it will take five years of experimentation at many colleges and universities and with many field settings before several good models of training emerge. And obviously, a social change model of training should begin at home; new social policies will be needed for universities, which often contain centers of research about, and action on, changing social policy. Such activity, based in the university, will provoke conflict and controversy with the larger society. When the attention of such a group focuses on the social problems of the university itself, the anguished cries will be loud indeed. New policies will be needed for creative response, and the community psychologists should be at the center of such policy-setting dialectic.

The discussions ended on a somewhat positive note. The group recognized that a social change model for community psychology involves a moderately high-risk strategy in that the spirit of the times must be right for such an enterprise. However, there was agreement that within the next two to three years we will see the shape of any emerging attempt to cope with such issues as the bringing of the economic system back into the service of human, as opposed to corporate, needs, or the valuing of public over bureaucratic and private purposes. With fingers crossed, the members believed that there was some good evidence, and some intuitive juice, that justified community psychology in readying its practitioners and, perhaps more importantly, its students for participation in a broad effort at national renewal. If such an effort is not forthcoming, we can take comfort in the words of a member of the colonial Connecticut legislature who, in opposing a motion to adjourn because of a widespread hysteria that the world was about to end, said to his colleagues,

One of two things will happen; either the world will end, or it will not. If it does not, we will have wasted valuable time. If it does, I prefer to be found at my desk doing the Lord's work until the end.

REFERENCES

Edelman, P. The rights of children. *Harvard Education. Review*, 1973, *43*, 639–652.
Galbraith, J. K. *Economics and the public purpose*. Boston: Houghton Mifflin, 1973.

13 Social Change

II. Systems Analysis and Intervention

Margaret Gatz and Ramsay Liem

The output of this work group is not by any means a finished product. Rather, it is directed toward the identification of important questions, the examination of basic assumptions and ideology (with the belief that this effort is critical to a community psychology of social change), and the development of a base on which to build. This report reflects points of tension in that sorting out process.

IDEOLOGY, VALUE BASE, AND SOCIAL ETHICS

There was broad agreement in the group that inequality is a basic element in our society today. Inequality, racism, sexism, oppression, and exploitation are reflected by such statistics as the high percentage of blacks in negative institutions (e.g., prisons) and the correspondingly low percentage of blacks in positive institutions (e.g., universities). This assumption led to the formulation of a goal of distributive justice with regard to power, services, opportunities, options. It was recognized that this goal implies a set of values and that these values threaten values held by other people in the society. Clarification of values and ideology is crucial, as they inevitably shape the definition of social problems, which in turn impose limitations on solutions to those problems.

The group spent a long time sorting out the target and definition of social change. It was suggested that *social change* might be defined as the manipulation of social networks to achieve a goal, inasmuch as inequality is contained in the very structure of American society. What is called for, then, is a new conception of intervention—the rejection of a professional requirement simply to deliver service to those in need, focusing instead on system dynamics and on the professional's responsibility and expertise to identify, analyze, and promote positive forces of change. One critical force consists of people in general, in contrast to those who are formally charged with the provision or planning of services. A point of tension within the group centered on the question of whether real and meaningful social change can take place within

Participants in this model: Dan Adelson, Sally Andrade, Margaret Gatz, Josue Gonzales, Margie Leidig, Ramsay Liem, Thom Moore, Anne Mulvey, Ernest Myers, Richard Price, Eileen Raffaniello, Eduardo Rivera, Stan Schneider, Dalmas Taylor.

existing institutions, or whether their continued existence in present form insures the perpetuation of inequality. There was general agreement that the level of the problem is systems, and that social change involves systems intervention and structural change (whether by radical incision or by facilitation or development). Service objectives, therefore, need to be shaped by considerations of systems change. Changing social structures will also create change in patterns of service needs and service delivery. Thus, service planning is not, in the long run, the way to meet current service needs. Goals and strategies must be considered on both a short and a long term basis, with the short term guided by the long term.

Finally, social change is not inherently good. With each change one necessarily gives up something, as well as potentially gains. To the extent that it is possible, community psychologists should attempt to define costs and benefits before intervening and should evaluate the activities and effects afterwards.

More broadly, analytic and conceptual work needs to precede and to go along with informed change programs that seek to address basic social structure. One cannot intervene without having some idea where one is going and without assessing what one has done. Awareness of the historical and sociocultural context is one aspect of this analysis. A second aspect is understanding the relationship between individual behavior and social structure.

These considerations lead to one way of thinking about the role of the community psychologist mentioned by several group members; namely, that the special expertise and special role of the community psychologist centers on his or her functioning as one who both acts and conceptualizes, who engages in research as part of any program of intervention and change, who uses research as a tool of social action, who integrates the results of research and evaluation into long-term practical change efforts, and who constantly seeks to clarify and articulate values, interests, and assumptions that inevitably shape these activities. This role, then, implies a sort of radical scientist-practitioner model.

The group affirmed the importance of asking: Who are we, as community psychologists, to define the objects of change and how to go about effecting change? Keeping this question in mind, group members proposed the following set of considerations:

1. People, and the community, must be treated with respect, and in ways that build on integrity, strengths, and culture.
2. People must have a leading role in defining and solving their own problems.
3. The community psychologist does not have a monopoly on expertise and knowledge. Rather, both the psychologist and the community have knowledge and skills in a variety of different areas. This perspective leads to a collaborative model. In this way, as well, the community psychologist is both teacher and learner.

4. Professionals are accountable to the community they serve and are responsible for asking who their constituency is. Representativeness is an important consideration, with a broad organizational base being critical for true representativeness. Combating the elitist instincts of academics and professionals requires more than awareness on the part of community psychologists.

A final important principle is reflexivity. It is always more comfortable to talk about social change when it is in someone else's system. But we all are part of the system we are trying to change. In changing the system we will thereby also be changing ourselves and exposing ourselves to the risks inherent in social change.

GOALS AND OBJECTIVES

The roles emphasized by the training program follow from the considerations listed. Rather than training for a single role, a range of roles is suggested. This diversity reflects both the range of opinions of group members about roles and an opinion that a range of roles is appropriate for a community psychologist within a model of social change. Further, given that systems are the primary target of change, direct involvement with structural issues and with individuals is important.

First, one set of activities of the community psychologist may be described in terms of systems intervention, incorporated in the role of catalytic agent. Second, the community psychologist may be a systems analyst/modifier and an organizational change agent working with community networks. Third, training in basic clinical skills, both individual and group, may receive emphasis. Systems-level change, as mentioned earlier, can be an appropriate objective of interventions at the level of individuals or small groups.

The collaborative model instructs community psychologists not to regard themselves as helpers, bringing problem solutions to the community. Rather, they function as facilitator-activators, using skills to promote change processes and to foster others' becoming facilitator-activators. At the individual level this approach would lead, for example, to concerns for the democratization of skills and knowledge.

Finally, the community psychologist is a socially responsible scientist-practitioner (or action-researcher). The collaborative scientist-practitioner model might be diagrammed:

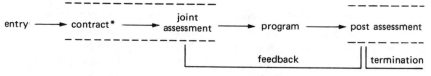

*Specify what action will be taken, who gives the mandate, and what responsibilities reside with whom.

LEVEL OF OPERATION

Group members felt that it was important to distinguish between:

1. change from within versus change from without
2. reform programs versus radical critique
3. developmental or evolutionary change versus radical, qualitative change
4. improvement of current social institutions: facilitation and proactive approaches, making the system work better for people, versus inequality so built into our structures that real pragmatic social change must involve an informed reconstruction of society

At the same time, it was also pointed out that we are all presently "within the system" and conditioned in our thinking and action by that fact.

An additional distinction may be drawn between long-term and short-term change goals. (This distinction needs to be separated from the within/without distinction, as both of these perspectives may be concerned with long- or with short-term change.) Short-term goals were referred to both pejoratively—as "bandaids"—and approvingly, as a sensitivity to dealing with immediate and real human service needs, which cannot be laid aside entirely while structural change is taking place. The inclusion of long-term change goals and their primacy was endorsed by the group, but the precise balancing of long- and short-term objectives was not fully developed.

A third area of discussion related to individual and systems levels of change (again, it helps to make this distinction separately from the two previous areas). On the one hand, there was the realization that a community psychologist in fact does work with individual people within an organization, system, or society. On the other hand, primary emphasis was placed on organizations, community networks, and social structures. An individual-systems conceptualization begins to bring these two positions together; to wit, people must always be considered in their social systems context. Then, the level of operation includes simultaneous consideration of individual and system in their interaction.

RESEARCH AND KNOWLEDGE BASE

The following substantive areas begin to describe an interdisciplinary knowledge base. Research should be emphasized, but it should be conceptualized in a new way, as a collaborative activity integral to all intervention and at the same time as an activity in which the psychologist may have special expertise. Research is social action. Research should meet needs. Research projects should not be undertaken without asking the question, "By whose authority and on whose behalf?" Research should address the same levels of operation described in the previous section.

Substantive Areas

- Individual and systems perspectives, focusing on the systems-person interface (drawing on ecological psychology)
- Individual (clinical) and systems assessment and intervention strategies
- Social sciences analysis and methodology—field sociology, anthropology, political science, urban and regional planning, public health (focus on social issues and on the comparison of different analyses and methodologies)
- Organizational psychology, social psychology, group process, community organization, social policy analysis and planning
- Lifespan development, definition of individual and community competence, personality theory, learning theory, the several literatures of oppression
- Experimental and quasi-experimental research design, program evaluation
- Political and social theory, economics, history, epistemology, and philosophy of science (these areas constitute the substantive and methodological basis for conceptualizing contemporary social structure)

Finally, various approaches to systems change should be examined critically. For example, how useful, appropriate, and effective is a sociotechnological approach?

Technology and Skills Required

- Substantive, methodological, and professional skills (including both individual and systems perspectives and techniques)
- Assessment and intervention strategies, from traditional clinical skills in general, to process consultation skills in particular
- Special strategies: consumer education, media skills, advocacy and broker skills, familiarity with lobbying and with legal processes
- Sophisticated, creative research skills: design, statistics, naturalistic research methods, evaluation skills
- Flexible problem-solving skills; that is, having a grasp of when and how to shift from one problem approach to another versus being tied to particular techniques. This quality is developed through each individual psychologist (and every student) being given the responsibility (and the encouragement) for developing an integrated pattern of perspectives, skills, and experiences. This pattern, along with a problemsolving approach, is what the psychologist brings to any change effort.

CAREER LADDER AND CAREER LATTICE OPPORTUNITIES

A social change model sensitive to cultural relativity is inconsistent with professional elitism. Students, faculty, all levels of agency staff, and community residents are all colleagues in the enterprise of change. Change might thus be thought of in the context of mutual education. This perspective means that a social change model is committed to eliminating elitist professional structures and to fostering continuing education and employment opportunities equitably.

FIELD WORK EXPERIENCES

Training must take place on the turf where problems are to be solved. The importance of placement for 5 to 20 hours per week, beginning in the first year, was stressed. Placement settings would include, among others:

- Traditional clinical: hospital, clinic, community mental health center
- Community service center: schools, day care, family planning, legal aid, senior citizens, police, clergy, halfway houses
- Community groups and organizations: labor unions, alternative schools, interagency groups, nonaligned interest groups
- Policy-making: governor or mayor's office, state departments of mental health, education, juvenile service, social service, APA
- Educational: community colleges
- Informational: public television and other media forms

These field training experiences should require students to negotiate entry and contract; to assess their interpersonal, theoretical, and methodological skills in a variety of sociocultural situations and structures; and to focus on concepts of systems dynamics, program development and evaluation, and the problems and potential for institutional change. The emphasis must not be on delivery of services, but rather on systems analysis and modification.

It is important to integrate fieldwork and coursework, with coursework providing the conceptual, organizing framework necessary for innovative action, and with fieldwork constituting the basis for creative thinking. Their integration permits simultaneously doing and standing back in order to understand what is going on—perhaps one of the most important skills of the community psychologist (referred to as the "participant-conceptualizer" role by Forrest Tyler at the Swampscott Conference).

Accomplishment of these objectives may be facilitated by faculty serving as role models. Then, rather than placing a student at an agency, a joint faculty-student "action team" would be involved in a field activity together. This collaborative experience might then constitute the practicum portion of a combined, integrated academic-fieldwork course. The action team, further, could become a major way in which the university responds to concerns in the community. Such a collective effort is an important model in itself.

14 Social Ecology

Charles J. Holahan

GUIDING PERSPECTIVES

Rather than conceptualizing social ecology as either a model or a program, the social ecology and environmental group perceived ecology within community psychology as representing essentially a perspective, or a viewpoint. As a perspective it is relevant to a number of different content areas and problem types. For example, an ecological viewpoint might be applied in conceptualizing urban problems, in analyzing the relationship between a community mental health center and its surrounding community, and in analyzing the internal forces operative in a school or a school system. The ecological perspective is also applicable across different levels of problem analysis. Under its umbrella it might include social system relationships within an organization, the effects of physical environment on behavior, or the pervasive influences of culture and history on human process in the sense discussed by Seymour Sarason (see Chapter 3). All of these represent opportunities for an ecological perspective or orientation within the broader framework of community psychology.

In one sense there is a weakness in that ecology is not a tangible package that can be tied with a ribbon and handed out at a conference. Yet, there is also a strength in ecology's potential for making an impact in a wide range of different spheres. A core conceptual concern of community psychology is to go beyond simply casting aspersions at an intrapsychic or exclusively clinical approach and to offer something new, something that unlocks the door to viewing both human behavior and the environment in a new way. The ecological perspective offers this opportunity in terms of the issues it raises, the conceptual categories it permits, and the kinds of training programs it encourages.

The broader issue can be approached in terms of what the group labeled as a number of core perspectives within the overall ecological approach. Three of these are explained briefly; the rest of this discussion follows naturally from each of these core perspectives. The first perspective is *interdependence.* It stresses the systematic notion that people, as they relate to the environment and to one another, are always intimately interrelated. Changing one element within a system will result in consequences in another part, and thus it

Participants in this model: Dennis Andrulis, Emory Cowen, Ursula Delworth, Ben Gottlieb, Regina Hilbertz, Sherman James, James Kelly, Toby Klass, Tim Kuehnel, John Monahan, Mimi Nesbit, Bob Newbrough, Maureen Pierce, Julian Rappaport, Seymour Sarason, David Stenmark, David Todd.

necessitates analyzing any problem at more than one level. A second core perspective, which again sets a framework out of which other issues will flow, is the emphasis on *person-environment transaction*. The concern here is with the "mesh" or goodness of fit between the individual's skills and capacities for action on the one hand and the setting's demands and opportunities on the other. A third core perspective stresses *evolution* or development. All environmental systems are constantly changing over time and can be adequately understood only in terms of both their histories and their futures.

VALUE BASE

Values, as they relate to an ecological perspective, may be viewed at two levels. First, there are no inherently ecological values in the sense that anyone who is an ecological psychologist will necessarily represent these values. There is always the personal challenge and commitment of value decisions as they emerge in dealing with a particular problem or a particular group of people. When power is shifted from one level of a system to another, who is going to acquire the power, who is going to lose it? Nevertheless, if one looks across ecologically oriented community psychologists, a number of values that are commonly shared do emerge, and these may be thought of as "overarching" values. Primary among these is effectance or empowerment. The ecologically oriented community psychologist is concerned with giving people a feeling of power, potency, and competence in transacting with their environments. A further overarching value might be labeled a commitment to the primacy of human experience. In dealing with an environmental system, the primary focus is on the importance of the individual and enhancing the individual's capacity for effective coping.

COURSE CONTENT

A number of derivatives or focuses of investigation flow directly from the core perspectives that characterize the ecological viewpoint in community psychology. These include conceptualizing the community as a social system, adopting an environmental emphasis, and developing research strategies appropriate to natural settings. While both ecology's newness and the fact that it is essentially a perspective make specific course recommendations at this time premature, some tentative course possibilities can be oriented around these derivatives. For example, the systemic viewpoint would support coursework in measuring and analyzing social system networks, organizational functioning and development, and community organization. The environmental emphasis would encourage courses in Barker's behavior setting theory, the developing fields of environmental and architectural psychology, urban issues, and regional planning. The concern with natural settings would dictate coursework in field research methods, quasi-experimental designs, evlauation of on-going social policy, and Lewin's model of action research.

POSTURE OF THE TRAINING PROGRAM

Particular emphases in training also flow naturally from the derivatives and values of an ecological framework. One of these is that not only is training important in the sense of content—teaching particular courses or particular skills—but the very structure and framework of an ecologically oriented program should itself reflect some of the principles and perspectives we have discussed. For example, a truly ecological training program should itself be interdisciplinary. This might be partially reflected in the diversified backgrounds of faculty and students, but, just as important, it should lead to encouraging an openness to diversified approaches to common problems and to different goals and objectives by people from different disciplinary backgrounds. An ecologically oriented training program should itself be an open system in the sense of demonstrating an open and free transaction with the surrounding natural environment. There should be responsiveness to community feedback to the academic institution and a concern toward developing field institutes such as an urban laboratory.

In addition, an ecologically oriented training program should reflect an emphasis on tactics, skills, and concepts responsive to temporal processes. A practicum student would be encouraged to spend sufficient time within an institution to watch it grow, change, and cope with natural crises over time. A further temporal emphasis would be on futurism, future environments, and future human problems. An ecologically oriented psychologist should possess a range of appropriate skills. There will not be any one skill to solve all the problems, precisely because human problems in the real world reflect system factors at a number of different levels—social-psychological, environmental, cultural, and historical.

CASE EXAMPLE: A TRAINING PROGRAM

This might become slightly more tangible through a description of one specific training program that represents the implementation of a number of these objectives—the Social Ecology Program at the University of California, Irvine. The program grew up in response to social problems and to the needs for social development in community settings. Since it began four years ago with only three faculty members, it has grown to 27 faculty members and has become UC Irvine's largest undergraduate major, with 1,200 students. Clearly, societal response and support is there. The program also represents a truly interdisciplinary framework. The psychologists are from social, clinical, environmental, and developmental backgrounds. In addition to psychologists, there are lawyers, urban planners, architects, and criminologists. An important interdisciplinary success is that faculty are not categorized according to their particular academic backgrounds; rather, they have learned to relate to one another on the basis of the particular theoretical and research issues they have in common. An additional aspect of the Irvine program is its commitment to field research and to field-based experience.

CASE EXAMPLE: A SOCIAL INTERVENTION

One particular social intervention also reflects an ecological viewpoint. On The University of Texas campus, an action research project has been initiated that is concerned with students' psychological coping mechanisms in dormitory living. First, project staff differentiated types of environment in terms of size of dormitory and a number of physical design features. Next, they examined some intervening factors in terms of the social networks that develop within each type of dormitory. They have also measured how people differ in terms of their desire for different types of social milieus and their ability to cope with them. A particular focus of the project is on the match or mismatch between individuals and the social milieu that is characteristic of the setting in which they reside, with concern for both overall adjustment and level of satisfaction in the living environment. A longer-term objective is to attempt on an experimental basis to develop a cohort of about 50 students for whom an ideal living environment can be planned by permitting the students to select their living setting, based on feedback about their own personality needs and specific information about the social milieu characteristic of each dormitory environment. There are plans to compare this group of students with a group that goes through the usual bureaucratic procedure. In this way the effects of the ecologically-based planning program for university living can be evaluated.

15 Applied Social Psychology

Barbara S. Dohrenwend

This committee was originally mandated to develop an applied social and urban psychology model of training in community psychology. However, the group decided that the two components in this mandate, *applied social* and *urban*, had quite different relations to a training model. Whereas applied social could provide the conceptual and methodological bases, urban designated only one kind of community setting in which the model might be implemented. One might, for example, equally well implement an applied social psychology training model in a rural setting or in the setting of an ethnically homogeneous community. The group agreed that community psychologists working in a particular type of community setting would be expected to relate their training program to that setting in terms of course content and field experience. However, other than making this expectation explicit, no attention was paid to the question of how a program set in an urban community would differ from a program in some other community setting.

The Guideline for Training Model Construction was followed loosely. No attempt was made to deal with each topic separately, and some topics were not discussed at all. However, insofar as they are applicable, the headings in the guideline are used in this report so that the material can be related to the standard set of topics.

LEVEL OF STUDY

The program was designed to provide training at the level of the PhD for a person who would be called a *community psychologist*. Discussion of training programs at the MA and BA levels did not extend beyond acknowledging that they would embody the same general orientation toward formulation of social problems and understanding of social processes as at the PhD level but with less extensive training, particularly in research design and technology.

RESEARCH AND KNOWLEDGE BASES

The committee decided that the research and knowledge bases of community psychologists could best be described in terms of questions that they must be

Participants in this model: Rodney Carman, Robert Czeh, Barbara Dohrenwend, Cheryl Gaudreault, Terry Gilius, Faye Goldberg, Stanley Lehmann, Brenda Rutherford, David Terrell.

able to answer in order to function effectively in the community. Five of the most important of these questions follow.

1. *What are the characteristics of the target population with whom the community psychologist intends to work? What are their strengths and their weaknesses?* In discussing this question it was noted that even when community psychologists have had previous personal experience in the type of community in which they propose to work, for example a black urban or white rural community, explicit efforts must be made to prevent normal leveling and sharpening processes (cf. Allport & Postman, 1965) from generating a stereotyped conceptualization of the community and its members during extended planning discussions by a university group. The preventive measure indicated is regular interchange with members of the community, who should participate at every stage of a project, including the earliest planning stage.

2. *What are the characteristics of the social and political systems with which the community psychologist will be working?* This question relates not only to local systems within the target community but also to larger political systems, such as state government, which may be expected to have important impact on the community.

3. *What are the effects of social and political systems on individuals?* With this question a basic position of this training model was articulated concerning the locus of forces that must be understood in order to formulate meaningful research questions and useful strategies of intervention for a program in community psychology.

4. *What are the historical processes that affect the public definition of social problems?* This question calls for recognition and understanding of the way in which the goals and activities of the community psychologist are embedded in and generated by the social system and may change in response to that system.

5. *What are the possible consequences of the community psychologists' activities?* This question points up the issue of the accountability of community psychologists to the groups and individuals with whom they intend to work. It also emphasizes their responsibility to act only after assessing the possible consequences of their actions, including potential personal and political ramifications.

To answer these questions, community psychologists and their students should begin by using whatever knowledge is already available. In so doing they will cross disciplinary boundaries into history, political science, and other social sciences. When they reach the limits of existing theory and findings, they should be prepared to design and execute research to provide fuller answers to these questions.

CONTENT AREAS AND COURSES

The content areas of a community psychology training program based on applied social psychology were defined in terms of courses, which were divided into two categories: those considered essential, and electives from which students would be urged to make choices consistent with their particular interests. These lists of courses were formulated on the assumption that students in the program would enter with an undergraduate major in psychology or its equivalent.

Essential content courses, which should probably be required of all students, are:

Proseminar in community psychology
Social psychology
Personality theory
Socialization and learning
Minority groups in American society

Courses that students would be urged to take if they were consistent with their interests are:

Epidemiology
Organization theory and public administration
Social stratification and demography
Political institutions, particularly local government
Anthropology
Economics

The content of these courses should be influenced by the community setting of the program, which might, in addition, be reflected in special courses concerned with, for example, urban or rural communities.

TERMINOLOGY AND SKILLS

The technical training of the community psychologist should emphasize breadth. Because community psychologists are problem oriented, they must be competent enough to utilize whatever techniques are appropriate to a particular problem. This need for flexibility dictates, however, that the training program recognize the difference between the level of mastery necessary to be an effective user and that needed to become a creative producer of new techniques. Thus, for example, the community psychologist should be a sophisticated user of packaged computer programs but should not be expected to develop facility in writing programs. To make possible the necessary breadth of training, community psychology students should not take courses designed for students specializing in a particular technique or skill; if necessary, user-oriented courses should be developed especially for community psychology students.

Within this frame of reference, community psychologists should be trained in two general categories of techniques and skills: research and interpersonal relations. Research training should include

Statistics, including multivariate analysis
Psychometrics (that is, techniques of test construction, including assessment of reliability and validation of tests)
Survey research
Experimental research in field settings
Use of computer statistical packages
Evaluation research

This list was not conceived as a set of courses but as an overlapping and interlocking set of techniques and skills, which could be packaged in various ways to suit the interests and convenience of faculty and students in different institutions.

To develop skills in interpersonal relations, community psychologists should be trained in

Interviewing skills for effective information gathering
Group process
Consultation skills

Again, this list does not designate courses, but the skills could be taught in whatever way seemed most effective in a particular training setting.

It should be noted that the student is trained to use the interview as a tool for gathering information, but not as a therapeutic technique. Therapeutic training, with its focus on intrapsychic processes and problems, is based on assumptions that seem incompatible with the training model proposed, as indicated particularly by the third question under "Research and Knowledge Bases."

The training in group process and in consultation skills is designed to enhance students' sensitivity in interpersonal relations. It is aimed also at developing their ability to understand and take a cooperative problem-solving role in working with community members. In this role they freely share their knowledge with community members and expect to learn from them as well; they expect to derive benefits from the relationship in terms of expanding the body of knowledge of community psychology and to contribute to benefits derived by the community in terms of its needs and interests. Community psychologists learn, in short, to deal with community members as equal partners in mutually beneficial relationships.

FIELD PLACEMENT

It is considered essential for the students to work in a field placement during most of their training. If possible, this placement would be selected by the students throughout their training. After the first year or so, however, they should be required as part of their training to negotiate their own placement, preferably obtaining a paid position in order to maximize the commitment of the setting to the student and the student to the setting. One committee member expressed doubts about this arrangement, however, fearing that supervision and the opportunity for training would be poor in a paid position.

In a field placement the student should work under the joint supervision of a person in the field setting and a faculty member. The supervisor in the field need not be a psychologist; in fact, the student should get experience working with members of other professions.

The purpose of the field placement was formulated as a series of objectives:

- To learn to collaborate with other professionals and with nonprofessionals
- To develop sensitivity to people of classes and ethnic backgrounds different from one's own
- To learn to diagnose social problems, including assessment of needs
- To develop opportunity for action research and carry it out, if possible
- To develop awareness of one's own strengths and weaknesses and learn how to use and compensate for them

FORMAT

The program should be located in a university, either as an independent PhD program or as an optional component in a social psychology program. Given the difficulties of establishing credentials for community psychology outside the university, it does not seem wise to attempt to innovate at the organizational level within the university as well. For this reason, despite recognition of the value of other disciplines to the community psychologist (see "Research and Knowledge Bases," "Content Areas and Courses"), for strategic reasons the group did not think that the program should be interdisciplinary.

FINANCIAL SUPPORT

Currently, financial support from NIMH is restricted. New awards cannot be made now, so this source of support is available only to supplement and improve existing NIMH training programs that may not have a community psychology component at the time that they are up for renewal.

As noted in the discussion of field placement, advanced students would probably be urged to obtain placements that would pay for their services. This procedure was urged as part of the student's training in negotiating a contract in a community setting. It would, in addition, provide a supplementary source of financial support for the training program.

IDEOLOGY, VALUE BASE, AND SOCIAL ETHICS

Underlying the model of training proposed here is the assumption that the community psychologist's goal is to change the social system so that it will be of greater benefit to individuals, rather than changing individuals so that they can adjust more effectively to the existing system. Further, experience indicates that the social changes envisioned within this framework are sufficiently profound to create the potential of conflict between the community psychologist and those who hold power in the existing system. At the same time, individual community psychologists are not ordinarily prepared to sacrifice their own comfort for the sake of their work. Community psychologists, as professionals, enjoy the material and social benefits of middle-class status. They are, therefore, chronically threatened by conflict between their ideals and their self-interest. In warding off this conflict, community psychologists attempt to avoid critically compromising either ideals or comforts. This chronic ethical dilemma appears to be an unavoidable condition of the practice of community psychology.

REFERENCE

Allport, G. W., & Postman, L. J. The basic psychology of rumor. In H. Proshansky and B. Seidenberg (Eds.), *Basic studies in social psychology.* New York: Holt, 1965.

16 Commonalities in Models and Approaches to Training in Community Psychology

Ira Iscoe

The diversity and complexity noted by Glidewell in his insightful critique of current training programs in community psychology (Chapter 6) is echoed in the approaches to training that were considered at the conference. It is apparent that there is a varied range of activities presently encompassed and projected under the rubric of *community psychology.*

Despite the diversity, there are a number of trends that are common to most of the proposed approaches to training in community psychology. In terms of basic values, there is, for example, general agreement that community psychology should move away from mental illness, and should focus on more positive concerns with well-being, a sense of belonging, and the enhancement of competencies of both individuals and groups. While community psychologists accept working with individuals on a one-to-one, face-to-face basis as sometimes necessary and desirable, most would agree that greater emphasis should be placed on indirect services implemented at the highest feasible level—the group, the institution, the organization, or, ideally, the entire community.

General recognition of the need for orderly progress that will benefit the entire community suggests that the revolutionary fervor of the '60s has dissipated. Community psychologists are now less inclined to direct attacks on established community institutions, perhaps as a result of their adverse experiences in this sphere. The need to insure the continuity of programs once they are initiated has replaced unrealistic and unsuccessful efforts to bring about radical change. Constructive evolutionary change is becoming the accepted approach, and this implies an increased emphasis on sociopolitical sophistication and knowledge of community processes. Emphasis in graduate training programs on these approaches was stressed with the realization that this will require new interfaces between training settings and communities.

Another important commonality may be noted in the expressed need for further research as a high priority for community psychology. A cohesive body of knowledge must be established as a foundation, drawing on relevant areas in psychology and other behavioral sciences to develop methodologies appropriate to community-oriented research. The research methodology currently taught in most graduate psychology programs is not well suited to the investigation of complex community problems. Quasi-experimental designs and multivariate statistical procedures would appear to be essential tools for community psychology research.

Related to the issue of research methods in community psychology is the question of where academic training should take place. Different models and approaches may well require that training take place in different settings. While some dissatisfaction was voiced about the commitment of psychology departments to training in community psychology, there was clear recognition of the need to maintain a solid academic base for the area. Several groups voiced their preferences for interdisciplinary programs and free-standing professional schools, but the rationale for locating community psychology training programs in such settings and the specific conditions that would be required for them to survive and flourish were not clarified.

The integration of theory and field work with dissertation research was viewed as essential to the training of community psychologists, but there was concern that community psychologists might be prevented from doing dissertations that involved, for example, empirical naturalistic observations. Apprehension was expressed that the need to be "scientific" might discourage dissertations dealing with genuine community problems. Community psychology might go the way of clinical psychology, where the need to maintain academic respectability frequently took precedence over the relevance of the topic being investigated. It was feared that the demand for elegance in experimental design might detract from admittedly less rigorous but more flexible approaches needed in the initial stages of research in community psychology. These concerns were voiced more frequently by graduate students and younger faculty members facing the realities of promotion in psychology departments. The prevailing reward structure within academic departments is thus a key issue to be faced by community psychology.

Several groups were not ready to deal with the problem of continuing education; others considered it vital and offered specific suggestions for implementing programs. In such programs, the recommended flow of activities basically remained one way—from the university to the community. The avenues for providing continuing education were consultation, workshops, and symposia in which university personnel "train" community psychologists in field settings. In some models, however, there are at least tentative provisions for input from field-based community psychologists.

A critical factor in any training program is its source of financial support, and here a clear trend emerges. The concept of pay-for-services to groups, agencies, organizations, and institutions was emphasized in contrast to the present practice of remuneration for services provided on a one-to-one basis. It was proposed that agencies should compensate community psychologists for services in such areas as consultation, evaluation, program planning, research design, and data analysis, among others.

The desirability for both academic departments and training agencies to fund training programs was strongly affirmed. It was also noted that agencies, both public and private, should receive "pay-back" in services performed by the trainee. However, as suggested by one of the working groups, "people go where the money is," and where the money is or may be, may not be where there is a good community experience for the trainee, or potential long-term beneficial effects for community psychology training programs.

Traditional service settings are more likely to have demands for traditional services such as diagnostic testing and psychotherapy, and such agencies are less likely to want consultants, evaluators, participant conceptualizers, program planners, and all of the other heady activities PhD community psychologists supposedly stand ready to deliver. Should community psychologists be trained in traditional clinical skills in order to gain access to agencies and institutions, and then branch out? While the clinical/community and community mental health approaches advocate training in traditional clinical skills, the intervention/prevention, social-change, social-ecology, and applied social psychology approaches do not. Sources of financial support for training in community psychology will have profound implications for the future of the field, and will undoubtedly have important impact on the orientation and direction of individual training programs.

Related to the question of financial support are implications for training in nontraditional settings such as city and state governments, departments of welfare, human resource planning, programs for the aged, educational and criminal justice settings, and the like. While the desirability of working in such settings is apparent to most community psychologists, there are also many problems and concerns. For example, personnel in these settings often have stereotyped attitudes toward psychologists as testers or therapists, and do not know how to use the skills of community psychology. Furthermore, most trainees do not have the experience or skill to sell their services in nontraditional agencies, and qualified psychologists are generally not available as supervisors. It seems clear that sources of financial support and access to community agencies pose issues that cannot be easily separated in providing field training and practicum experiences for community psychology students.

Another area of strong agreement was that the base for practicum and internship training in community psychology should be broadened. Most of the working groups at the conference faced up to the challenge and the difficulty of working out fees-for-service arrangements in nontraditional settings. However, questions relating to the desirability of an internship were not clarified and differentiated from other forms of advanced field training experiences.

With regard to the question of level of entry into community psychology, no clear consensus emerged among the conference participants. There was substantial agreement that community psychologists with the PhD should have a broader range of competencies and skills, and that persons with MA degrees and, especially, graduates of BA programs, will have narrower, more specialized skills that may require them to work under supervision. It was further recognized that community psychologists with a PhD are best qualified to conceptualize the field, and that advances in the conceptualization of community psychology, and in the development and evaluation of techniques for practice and research are required if subdoctoral programs are to train persons who can contribute effectively to the solution of community problems.

As previously noted, there appears to be a strong desire among community psychology programs to move away from community mental health centers, where the delivery of clinical services is emphasized, and to work more directly within the mainstream of organizations and institutions such as schools, police departments, housing, rehabilitation and welfare programs, and in the offices of state and local planners and city managers. It is further envisioned that working with private agencies may take on a new emphasis as public funds are drying up and previously supported governmental activities are being shifted to private agencies on a contract basis.

The presence of a significant number of graduate students and younger community psychologists served to infuse the deliberations with more concern about practical issues and the relevance of the content of training programs than was the case with most previous training conferences that were described in Chapter 1 of this volume. The difficulties experienced by the conference participants in following the guidelines that were suggested by the planning committee clearly reflected the complexity of the task, and the great need for clarification of the goals, roles, and functions of an emerging discipline. While the diversity in approaches to training in community psychology led to considerable frustration of those who would like to articulate and implement specific training models, this diversity would seem to be an accurate reflection of the current status of training in community psychology.

How well did each of the working groups accomplish its purpose, and what are the implications of these diverse models approaches to training? Veteran observers agreed that this was one of the hardest working conferences they had ever attended. The complexities of the field and the need to structure the conference agenda, while avoiding the dangers of dogma and premature crystalization, were evident throughout the conference proceedings. The amorphous nature of the field and the lack of well-established, widely accepted training models contributed to the challenge, and perhaps to the frustration of the participants, as well.

IV CENTRAL ISSUES IN COMMUNITY PSYCHOLOGY

INTRODUCTION

Emory L. Cowen

This prologue will illustrate some of the things that go wrong when a nonhistorian is invited to write a historical introduction.

Austin '75 was a multifaceted, many-splendored convocation. Stimulating invited talks, diligent work groups, formal and informal plenary sessions, interstitial caucuses, and well-lubricated evening pool-side collectivities all were part of the stuff from which the final fabric is fashioned. A series of models-subgroups, designed to flesh out the values, strategies, and operations of phenotypically diverse approaches that compose the extended community family, were the conference's backbone. Each of the participants was attached to such a subgroup, taking part in its processes and dialogue, and contributing to its reports and recommendations. The models' strand is visible from preconference planning and materials, through the conference, and here again in the final report.

Yet because several key conference focuses, as gleaned from the preconference materials, cut across the several models, a different type of cross-sectional slice was needed to keep the separate pieces of the models' groups optimally glued together. Exactly when, and how, that initially subliminal awareness reached threshold is a story that calls for a more able historian than I. My personal involvement in the process was more back-doorish and catalytic than planned. Although I was not at the time a member of the Conference Steering Committee, through a defect in the democratic electoral system, I *was* president-elect of Division 27. The worst millstone, by far, around the neck of a president-elect is being chairman (by default) of the division's APA Program Committee. That is the land-mined route by which I got into the act.

The division's Executive Committee had agreed at its January 1975 midwinter meeting to reserve some program time at APA for a symposium-style conference report. Little was specified about the exact format of that session except to vest responsibility for the decision in the Conference Steering Committee. Because at that time the Steering Committee was in a work-swamp and up to its gluteus maximus in snapping alligators (that is, urgent nonpostponable decisions about conference formats, preconference materials, attenders, budgets) it had, to mix a metaphor, more immediate fish to fry than an APA symposium to be held on September 1, 1975. But, since I was a (very nervous) program chairman who had to submit a specific symposium title and the names of participants by April 1, 1975, and because there was a big blank space next to "Austin Symposium" on my nifty master-chart, each further day of nondecision made the cattle-prod look better and better to me as a motivating device.

There ensued, in typical random, frenetic sequence, a series of long-distance phone calls between myself and Steering Committee members, and among various permutations and combinations of those members, that served, if nothing else, to notably improve AT&T's position on the "Big Board." By mid-February '75 the (substantial) compulsive side of me could no longer bear the stress of nonclosure. The angst prompted me to frame a desperation letter with an initial, rough mark-up of a plan for a cross-sectional approach to key conference-relevant areas, that might help shape the conference itself as well as the later APA symposium report.

The basic idea was this: Let's designate five key, face-valid areas of interest to community psychology that are relevant to, and cut across, models, and let's put each under the tender loving care of one person to track and report on during the conference and again at APA. The basic concept "grabbed," leaving only the specific areas of chief honchos to be designated. These matters were resolved in a further frenzied round of long-distance calls, the main astonishment of which was that it did *not* result in an AT&T stock split.

Promising leads about crosscutting topical areas came from the preconference survey materials that Bloom had collected. On that basis the following five were selected: (1) Entry Levels and Subprofessional Personnel, (2) Field Training and Placement, (3) Future Conceptual Directions, (4) Knowledge and Research Base, and (5) Alternative Conceptual Models.[1] Next, the people! At that time (and still today), there was a strong feeling that Division 27's past destiny had largely been shaped by a very limited number (and closed group)

---

[1] To illustrate Robbie Burns' prophetic quote, "the best laid schemes o' mice and men gang oft a-gley": Although in the original, abstract (i.e., not constrained by reality) view from atop the mount, it seemed attractive to have a "king of the models" to put it all together, it became clear by day 1 at Austin that this role was neither realistic nor workable. By mutual consent, the role shifted to that of summarizing conference themes (i.e., "the pulse" of the conference), and was so handled: a) at Austin, b) for the APA symposium, and c) in this final report.

of founding fathers, this notwithstanding the fact that an exciting second generation had evolved and become quite visible by spring of 1975. This seemed to be the ideal moment to break out of the closed circle and to get important future-shaping inputs from people other than the division's senior citizens. Hence, a decision was made to invite as chairpersons only individuals who were less than 10 years beyond their degrees. Five such people were identified from the list of tentative Austin participants, and I was asked to be the division's formal "inviter."

With very little time before the APA program deadline, and with a Portnoyesque ability to anticipate all imaginable false steps and breakdown points, I approached this task with substantial ambivalence. On the one hand, there was the excitement of being associated with a good concept that rang true. On the other hand, there was the lurking, foreboding surety that the negotiative steps would be frustrating and time-consuming, with the necessary pieces not falling into final place for at least several weeks—if indeed they ever did.

With that "Joe Brfyzstlk cloud-of-doom" over my head, I prepared to rejoin Alexander Graham Bell's most famous invention for another long siege. Having been that route before, I knew in my bones what would happen. Secretary A would tell me that Dr. X was on safari taking pictures of wildebeasts in the Serengetti game preserve, not to return for three weeks, and that Dr. Y was shelved indefinitely with mononucleosis. If I was lucky enough to reach Dr. Z, he'd surely have to review his Merrill-Lynch portfolio and consult his astrologer before being able to make the decision. And if I had the temerity to suggest that he should be our apple specialist, no doubt he's say avocados. (An optimist, I'm not!)

What really happened, though, wasn't at all like that. Each of the five people was "hit" amidships on the first phone contact—no wrong numbers, no busy signals, not even a coffee break! Each listened graciously to my droning, structuring spiel. Each agreed to participate cheerfully and willingly—no ifs, ands, or buts. And, in a system with zero degrees of freedom—that is, five people and five jobs—each indicated that the specific area tentatively proposed for him was exactly the one he himself would have chosen. With that critical logistic step so effortlessly and painlessly negotiated, we could all go down to the seashore (Melina Mercouri, 1961).

By late February, then, we had an evolving structure, our five topical areas, and a person to ride shotgun in each. The roster was as follows:

Entry levels: Steven Danish (Pennsylvania State University)
Field training: David Stenmark (University of South Carolina)
Future conceptual directions: Julian Rappaport (University of Illinois)
Knowledge base: Edison Trickett (Yale University)
Models (to become conference themes): Jack Chinsky (University of Connecticut)

In fact, by that time we had just about everything but a name for the fearsome fivesome. In conversations immediately preceding the action period they had been variously referred to by such pedestrian titles as *group leaders, chairpersons, trackers,* and *recorders.* The least lacklustre designation mentioned to that point, in obvious deference to the fact that the conference was to take place in the Great Southwest, was *chief honcho!*

Because I had been (defensively, but necessarily) vague in my phone contacts with the new appointees, I promised to write them a fuller structuring, summarizing letter, laying out whatever concretes I could describe. That part of history I can accurately recapture, because, disorganized files notwithstanding, I succeeded in locating my launching document of March 3, 1975. It began by enshrining a new title for the leaders. I was, at the time, rereading an all-time favorite, Leo Rosten's *The Joys of Yiddish* (New York: McGraw-Hill, 1968), in preparation for a graduate seminar in community health that I teach. The belly-laugh ratio was as high as ever. And suddenly from page 223 a name for the five leaders leapt into figure: *Mavins.* Rosten's exact definition is:

mavin (May-vin)—pronounced maven, to rhyme with raven. Hebrew: 'understanding.' An expert: a really knowledgeable person; a good judge of quality and a connoiseur. 'He's a *mavin* on Mozart.' 'Are you a real mavin?' 'Don't buy it until you get the advice of a mavin!' *Mavin* was recently given considerable publicity in a series of newspaper advertisements for herring tidbits: 'The herring mavin strikes again', proclaimed the caption, and the picture showed an empty jar. (p. 223)

It sounded a lot better than *chairperson.* It had pizzazz. As a five-letter word beginning with "m," it fit very well with "model." Models' groups, mavins' groups-it all had a very nice ring.

There were, to be sure, a few minor problems with the term. Several colleagues (with some reason) perceived it as chauvinistic and, implicitly, hostile. But then again, since I am both chauvinistic and hostile (not to mention insensitive), I duly noted the accusation without being overly ruffled by it. Several mavins were themselves less than overjoyed with the title because both their self-concepts and their educational styles went in more catalytic than mavinistic directions. One remarked that it made him feel like a used-clothes salesman. But by that time the damage had been done. Over the intervening months, during the conference itself and since, the term *mavin* did, indeed, become etched in bronze. If nothing else, Austin aficionados left the meeting with a richer understanding of that concept.

Officially (for purposes of program and record) the mavins' groups were called Special Interest Groups (SIG). Structural steps needed to facilitate the operation of such groups were taken both before and during the conference. Thus, each mavin wrote a one-paragraph description of his designated turf. These descriptions were distributed with preconference materials, and participants were invited to sign up for one of the five groups. Two within-conference, late-afternoon times were designated for SIG meetings. Since participants were free to sign up as they wished, SIG membership cut sharply across models-groups and was quite diverse. Mavins themselves further encouraged a broad input base by attending different models sessions, by speaking with as many people as possible, and in some cases by tape-recording meetings and going over the output in the wee hours of the morn.

One further structural change in the original game plan was needed. Whereas it was first felt that there should be a mavin for "models," the fact that there already were seven such group leaders led the Steering Committee to conclude that to have still another would add to, rather than reduce, the confusion. Thus, Jack Chinsky, the originally designated "modelist," became "Lucky Pierre." His key role within the mavin's framework was the challenging one of trying to develop an overall tonal and thematic summary of the conference. During the conference it was agreed that he would lead a second subgroup of the most heavily oversubscribed of the remaining four SIGs; that turned out to be "future conceptual directions."

A major (two and one-half hour) time bloc on the final afternoon was reserved for preliminary mavins' reports to a plenary session of the conference. Chaired by this "historian," the meeting began with (approximate) 20-minute summaries of each area by its respective mavin, followed by comments and observations first from Kemba Young, Brian Wilcox, and Karl Slaikeu, and then by three of the distinguished keynote speakers: Jack Glidewell, Jim Kelly, and Bob Reiff. Next came an open question-and-comment period involving all conference participants. The session ended with a summation by Charles Spielberger, division president and member of the Conference Steering Committee.

In the four months between Austin and Chicago (APA), mavins continued to work on and refine their products. Verbatim transcripts of the proceedings became available in late June. Additional feedback from participants was sought and received. Gray cells fired. The three-hour APA symposium for the conference report was chaired by Ira Iscoe. Each mavin presented a refined report for his area, followed, again, by a discussant's panel and comments and questions from the audience. The symposium was very well attended. It drew active audience involvement and received widespread approbation. Area summaries had evolved one significant further step.

The final polishing steps were taken after APA. The product is reflected in the five chapters that follow this introduction. The areas considered are fundamental to community psychology. How they are represented will, in all likelihood, help significantly to shape its future. The five mavins have brought much ability, dedication, thought, and imaginativeness to the task. They are one major facet of Austin. Moreover, because they are *who* they are, they also reflect, and auger well for, community psychology's future.

17 Human Development and Human Services

A Marriage Proposal

Steven J. Danish

Historically, entry-level issues have involved a specific emphasis on paraprofessional manpower—their needs, roles, interests, and career advancements. However, these issues extend well beyond entry into the human service system to an examination of the kind of system being entered. Examination of the conceptual posture (Cowen, 1973) underlying the system is essential. Such an examination provides a framework for analyzing what services entry-level personnel should deliver, how the services should be delivered, and how the personnel should be trained (Rappaport & Chinsky, 1974).

This chapter examines the conceptual underpinnings of the present human service delivery system and several consequences of this system. In addition, an alternative conceptual framework for delivering human services is proposed. The general approach is to raise questions about the present system and to propose a perspective for a new model that provides a broader context for considering entry-level issues.

THE CURRENT STATUS OF SERVICE DELIVERY: A REMEDIATION MODEL

Despite attempts by community psychologists to institute preventive and enhancement models of service delivery (see Cowen, Gardner, & Zax, 1967; Zax & Specter, 1974), the delivery of human services is still generally characterized by a psychological remedial model emphasizing problems and dysfunctions. Cowen (1973) has described in considerable detail the assumptions inherent in such a model and its problems. However, two implications of such a model have not received sufficient attention: the emphasis on professionalism and the parochialism of psychology as a discipline.

The author acknowledges the continual collaboration and stimulation of Anthony R. D'Augelli throughout the writing of the chapter. His perspective on the intervention process is embedded throughout. The contributions of Paul B. Baltes and Carol Ryff are also appreciated. The suggestions and critical comments of Judith Frankel D'Augelli, Rayman Bortner, David Hultsch, John Nesselroade, and Ted Huston were particularly helpful.

Professionalism

Because of the emphasis on problems and dysfunctions, the system has stressed the need for professionals to deliver the services. Society has accepted this decision to the extent that the dictum "only doctors can really help" has become widespread. Therefore, most of the direct delivery of human services is done by doctors, be they medical doctors or PhD-level psychologists. Indeed, when less than doctoral-level personnel provide services, it is usually done under supervision and may even be seen as an adjunct to the "real" help being offered. The result is a system of licensure essentially directed toward licensing PhDs who can pass academic tests. How well they can help is not considered. Also, the restrictions of third-party payments to other than licensed PhD-level psychologists further widens the breach. Paraprofessionals have become an important manpower source only because they are cheaper, more plentiful, and often able to work with clients who do not fit the YAVIS profile. Thus, they relieve the demand on the "professional" so that he or she can continue to work with the intrapsychic problems of his or her clients.

However, the reason why direct services are delivered by professionals goes beyond society's pressures and, in part, can be explained by the personal needs being met by the delivery of direct services. Helping people directly has many benefits, not the least of which is the prestige given the professional by society. In addition, it provides opportunities for people to see themselves as making a significant impact on others, perhaps meeting their own needs to be rescuers. As opposed to more indirect forms of helping, direct services also permit one to develop and maintain intimate relationships that may contribute to self-esteem and relationship needs. Thus, the fact that we find ourselves performing primarily direct services is probably an interaction of our own needs and society's pressures.

The view that the professional is more effective than the paraprofessional is an implicit, if not always explicit, belief. This view is based on the assumption that degree equals competence, a position difficult to support given the data on the efficacy of direct professional service. The assertion that professionals are more effective direct service providers has become a major point of contention among various segments of the human service system and even within the APA as a whole. The Austin Conference was concerned with this issue as well and, as part of the discussions of entry-level issues, adopted three propositions:

1. Master's-level psychologists should be made full members of APA.
2. An effort must be made to separate membership in APA from the implication that such membership represents an endorsement of competence as a community psychologist.
3. The term *paraprofessional* is a poor one; it connotes "less than." At present, while a variety of other terms are used to describe Bachelor,

Associate of Arts, and high school trained personnel, no term is totally acceptable. Personnel should be defined, not by their degree, but by their competencies, and a system for defining the necessary competencies and determining how to evaluate them should be a major project of Division 27.

Whether or not these propositions are implemented, their impact will be analogous to attempting to demolish a building with a hammer. It will be a slow process, and we will probably quit before we finish. The problem with these proposals is that they direct their attack toward a by-product of the human service system, professionalism, rather than toward the structure of the system itself. True reform will require a new conceptual position to replace the elitism of professionalism and its service delivery system.

Parochialism

A second by-product of the remedial delivery system is a restricted view of what constitutes help. Help is often confined to interpersonal or psychological rehabilitation such that it becomes offered as part of the exclusive domain of psychologists. Although recently the definition of a helper has been expanded to include parents and teachers (for example, Guerney, 1969), most of these helpers still consider their primary role as helping in a psychological or interpersonal sense. Such people as police (Bard, 1969, 1971; Danish & Brodsky, 1974; Danish & Ferguson, 1973); dieticians (Danish, 1975); food service personnel (Powers, Note 1); community service and public affairs personnel (Kelly, Note 2); and lawyers (Danish & Katkin, Note 3; Greening & Zielonka, 1971/1972) play an important part in the helping process in our society. For example, police often find themselves involved in situations requiring human relationship skills. In fact, as much as 80% of their job may entail the application of such skills (Cumming, Cumming, & Edell, 1965; Sterling & Watson, 1971). Given the widespread need for helping personnel in our society, the human service system must expand its view of what constitutes help. Again, a reconceptualization of the assumptions underlying the delivery of services is required. Some suggestions about how one might expand the system are presented in a later section.

The idea has been developed that we need to consider the conceptual system behind the delivery of services and the assumptions derived from the conceptions rather than to focus narrowly on issues in entry level. The suggestion has been made that our present remedially-oriented system produces several negative consequences. A framework for an alternative model follows.

HUMAN DEVELOPMENT AS A FRAMEWORK
FOR HUMAN SERVICE DELIVERY[1]

In an analysis of social and community interventions, Cowen (1973) proposes a preventive model as an alternative and describes a number of thrusts derived from such a model. Both the model he discusses and an enhancement model (D'Augelli, Note 4) are positive alternatives to the remediation model previously discussed. However, while some of the implications of such models are delineated, the conceptual framework has not been as well developed. Prevent what? Enhance what? At present we do not possess a framework whereby we know what to prevent or enhance with regard to either individuals, families, small groups, or communities. Thus, we often go around "preventing" or "enhancing" on the basis of personal preference. What should a preschool child be able to do socially, cognitively, physically at age 4; an adolescent at 13; a young adult at 27; a person at 45; and older adult at 70? What are their motivations, hopes, dreams, etc.? Can we intervene, will our interventions make any difference, or is development so sequenced that the maturational progress and day-to-day living together account for any changes taking place? In other words, what is the range of modifiability of human development, and does this range change as a function of what one wishes to modify and where the individual is in her or his lifespan (Baltes & Willis, 1976)? Further, what are the ethical implications of our enhancing or preventive interventions? Whose needs are being met if we "help" a 65-year-old man realize that his expectations for continued professional success run counter to society's needs and that he should instead prepare for death?

What becomes evident, then, is that what is lacking is an adequate knowledge base and foundation from which to intervene. A model of behavior is required which: (1) incorporates statements about desirable goals or end states of behavior, (2) focuses on sequential changes, (3) emphasizes techniques of optimization, (4) considers the individual or system as an integrative biopsychosocial unit (Ford, 1974) and therefore is amenable to a multidisciplinary focus, and (5) looks at the individuals or systems as developing in a changing biocultural context. One specific model that meets the above criteria is a human development perspective (Baltes, 1973; Harris, 1957; Riegel, 1973).

Traditionally, developmental psychologists have restricted their study to young children and adolescents, with the major focus on cognitive and social behaviors. The proposed human development perspective differs significantly from that approach.

While this section does not purport to examine substantive controversies in the field of human development, the proposed perspective is intended to go

---

[1] While many of the examples and much of the language in the chapter focus on the implications of intervention for individuals, the human development perspective applies equally well for systems such as families or communities.

beyond traditional psychological conceptions of development. The framework presented herein is oriented toward a multidisciplinary view of the individual throughout the lifespan. It presupposes an upward progression in which an intervenor recognizes higher levels of development and, more important, seeks to achieve them. While behavior is ordered, the progression is not smooth since it takes place within an ever changing social context. Riegel (Note 5) has stated that:

developmental leaps are brought about by discordance, asynchrony, or conflict between these [inner-biological, individual-psychological, cultural-sociological, outer-physical] planes of progression. But rather than regarding these critical episodes in a negative manner or from a fatalistic point of view, they provide the very basis which makes the development of the individual and of society possible. (p. 10)

Thus, contrary to the view that critical episodes are destructive events, they may in fact serve to intensify a restructuring process and marshal resources toward further growth. The events may be precipitated by forces within the environment (nonnormative events such as natural disasters) or may be a result of the interaction between the individual's developmental process and the social context (normative life events such as leaving home, loss of a loved one). The term *normative* does not suggest that all individuals go through all events, just that some events are more frequently applicable for all individuals.

There are a number of major implications for human services that can follow from a human development perspective. The first pertains to viewing a taxonomy of critical life events as a guiding principle on which the human development framework is based. The second involves assessing the conceptualization of normative and nonnormative critical life events. The remediation model seems to adhere to an implicit homeostatic view of humanity in which everything should be done to assist persons to return to their prior level of functioning. Thus, critical life events are viewed as detriments to people's balance that should be overcome as quickly and painlessly as possible. This is known as *remediation*. If possible, these crises should be prevented.

On the other hand, if a human development perspective is adopted, our intervention goals go beyond maintaining the status quo and involve facilitating others to move toward "optimal development." We may do this by intensifying or speeding up the process of development or by enabling individuals to achieve higher levels of development. In this way we assume an enhancement posture. Enhancement, in this case, might begin by assisting individuals to optimize their resources during critical life events. However, the eventual objective is to enable individuals to gain control over their life events by providing them with the skills to direct their own future—life management through planning.

At the beginning of this section it was suggested that a model of behavior that adopted a human development perspective would need to meet five criteria. The proposed model does not adequately answer two of the criteria: statements about desirable end states and an emphasis on sequential changes. If a fully functioning model is to be implemented, it will be necessary to determine if end states can be identified and if behavior is in fact sequenced. These are questions that at the present time must be left to lifespan human development researchers and theorists.

FROM THEORY TO PRACTICE: ENHANCING HUMAN DEVELOPMENT

With the adoption of a human development perspective, the human service system has a framework from which to implement an enhancement model of service delivery. One means of implementing services derived from this model is to develop a life skill orientation.

Delivering Life Skills

The framework proposed stresses the importance of critical life events as periods in which significant changes take place for individuals, families, communities, and the like. While many of them are normative, likely to occur for most individuals and probably correlated with age, they are not causally related to age. Thus, one cannot predict their occurrence nor be sure of the age when they may happen for any one individual. Further, we cannot predict the manner in which these events will happen. Therefore, extensive preparation for a specific life event has limited value. An alternative to preparation for any one specific event is the teaching of life-enhancing skills (D'Augelli, Note 4) that have value for a number of the life events. Such skills might include goal planning, decision making, value clarification, risk taking, environmental assessment, relationship development and maintenance, assertiveness, and self-control. These life-enhancing skills need not be anchored to any one situation but can be applied to a number of situations. Therefore, if one is taught this armament of skills, one can use them as needed. In addition, three more generic skills would be taught: (1) choosing the appropriate skill, (2) planning, developing, and implementing one's own life skills for a specific event, and (3) a process by which one can examine consequences of and alternatives to various responses, a form of behavior rehearsal. These three might be considered skills to prepare one for coping with any of the specific events.

These skills are not situation specific and can be used in response to a number of life events. However, since the events occur across the lifespan, the skills may have to be taught or reviewed several times to account for changes in cognitive development. For example, the process of learning a decision-making skill would differ depending on the level of abstraction the learner could handle. The program developed by Branca, D'Augelli, and Evans (Note

6) to teach decision making for elementary school children and one developed by Wakshul (1975) for college students use the same principles yet differ in the degree of complexity required to learn them.

While the intent here is to describe the dissemination of such services, a word about teaching skills seems appropriate. Life skills are taught by intervenors enacting the role of teacher rather than the role of therapist. Principles of instructional design (Gage, 1963; Gagne, 1970) appropriate for a skill-learning format should be used. Such a format would include: (1) identifying explicit behavioral objectives, (2) practice or application of skills to be learned, (3) self-learning by group discussions, (4) rationale for learning (understanding of importance of certain skills), (5) sequential presentation (learning concept A before concept B), (6) active trainee participation, (7) the use of modeling, and (8) the use of immediate feedback concerning the appropriateness of trainee responses.

Delivering Multidisciplinary Services

In addition to a focus on life skills, a second set of services implied by a human development framework includes services derived from the multidisciplinary perspective. While these services might not in themselves act to enhance development, they would provide an atmosphere in which development might proceed in a more orderly fashion or achieve higher levels of attainment.

Earlier it was noted how parochialism seemed to be a characteristic of the remedial model with psychological remediation. A human development framework would view individuals from a biopsychosocial perspective and recognize the likely interaction among these three spheres. Thus, while there might be service providers from different orientations, such as mental health personnel, community caregivers (Caplan, 1964), medical or nutritional personnel, or urban agents (Kelly, 1964), their purpose would be similar, and one could expect the delivery of one type of service to affect the others.

Reorganizing Human Services for an Enhancement Orientation

Although some have proposed an emphasis on preventive or enhancing interventions, the human service delivery system is still organized and funded to offer remedial services. The community mental health center (CMHC), the major vehicle for service delivery, typically operates as a traditional psychological clinic. However, if it is located in a depressed part of town, it has a "community" orientation. Clients with problems are seen by professionals in offices. Occasionally, to emphasize the center's new look, clients are seen in groups in larger offices. Many centers have consultation and education (C&E) units. These units are the most theoretically consistent with community psychology. They usually are seen as the black sheep of the CMHC and receive little funding. From the center's point of view, the role of C&E is to find more clients for the professionals to help. Thus, its purpose is to refer, not to divert, clientele. Preventive or enhancing interventions are most often conceived and implemented by university personnel on small-scale levels for limited time periods. In other words, when nonremedial interventions take place, they are conducted mainly on experimental bases.

A Method for Enhancement: Developmental Education

The search for a methodology that will permit an enhancement orientation finds a most promising direction in the developmental educational approach described by Guerney and his colleagues (Authier, Gustafson, Guerney, & Kasdorf, 1975; Guerney, Guerney, & Stollak, 1971/1972; Guerney, Stollak, & Guerney, 1971). This approach uses the school as its model and instruction as the means for enhancement. The intervenor becomes a teacher rather than a therapist. Adopting such a model allows the intervenor to be a skill trainer who teaches the client the life skills previously proposed and facilitates the retention of the skills through the lifespan.

The potential for the developmental educational intervention model would result in an exciting revolution in the delivery of human services. Services would be delivered in a more widespread fashion. As an educator, the intervenor could become an integral part of the academic curriculum from preschool through continuing education. Such services and the people providing them would no longer need to hide in guidance counselors' offices. They could rightly take their places in the classroom (and in the teachers' lounge). Goals for social and interpersonal development could be identified in the same manner as they are for reading and writing. Continuing education courses for adults, usually restricted to gardening, conversational French, or pottery making, might now include generic life skills or specific skills such as parenting or using leisure time. But the schools are not the only place the life development specialist could be employed. The traditional community mental health center would be replaced by individual and community development centers, where YMCA/YWCA-like programs could be implemented for life development just as they presently are for physical and recreational enhancement. Finally, the life development specialist could become involved in training volunteers to teach some of the more basic skills to others. These volunteers—the Big Brothers, Big Sisters, and Foster Grandparents of today—would not only give love and attention to others; they could also teach the coping skills that many of these youngsters need (Goodman, 1972). We could then truly develop the pyramid system for delivering services that community psychology has talked about since its inception.

IMPLICATIONS AND PROPOSALS
FOR TRAINING

A General Assumption

To perform the described roles, specific training programs need to be developed. While there is no need here to delineate an entire curriculum, an overview seems useful. The focus of the overview is directed toward identifying the necessary skills; the required knowledge base, a human development perspective, has already been outlined.

A major assumption that underlies the proposed overview is that training is necessary. Many of the early human service personnel (paraprofessionals) received little formal preparation for their jobs. It was often assumed that careful selection would result in effective personnel (D'Augelli & Danish, 1976; Durlak, 1973).

While this view may no longer predominate, questions do arise as to how one should conduct the training needed to teach human service delivery skills. In part the answers to these questions are embedded in the confusion that exists between training goals and training processes. Earlier, the adoption of a new framework for viewing human problems and the implementation of a new methodology for working with these problems was proposed. But how does one learn this methodology? It would seem that the same procedures used to learn other skills are applicable to learning human service skills. Too often, training consists of a series of lectures about the importance of various skills (Danish, 1975), or the assumption is made that the behaviors associated with the skills are something one either has or does not have and that they cannot be learned (Danish & Ferguson, 1973). Thus, one is told, for example, "Remember, don't forget to listen." Such prescriptions are not effective. Skills are learned through lecture, practice, and demonstration (Danish & D'Augelli, 1976).

Neither careful selection nor lectures about skills are sufficient to assure quality personnel. Training must take place. It is proposed that the training be a series of competency-based modules. The modules would begin with generic skills required for all service deliverers, regardless of whether they provide direct or indirect service or what type of direct services they deliver. On completion of these generic skills, many individuals would stop. However, some individuals might choose to become specialists in a certain phase of service delivery and thus learn additional skills.

The modules could be taught in institutions of higher education but might just as easily be taught as a part of preservice education programs or in a continuing education format. This format, in which training becomes an integral part of the job, would serve to keep motivation high and generally keep individuals moving toward professional fulfillment. Further, it would offer a much more feasible model of professional growth than does the Vail

Conference report (Korman, 1974), which recommends that personnel have two months for professional growth every two years.

Rapport Building: The First Step

Prerequisite to the delivery of most services, whether direct or indirect, biological, psychological, or social, is the development of a trusting relationship between the deliverer and recipient of the services and an understanding of the recipient's situation, goals, and problems. This relationship is requisite whether it is between individuals or between an agency and the community. Some theorists, for example Rogers (1957), have suggested that the behaviors associated with rapport and understanding are the necessary and sufficient conditions for helping others. Whether or not one agrees with this view, responsiveness does facilitate exploration of relevant concerns and goals and helps one talk on a more personal level. While this exploration and openness cannot be equated with help in most cases, it does encourage the development of trust and allows the service provider to better understand the recipient's situation and goals, regardless of their nature. In other words, rapport facilitates understanding whether the area of concern be biological-physical, psychological, or social in character. Furthermore, rapport enables the indirect service provider to better establish training, consultative, and supervisory relationships.

A number of programs have been developed to teach rapport-building skills (Carkhuff, 1969; Danish & Hauer, 1973; Ivey, 1971; Kagan, 1972). A brief description of these programs, including the specification of program goals and processes, attempts made to "trainer-proof" the programs, and issues involved in delivering each program, is presented by Danish and Brock (1974). For example, the Danish and Hauer (1973) program, *Helping skills: A basic training program*, is designed to train six rapport-building skills. These skills, presented as self-contained "stages," are: Understanding Your Needs to be a Helper, Using Effective Nonverbal Behavior, Using Effective Verbal Behavior, Using Effective Self-Involving and Self-Disclosure Behavior, Understanding the Communications of Others, and Establishing Effective Helping Relationships. The same training procedure is followed in each session. The process of skill training entails several steps: (1) the skill is defined in behavioral terms, (2) the rationale for the skill is presented and discussed with the trainees, (3) a skill attainment criterion is specified, (4) trainers model effective and ineffective skill performance, (5) trainees practice the skill under intensive leader supervision, (6) homework emphasizing continued behavioral rehearsal is assigned, and (7) during the subsequent session an evaluation of trainee skill level is conducted, using behavioral checklists and other evaluation tools.

Data collected on the program indicate that trainees can learn rapport-building skills (Danish, D'Augelli, & Brock, 1976) and maintain their skill level fairly successfully over a seven-month follow-up period (McCarthy, Danish, &

D'Augelli, in press). In addition, it was found that appropriate use of these skills was positively correlated with the amount of time the client talked (D'Augelli, Handis, Brumbaugh, Illig, Searer, Turner, & D'Augelli, Note 7). Therefore, rapport-building skills can be identified and taught effectively.

Training to Teach Life–Enhancing Skills

While training in rapport-building skills has become an accepted part of many programs, especially those for counseling and therapy, training for teaching nonacademic, personal-psychosocial, life-enhancing skills is essentially non-existent. Because such skills are not a regular part of the services delivered, no such training program has been developed. Such programs would focus on teaching the competencies that would enable the intervenor to act as a skill trainer-consultant to others. Experience in applying generic education programs to specific critical life events is needed. Also called for are exposure to and practice in designing life-skills training packages.

D'Augelli (in press) has described a program being developed and piloted for training direct intervenors to deliver life-enhancing skills.[2] The program begins with training in assessing the goals of others. This skill (actually, a set of complex skills) sidesteps the problem orientation and focuses on identifying the direction that the skill-recipients wish to go, that is, what their personal and interpersonal goals are. Basic to this skill is teaching the intervenor (and therefore the recipients) to reconceptualize problems in goal terms. In other words, the focus is not on what one cannot do and why but on what one would like to do. The helper must work at behaviorally specifying the person's goals, the importance of the goals, and the roadblocks that are impeding the achievement of the goals so that the deliverer and recipient(s) can develop a specific intervention program to accomplish these goals.

Other skill training would be consistent with the life-enhancing skills previously mentioned, such as decision making, risk taking, and self-change strategies. Although theoretically it would be possible to provide training in teaching all life-enhancing skills, it is clearly not feasible. Thus, training is provided in program development. We have developed a skill entitled "Designing Self-Development Programs" that involves teaching the intervenor the general format used to define life skills and how to design the learning experiences required to attain competence in these skills. In other words, we are "giving our psychology away" (Miller, 1969) so that eventually the recipient can learn how to develop her or his own skills training program.

The basic strength of this model is in the dovetailing of training and service. In the training itself, a structured, systematic model similar to that employed by Danish and Hauer (1973) is used. This same model is used in the

---

[2] Information about the training program in life-enhancing skills is available from the author.

delivery of the life-enhancing skill. Thus, the skills-oriented approach to training is carried through to the service itself.

BEYOND FANTASY: SUGGESTIONS
FOR IMPLEMENTATION

This chapter may appear to be another in a series of harangues about prevention/enhancement. Its implications range from the development of new roles for entry-level personnel to the questions about the value of professionals doing direct service. Suggestions are included about the implementation of a new system for delivering human services that have relevance to the whole concept of how one should view the nature of man.

With such a diverse set of implications, the material can be seen in a number of ways. One could view the proposals as the fantasies of an "ivory tower intellectual." It could be posited that entry-level issues and problems have not been dealt with directly enough. Or one could consider the steps necessary to train Life Development Specialists and the changes that must occur in higher education and continuing education systems to begin such training. It would seem that as new personnel are trained, they will help in the initiation of the new delivery system being proposed. However, we do not need to wait for the change to come from within; there are interventions we can make now to facilitate the development of the new system. For it to be successful, there must be changes in the way human services are funded. Since the efficacy of present-day services are questionable, any program that proves effective by almost any standard of accountability would be viewed favorably. Most important, however, changes must take place in the way human services are viewed by the public. Such services are viewed now as "helping sick people." Present public service announcements emphasize remediation, not prevention or enhancement. We must emphasize development, not health or sickness. The adoption of such an emphasis would alter the public's impression of what constitutes mental health and mental illness.

Evaluation and administration/public relations are some of the roles appropriate for the PhD-level community psychologist. The focus here has been on entry-level personnel as the direct service providers within the new system; the "professional" has been virtually ignored. With the direct service being done by human service personnel who are not professionals, the professional can either support the continuance of the remedial system, drop out of the system, or find new roles. The new roles would be as indirect service providers—trainer, consultant, supervisor, program planner and developer, administrator, or evaluator. It is in keeping with the purpose of graduate education to train professionals to enter these positions rather than direct service positions (Danish, 1974). Unfortunately, little or no training is presently available to teach one to perform indirect service, and an implication of the initiation of this new service system is the chaning focus of graduate education.

Despite the feasibility of the proposed new system, it is the fancy of a dreamer to assume that one system will replace another. Furthermore, it may be harmful for the remedial system to disappear. Regardless of our efforts to prevent or enhance development, there may always be individuals who will need more traditional psychological services. Also, some may always "need" the help of "doctors." Two parallel systems could exist, with funds being distributed on the basis of accountable performance. Yet, the day may come when the new system has become so effective that the doors will open to the remedial-oriented community mental health centers and no one will be there. It is toward this end that we must work.

REFERENCE NOTES

1. Powers, T. F. *The future of food service 1985-1990.* University Park: Food Service and Housing Administration, The Pennsylvania State University, 1975.
2. Kelly, J. G. *Careers in community service and public affairs at the B.A. level: The University of Oregon experience.* Paper presented at the annual meeting of the American Psychological Association, Montreal, Canada, August 1973.
3. Danish, S. J., & Katkin, D. *Training lawyers in human relations skills: A proposal for assessment, training and evaluation.* Unpublished manuscript, The Pennsylvania State University, 1974.
4. D'Augelli, J. F. *Early thoughts on primary prevention.* Working paper presented to the Prevention and Evaluation Branch of the Governor's Council on Drug and Alcohol Abuse, Harrisburg, Pa., April 1974.
5. Riegel, K. *Toward a dialectic theory of development.* Paper presented at Dialectics Workshop, Rochester, New York, May 1974.
6. Branca, M. C., D'Augelli, J. F., & Evans, K. L. *Decisions are possible: A skills training program for children.* Paper presented at the annual meeting of the American Educational Research Association, Washington, D.C., April 1975.
7. D'Augelli, A. R., Handis, M. H., Brumbaugh, L., Illig, V., Searer, R., Turner, D. W., & D'Augelli, J. F. *The verbal helping behavior of telephone center volunteers.* Manuscript submitted for publication, 1976.

REFERENCES

Authier, J., Gustafson, K., Guerney, B. C., & Kasdorf, J. A. The psychological practitioner as a teacher: A theoretical-historical and practical review. *The Counseling Psychologist,* 1975, *5,* 31–50.
Baltes, P. B. Prototypical paradigms and questions in life-span research on development and aging. *Gerontologist,* 1973, *13,* 458–67.
Baltes, P. B., & Willis, S. L. Toward psychological theories of aging and development. In J. W. Birren & K. W. Schaie (Eds.), *Handbook on psychology of aging.* New York: Van Nostrand Reinhold, 1976.

Bard, M. Family intervention police teams as a community mental health resource. *Journal of Criminal Law, Criminology, and Police Science*, 1969, *50*, 247–250.

Bard, M. The role of law enforcement in the helping system. *Community Mental Health Journal*, 1971, *7*, 151–60.

Caplan, G. *Principles of preventive psychiatry*. New York: Basic Books, 1964.

Carkhuff, R. R. *Helping and human relations*. New York: Holt, 1969.

Cowen, E. L. Social and community interventions. In P. H. Mussen & M. R. Rosenzweig (Eds.), *Annual review of psychology* (Vol. 24). Palo Alto, Calif.: Annual Reviews, Inc., 1973.

Cowen, E. L., Gardner, E. A., & Zax, M. (Eds.). *Emergent approaches to mental health problems*. New York: Appleton-Century-Crofts, 1967.

Cumming, E., Cumming, I., & Edell, L. Policeman as philosopher, guide and friend. *Social Problems*, 1965, *12*, 276–286.

Danish, S. J. Counseling psychology and the Vail Conference: An invited comment on training settings and patterns. *The Counseling Psychologist*, 1974, *4*, 68.

Danish, S. J. Developing helping relationships in dietetic counseling. *Journal of the American Dietetic Association*, 1975, *61*, 107–110.

Danish, S. J., & Brock, G. W. The current status of paraprofessional training. *The Personnel and Guidance Journal*, 1974, *53*, 299–303.

Danish, S. J., & Brodsky, S. L. *Manual for police human relations training*. Carbondale: Center for the Study of Crime, Delinquency and Corrections, Southern Illinois University, 1974.

Danish, S. J., & D'Augelli, A. R. Rationale and implementation of a training program for paraprofessionals. *Professional Psychology*, 1976, *7*, 38–46.

Danish, S. J., D'Augelli, A. R., & Brock, C. W. An evaluation of helping skills training: Effects on helper's verbal responses. *Journal of Counseling Psychology*, 1976, *23*, 259–266.

Danish, S. J., & Ferguson, N. Training police to intervene in human conflict. In J. Snibbe & H. Snibbe (Eds.), *The urban policeman in transition*. Springfield, Ill.: C. C. Thomas, 1973.

Danish, S. J., & Hauer, A. L. *Helping skills: A basic training program*. New York: Behavioral Publications, 1973.

D'Augelli, A. R. Paraprofessionals as educator-consultants. *Professional Psychology*, in press.

D'Augelli, A. R., & Danish, S. J. Evaluating training programs for paraprofessionals and nonprofessionals. *Journal of Counseling Psychology*, 1976, *23*, 247–253.

Durlak, J. A. Myths concerning the nonprofessional therapist. *Professional Psychology*, 1973, *4*, 300–304.

Ford, D. H. Mental health and human development: An analysis of a dilemma. In D. Harshbarger and R. Maley (Eds.), *Behavior analysis and systems analysis: An integrative approach to mental health programs*. Kalamazoo, Michigan: Behaviordelia, 1974.

Gage, N. L. (Ed.). *Handbook of research on teaching*. Chicago: Rand McNally, 1963.

Gagne, R. *The conditions of learning*. New York: Holt, 1970.

Goodman, G. *Companionship therapy: Studies of structured intimacy.* San Francisco: Jossey-Bass, 1972.

Greening, T. C., & Zielonka, W. Special applications of humanistic learning: A workshop on attorney-client relationships. *Interpersonal Development,* 1971/1972, *2,* 194–200.

Guerney, B. G., Jr. (Ed.). *Psychotherapeutic agents: New roles for nonprofessionals, parents and teachers.* New York: Holt, 1969.

Guerney, B. G., Guerney, L. F., & Stollak, G. E. The potential advantages of changing from a medical to an educational model in practicing psychology. *Interpersonal Development,* 1971/1972, *2,* 238–245.

Guerney, B. G., Stollak, G. E., & Guerney, L. F. The practicing psychologist as educator—An alternative to the medical practitioner model. *Professional Psychology,* 1971, *2,* 276–282.

Harris, D. *The concept of development.* Minneapolis: University of Minnesota Press, 1957.

Ivey, A. E. *Microcounseling.* Chicago: C. C. Thomas, 1971.

Kagan, N. *Influencing human interaction.* East Lansing: Michigan State University, 1972.

Kelly, J. G. The mental health agent in the urban community. In *Urban America and the planning of mental health services.* New York: Group for Advancement of Psychiatry, 1964.

Korman, M. National conference on levels and patterns of professional training in psychology: The major themes. *American Psychologist,* 1974, *29,* 441–449.

McCarthy, P. R., Danish, S. J., & D'Augelli, A. R. A follow up evaluation of helping skills training. *Counselor Education and Supervision,* in press.

Miller, G. A. Psychology as a means of promoting human welfare. *American Psychologist,* 1969, *24,* 1063–1075.

Rappaport, J., & Chinsky, J. M. Models for delivery of service from a historical and conceptual perspective. *Professional Psychology,* 1974, *5,* 42–50.

Riegel, K. Dialectic operations: The final period of cognitive development. *Human Development,* 1973, *16,* 346–370.

Rogers, C. R. The necessary and sufficient conditions of therapeutic personality change. *Journal of Consulting Psychology,* 1957, *21,* 95–103.

Sterling, J., & Watson, N. A. *Changes in the role concepts of police officers.* Mental Health Program Reports #4, 1971, 261–280.

Wakshul, B. *A description and evaluation of a personal decision-making skills program for college students.* Unpublished master's thesis, The Pennsylvania State University, 1975.

Zax, M., & Specter, G. A. *An introduction to community psychology.* New York: Wiley, 1974.

18 Field Training in Community Psychology

David E. Stenmark

The proposed community psychology field training model integrates the major concerns and realities apparent in the field today. These concerns are reflected by the academic community psychology programs surveyed by Bloom in the preconference materials, as well as by the conceptual models articulated at the Austin Conference. This model is the result of a group enterprise that crosscut the Austin meetings, with the group representing a reasonably well stratified sample of academic and applied community psychologists at all stages of professional development.

PREVIOUS THEORIES AND GOALS

The group enterprise had three basic goals: (1) to design a field training model suitable for implementation by all seven conceptual models, (2) to provide accessability for persons at all training entry levels, and (3) to construct a recommended, graduated sequence of competency-based, task-oriented field training experiences. The present model, then, differs from previous models in the literature in several important ways. First, although the literature contains numerous articles focused on training concepts and principles, they are primarily tied to the community mental health model or to the clinical-community orientation, rather than to community psychology. Second, the training literature on the whole has focused on separate approaches for PhD training, continuing education training, paraprofessional training, etc. In contrast, the present approach follows the recommendations outlined by Danish (Note 1), and is based on his notion that "the difference between a PhD-level community psychologist and another community psychologist regardless of level or degree, is not whether one is more competent than the other, but rather the number of competencies each should have and demonstrate." Third, the present field training model differs from existing programs and previously published descriptions of training in that it provides a sequence of field

Original paper presented at APA, Chicago 1975, in I. Iscoe (Chairperson), *Report on the Austin Conference: The Future of Community Psychology.*

F. T. Miller, Jeff Whiteley, Robert Williams, Steve Larcen, Sherry Payne, David Terrell, Eileen Rafeniello, Leonard Haas, and Mary Teague each made significant contributions to the development of this chapter.

The author especially thanks Jerri Munley-Foley for her support and development of the manuscript.

training experiences of graduated complexity, suitable for endorsement and implementation in all of the existing community psychology training programs.

At present, community training programs appear to be characterized by entrepreneurial and highly idiosyncratic academic training formats in which the progressive involvement in field training experiences is a function of the most recent community involvement of the program's head "honcho" or other faculty. No single planned system of professional development, common skill acquisition, or set of common training experiences has yet received endorsement and behavioral expression in the profession or in its training programs.

At the Austin Conference, Aponte (Note 2) reported the findings from a recent study on training in community psychology. The study was based on a 90-item survey that examined 341 MA and PhD psychology programs and 114 internship settings. The findings relevant to this model were that at the present time (1) there are a very limited range of field placements for community psychologists, (2) there are a limited range of jobs in which community psychologists have been placed, (3) community psychologists are being trained in a narrow range of skills, and (4) community psychology training programs still appear to be tied into the community mental health model. Reiff has noted that community psychology, and particularly community psychology training, has provided more of a reactive than a proactive response to social problems. This observation draws credence from the findings of Zolik, Sirbu, and Hopkinson (Note 3) in their graduate student perspectives on training in community mental health. Several of Zolik's comments focused on field training and seem appropriate here.

Survey comments by some of the students indicated that in many cases availability [of field training experiences] meant that obtaining these experiences was possible only through the student's initiative, rather than there being a planned field placement available as part of the training program ... community mental health/community psychology field experiences were more readily available than academic training ... concern was expressed over the need for academic courses to provide new integration of field experiences at the conceptual level ... and that the frontiers and innovations are to be found within university walls appears to be a myth as far as community mental health/community psychology is concerned; far greater advances on CMH/CP have been made out in the field.

In summary, a conceptual hiatus emerges with respect to goals, values, and overarching concerns of academic and field placement training of community psychologists.

Kelly (1970) predicted the present dilemma and suggested antidotes for its resolution:

The focus on training is not an emphasis on how to tinker with the curriculum, but refers to the socialization of a new profession. The initial premise is that since community psychology is different from other forms of psychology, then its socialization will need to be different. For the training of the community psychologist demands a critical period in which he learns the styles of work which are going to be relevant for his own future adaption. If the differences and requirements are real, training programs will need to be designed to reflect these varied conditions. The adaptive tasks of the community psychologists are not to accommodate to the university, his tasks are to follow the life course of the community and to adapt to the community environment.

Some of the more skeptical might view Kelly's suggestion as idealistic and not rooted in academic realities. The present training model was designed to satisfy both the psychologist's need to adapt to the community and the academician's need for structure and form.

The Proposed Model

The description of the proposed community psychology field training model covers more than the model itself. It focuses on a number of major concerns: (1) a definition of field placement, (2) some considerations of the field training site, (3) recommendations regarding the integration of the seven community models, (4) the manner in which entry levels relate to the model, (5) the description of the graduated sequence of training experiences, and (6) some specific principles and recommendations regarding field training.

Basic to an understanding of the model is an understanding of the use of the term *field training*. There are two kinds of training, one centered primarily in the academic setting and one that occurs in a variety of community-based placements outside the university. The data and research base, as well as the supervisory input, may be unidisciplinary and typically psychological in nature, or they may be multidisciplinary and task-oriented. The present model ascribes to the multidisciplinary training approach.

Field training in the present context would include the following kinds of activities: (1) course-related practicum, (2) practicum courses, (3) field training placements, and (4) field traineeships. The course-related practicum would be essentially didactic, or formal, academic courses with three to six hours a week of course-related field training experiences. The second level, the practicum courses, would involve eight to 20 hours a week of concentrated effort and field training activities; faculty involvement would consist primarily of direct supervision and placement coordination. The third level, field training placements, would involve a temporal commitment of 20 to 40 hours per week and might extend for a semester or a three- to six-month period. The fourth level, field traineeships, would constitute a year-long, fulltime, supervised experience as a functioning community psychologist.

The described model is designed around a minimum requirement of approximately 4,000 supervised hours of field training practicum placements for the PhD. The term *internship*, which over the years has generally referred to a year-long (2,000 hour), full-time commitment (and which is currently an

APA minimum requirement for university departmental accreditation for awarding the PhD in clinical psychology), has not been specifically retained or excluded. It is recognized that for many PhD clinical-community psychologists, either an internship or an alternative is needed. A number of year-long internships currently are funded and available throughout the field-training network in clinical-community settings. However, for PhD-level community psychologists who plan to practice in a community setting rather than on an individual basis, and who therefore need neither a license to practice psychological testing or psychotherapy nor an APA-approved clinical internship, both the term and the year-long internship experience should be replaced.

The proposed training model recommends a sequence of supervised field-training experiences that would begin in the first month of the first semester of graduate training and continue each subsequent semester throughout all four academic years. These experiences would involve a systematically increasing level of time commitment, skill acquisition and competency, functional responsibility, and trainee supervisory responsibilities. The total supervised field training would cover approximately 4,000 hours, the equivalent of two years fulltime professional experience. It should be noted that such factors as faculty time, staffing patterns, and other programmatic considerations would require some modification and reallocation of resources within the existing trainee structure before the model could be put into effect.

The selection of the specific field training sites should be congruent with the values and goals of the training program. In essence, the conceptual model endorsed by the training program should dictate the nature of the site, the skills to be acquired, the tasks to be performed, and the acceptable competency limits to be achieved. The field placement site should include, but never be restricted to, a university-based setting or community psychology center analogous to a clinical psychological services center.

An important issue frequently discussed by academic community psychologists focuses on minimum requirements or other criteria that qualify a person in the field placement setting to supervise or legitimize the training of graduate students. Must that person be a PhD? Must that person be a psychologist? Preferably not. Rather, the present model suggests that field training experiences be defined in terms of specific tasks to be performed or skills to be acquired. In this context, an appropriate field training supervisor would be any person, regardless of degree status, who is resident in the field placement and has exhibited competent performance on any given task or skill. Ideally, however, at least one person from each major field training site would be brought into the academic community as an adjunct professor.

BASIC CONCEPTUAL MODELS OF COMMUNITY PSYCHOLOGY

Seven conceptual models of community psychology were developed by subgroups of the Austin Conference: (1) the clinical-community conceptual model, (2) the clinical-community and community mental health model, (3) the community development and community systems approach, (4) the interventive-preventive conceptual model, (5) the social change model, (6) the social-ecology environmental model, and (7) the applied social-urban community psychology conceptual model.

A critical review of these models reveals that: (1) they are not yet definitive models, but rather are programmatic or conceptual focuses; and (2) considerable overlap and duplication exist in purpose, function, success criteria, entry levels, journeyman levels, academic and field site training procedures, and critical skill or task acquisition areas.

The seven conceptual models lend themselves to three kinds of task orientations for field training: Models I and II—clinical-community and community mental health—form a single cluster; Models III, IV, and V—community development and community systems, interventive-preventive, and social change—insofar as they are related to the delivery of mental health and other health services, form a second cluster; and Models V, VI, and VII—social change, social ecological environmental, and applied social-urban community—form a third cluster. In the last cluster, the turf or domain is expanded and generally applied to institutional and governmental events and functions. This division may seem overly simplistic. However, it should be noted that there is a general trend for these clusters to focus respectively on individual and small groups, agencies and organizations, and super organizations and institutions.

SEQUENCE OF COMPETENCY–BASED FIELD TRAINING EXPERIENCES

Four basic developmental or sequentially graduated competency-based field training experience levels are proposed in the present model. These training phases were born of compromise and were designed in an attempt to provide continuity across all the conceptual models and all training entry levels. The terms admittedly are not innovative. The four training phases are: (1) observer, (2) evaluator, (3) intervenor, and (4) conceptualizer-designer. These training phases are not time referenced, nor are they viewed as necessarily one-year experiences. Rather, the training-phase sequence is seen as an outgrowth of expressed behavioral competencies at each task level. In essence, the rising community psychologist would achieve a competency at a given training level, would demonstrate it, and then would move on to the next level.

Figure 1 graphically presents the integration of the conceptual models, the competency-based training levels, and the various professional and paraprofessional entry levels for the Austin field training model. For example, the PhD community psychology graduate student would be expected to master all four "competency-based training levels" for *one* conceptual model, as well as develop an awareness of the goals, purposes, and task orientations of the remaining conceptual models. An MA student would be expected to master two levels, a BA student one level, from any given conceptual model.

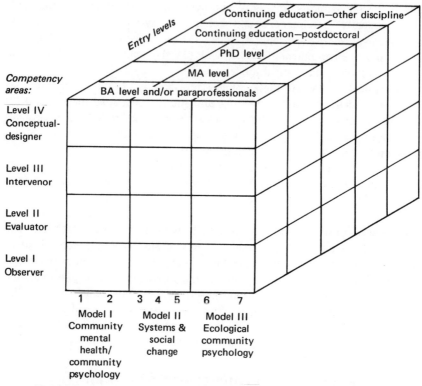

Models:

1 = Clinical community
2 = Clinical community & community mental health
3 = Community development & systems
4 = Interventive-preventive
5 = Social change
6 = Social ecology environmental
7 = Applied social & urban psychology

FIGURE 1 The integration of conceptual models, competency-based training levels, and various professional and paraprofessional entry levels for the Austin Field-Training Model.

Continuing education and postdoctoral students, however, would probably be encouraged to sample competency levels and conceptual models in accordance with their needs and professional interests.

Clearly, few community psychology training programs will have sufficient depth of resources to provide adequate learning experiences across all conceptual models, all entry levels, and all competency levels. It would appear that the hiatus in community psychology field training programs today is the result of a lack of clear focus and commitment by training programs to any given conceptual model or progressive sequence of competency-based training experiences.

Tables 1 through 4 provide a description of the goals, generic functions,

TABLE 1 Field training model, phase I: Observer[a]

Generic functions: All models	Conceptual model I: Community mental health/community psychology	Conceptual model II: Social action	Conceptual model III: Ecological-urban
1. Descriptive reporting	1. Description of client-family, client-employment, client-poor, client-agency, etc., interactions	1. Description of organizational structure of field placement (intended and operational)	1. Description of person × environment × institutional interfaces
2. Determination of relative frequencies of events	2. Description (frequencies) of behavioral baseline data	2. Identification and description of major functions, events, and activities in terms of relative frequencies	2. Recording of frequencies of diverse (classes of) individual, situational, and environmental forces upon community institutions
3. Determination of basic values, goals, assumptions, strengths	3. Description of basic values, historical perspectives, personal goals, assumptions, strengths, problem solving style of person in the context of family, peers, treatment-therapist, etc.	3. Description of agency's basic roles, stated goals, assumptions, and strengths	3. Survey of (collection of data on) community values, goals, attitudes toward the "quality of life" service providers, government responsiveness, etc.
4. Description of major conflicts, constraints, limits	4. Description of intrapsychic, interpersonal, and intraenvironmental conflicts, constraints, limits	4. Description of facilitative and obstructionistic staff behaviors, decision-making and power structures (real and paper, utilized and untapped)	4. Description of major (SES specific) conflicts, constraints, limits, core interests, and needs of the community
5. Description of known networks, interdependencies, power structures	5. Description of actual and potential networks, and interdependencies	5. Description of formal and informal agency and staff networks, interagency facilitative and obstructionistic liaisons	5. Description of information sources and impact; critical events, and environmental-personal chance events; example: marriage as an institution; what impacts on marriage; and what kinds of person × environmental events appear to support continued marriage or facilitate alternative choices
	6. Analysis of CMHC role in effectively dealing with nos. 1–5	6. Description of others' perception of agency and agency functioning: clients' view, funding agency's view, legislative, advisory board, press, community, other agencies' views	

[a]Goal: To develop a predictive understanding of human behavior from a data-based posture.

TABLE 2 Field-training model, phase II: Evaluator[a]

Generic functions: All models	Conceptual model I: Community mental health/community psychology	Conceptual model II: Social action	Conceptual model III: Ecological-urban
1. Psychometric and instrument development	1. Development of psychometric instruments designed to assess intrapsychic and interpersonal functioning of the individual in various contexts (i.e., individual and group testing, client-family behavioral assessment)	1. Development of tests and surveys that measure intraprogram functioning and relations and the community's evaluation of programs (e.g., staff views on attitudes toward agency, agency functioning, strengths and weaknesses, effectiveness, clients' views)	1. Invention of ways to assess the history; the routines and sequences of population behavior; the political relationships past and present; the norms and values of social groupings; the environment; the interaction of programs, technologies, and physical-environmental forces; and the strengths and weaknesses of the community
2. Statistical analyses techniques	2. Validation of psychometric instruments, interpretation of test results, and therapy outcomes	2. Utilization of appropriate statistical analysis techniques to evaluate agency functioning (e.g., validate organizational processes, prediction of trends to determine future needs)	2. Utilization of the appropriate statistical measures to analyze data concerned with historical context, routines and sequences, political relationships, physical-environmental forces, etc.
3. Research design	3. Development of research design methodology in order to evaluate the individual in his or her contexts, assessing the effectiveness-application-practicality of program implementation, outcome studies, differential effectiveness of services	3. Development of research designs conducive to evaluating the agency's staff effectiveness in the delivery of services	3. Development of research design to evaluate the basic aspects of the community; assessment of multiple interventions on the community
4. Preliminary bridge between data and action; development of recommendations	4. Remedial and preventive measures in dealing with the individual and the family, ongoing evaluation of interventions, referral skills, case load management, obtaining financial resources.	4. Formulation of recommendations for restructuring of organizational hierarchy and interagency functioning	4. Formulation of recommendations for restructuring the community, society, nation, in order to create a better life for all
5. Program evaluation techniques: develop management information systems; fiscal X delivery of services matrices; client data management systems; and program outcome-effectiveness systems	5. Use of computer technology and program evaluation techniques to monitor and assess psychothera-	5. Goal Attainment Scaling (Robert Sherman), Output Value Evaluation (Joseph Halpern), ATGON (automated informant oriented oriented—Nancy Wilson), manage-	5. Assessment of programs attemping to restructure life in the commun-
6. Introduction to data-based planning; survey techniques, community needs assessment, quality of life studies			
7. Epidemiological techniques			
8. Reality testing of community psychology conceptual models			
9. Active supervisory and teaching of phase I trainees (Observers)			

peutic and diagnostic services (e.g., recidivism rates, percentage of goals attained, client data management, fiscal × delivery of services, management information service)

6. Attempts to enhance the psychosocial opportunities of people (e.g., quality of life studies, family interactions survey, peer relationships survey, community needs assessment, treatment—therapy—planning, goals for groups—wards—units, individual needs assessment)

7. Evaluation of the community in terms of stress-producing stimuli that might precipitate mental illness (e.g., case histories, family studies, group characteristics, response to program surveys)

8. Development of experienced-based educational model, synthesizing with formal models presented in literature (e.g., evaluation of individual services delivery systems in terms of community effectiveness, practicum placements using previous evaluator skills in a mental health setting)

9. Arranging for students to get teaching experience and practical skills already acquired while helping others to learn

ment information system, fiscal × delivery of services, program outcome effectiveness

6. Center or organizational goals, survey techniques, agency needs (goal performance difference, semantic differential, MBO), staff versus leader, community needs assessment, quality of life

7. Identification of stimuli that could precipitate agency or organizational functioning (e.g., studying historical context)

8. Use of conceptual models to administer agency or organizational functions

9. Same as no. 9 in second column

ity to create a feeling of community independence (e.g., community form survey techniques, key informants)

6. Planning restructuring models based on analysis of community behavior in terms of routines and sequences, political and institutional relationships, topography, quality of life, community needs, etc.

7. Mapping of the problem areas in the community (e.g., skid rows, poverty areas, high crime areas, etc.) to pinpoint specific geographical areas of intervention (historical perspective, computer mapping, population characteristics, target populations)

8. Gross evaluation of the community concerned with whether or not change can be effected at the ecological-urban level; practicum placement using skills in a governmental, planning board setting

9. Same as no. 9 in second column

---

[a]Goal: Develop competency in data collection, analysis, interpretation, and data management systems designed to describe the interaction of: (1) persons, (2) organizations, (3) technologies, and (4) physical-environmental forces.

TABLE 3 Field-training model, phase III: Intervenor[a]

Generic functions: All models	Conceptual model I: Community mental health/community psychology	Conceptual model II: Social action	Conceptual model III: Ecological-urban
1. Systems theory applications	1. Application of individual remedial and preventive measures in community mental health settings (e.g., individual and group psychotherapy)	1. Implementation of recommendations following evaluations through an interagency interaction process, governmental agencies working in systems for the delivery of services	1. Change of the ecological environment via a multi-disciplinary action in order to enhance a "psychological sense of community" (develop systems for community assessment and action in preventive and interventive ways to improve quality of life)
2. Effective use of mass media (i.e., public service time, press release, etc.)	2. Increasing the community's awareness of existing mental health services (e.g., advertising centers, hotline numbers, mental health education programs)	2. Announcement of public meetings, inform public of existing services, inservice training	2. Use mass media to encourage public cooperation in ecological change; develop networks of communication for community involvement and awareness; inform and educate public and attitude change
3. Program development techniques	3. Participation in the development of a mental health facility or a historical and current analysis of an existing program, implementation of inpatient and outpatient services	3. Organizational development, improvement of delivery of services, involvement in a social action process or historical research of social action programs, analysis of program strengths and weaknesses	3. Development of specific recommendations for change (i.e., architectural structures, creating a "center of community life," multiclass of networks, and resources)
4. Grant-writing and foundation funding	4. Obtaining funds for CMH settings (new or existing programs)	4. Writing of grants with a focus on tapping governmental allocations	4. Participation in grant writing, funding, implementation, and evaluation to change the ecological environment
5. Attitude assessment and change techniques	5. Administration of attitude scales to measure mental hygiene-assessment of attitudes and development of subsequent actions in terms of results, community attitudes towards the delivery of mental health services	5. Attitude assessment skills; assessment of community attitudes towards government interventions and service organizations, keying on alternatives to existing biases and re-education	5. Assessing of community and neighborhood attitudes towards ecological change basing the direction of change on the attitudes
6. Community mobilization (group, organizational, and institutional dynamics)	6. Use of community resources through the training of indigeneous workers to function as salaried paraprofessionals and/or	6. Reorganization of staff functions, outline and implement staff training, interagency cooperation and communication, professional growth, institutional dynamics,	
7. Government, political systems, legislative change procedures			
8. Social action research			
9. Data-based decision procedures (e.g., develop DIME file for Human Services)			
10. Supervision and teaching of phase I (Observer) and phase II (Evaluator) trainees			

volunteers, localize community agencies and utilize client networks

7. The examination of past and present political networks and the education of legislators to create knowledgeable political change agents for mental health related issues (e.g., right to treatment, confidentiality, incompetence to stand trial, criminal responsibility)
8. Altering values of the community that inhibit the delivery of services and the successful treatment of the target population; erasure of false myths
9. Implementation of data-based decision rules to deliver mental health services; determining the environmental effects on client and the community resources to client
10. Same as no. 10 in first column

strive for community independence

7. Acting as a liason or lobbyist for government planners and legislators regarding social action issues; community input into social change; organize continuing education for judges, legislators, physicians, training legislators to be change agents; establish a Comprehensive Critic (1965)
8. Research that keys on the elucidation of social problems, definitions of social problems, and alternative methods of intervention
9. Use of DIME and tickler files to assess demographic characteristics and needs assessment, intervention through delivery of services
10. Same as no. 10 in first column

of the community; determination of community values; creation of methods to alter "closed community biases"

6. Organization of neighborhood power groups and political strengths into a community effort, evaluation and intervention teams, programs geared toward community needs, inject community psychology viewpoint into governmental planning; utilization of community movements in a socially acceptable manner (e.g., Black Panthers, Gay Lib, United Fund, SDS)
7. Consultation provided to politicians and legislators; change laws to provide ecological alterations; intervention into community political networks in order to develop a "community voice" in the legislative process
8. Research focusing on ecological deficiencies and problems of urban living in order to develop change strategies
9. Ecological change based on statistical analysis of urban interrelationships
10. Same as no. 10 in first column

aGoal: Action and implementation: integrate the observer and evaluator findings, determine systematic points of intervention and design social action research measures to assess the outcomes of interventions.

TABLE 4 Field-training model, phase IV: Conceptualizer-designer[a]

Generic functions: All models	Conceptual model I: Community mental health/community psychology	Conceptual model II: Social action	Conceptual model III: Ecological-urban
1. Design community research	1. Development of research that assesses individual-community needs and the delivery of services (e.g., identification of high risk populations)	1. Research assessing community needs versus demographic constellations oriented towards more effective agency intervention	1. Research assessing population X institution X ecological environment
2. Design system and institutional research	2. Testing the effectiveness of the mental health service delivery model in terms of the match between services, setting, and community needs	2. Testing the effectiveness of an agency problem-solving model; research that changes inter-organizational dynamics	2. Research testing the effectiveness of gross urban-ecological change and basic assumptions underlying the model; the consequences of legislation on ecological change
3. Integrate concept, theory, and model building with interventive action plans	3. Reconceptualization of CMH/CP model in terms of past evaluations of interventions	3. Reconceptualization of agency-interventive model based on past evaluations of community needs	3. Testing of underlying assumptions of ecological-urban model; develop interdisciplinary communications network; develop theories of how social and political organizations develop, function and dissipate (Murrell)
4. Administrate and formulate grant funding (under faculty directions)	4. Development of innovative methods for using administrative networks; the allocation of funds for maximum use of services in terms of priorities	4. Development of innovative methods of utilizing governmental and interagency networks for the procurement of grant funds	4. Develop innovative methods of utilizing neighborhood and urban political networks for procurement of funds (e.g., conduct grant writing workshops for agencies, etc.)
5. Formalize consultation skills	5. Interdisciplinary, peer, and "external critic" consultation (e.g.,	5. Institutional mangement (personnel, budget, community relations), grant writing, needs assessment, program evaluation and planning, crisis intervention	
6. Direct pyramid training structure for phase I, II, and III trainees			
7. Undertake extensive interdisciplinary training (e.g., business and institutional management, political science, law, journalism, and population geography)			
8. Prepare dissertation outline			

consulting mental health agencies using such skills as diagnostic training and behavioral assessments)

6. Same as no. 6 in first column
7. Law, medicine, sociology, business, institutional management, population geography
8. Use of dissertation to formulate a new conceptual model for mental health services delivery

6. Same as no. 6 in first column
7. Law, sociology, business administration, political science, management
8. As a weapon of social action and change, research of agency-community interaction

5. Consultation to neighborhood power groups, urban political systems, community groups dealing with CMH and social action, urban planners, water and waste control, utilities commission, transportation, etc.
6. Same as no. 6 in first column
7. Business administration, political science, architecture, transportation, urban planning, environmental control, geography, history, etc.
8. Dissertation as a historical analysis of the pathological and/or constructive developments of communities in order to determine the flow of ecological-urban change

[a]Goal: Journeyman functioning level; to serve as the primary source of conceptual development, model building, interdisciplinary consulting; and training of other trainees.

and sample task orientations and skills for each major community psychology conceptual model and each of the four competency-based training levels. The examples are offered to provide understanding of the Austin field training model, not as rigid constrictors to program planning and curriculum development.

Several recommendations of an ancillary or corollary nature were made at the Austin Conference:

1. *Written contracts.* The consensus of the Austin conferees was that there is need to have clear, written contracts to be negotiated by the faculty supervisor, the placement supervisor, and the student observer, evaluator, or intervenor. The contract should state the functions, time commitments, time constraints, task roles, functions to be performed, and supervisory commitments on the part of faculty, site supervisors, and practicum students. It was recommended that the faculty rank field placements and task roles in terms of the relative complexity of the placement.
2. *Reciprocity.* It was recommended that the notion of reciprocity be recognized in the relationship between academic and field placement settings. Issues related to what the field training site can realistically expect to get out of placements and training functions, as well as the university's expectancies, should be open and above board.
3. *Collegial versus student-faculty relationships.* The remaining three recommendations focused on the nature of the student-faculty relationships in relation to the field training experiences. Austin conferees recommended the endorsement of a collegial relationship.
4. *Facilitative versus obstructionist training interactions.* The group requested that an effort be made to utilize obstacles and failure experiences in field training as opportunities for learning and concept clarification.
5. *Pyramid supervisory trainee structure.* The final recommendation was that a pyramid-like supervisory and training structure be employed in a way that students in community psychology training would all be actively involved in the teaching of less experienced trainees. This recommendation has been implemented in the development of this recommended field training model.

REFERENCE NOTES

1. Danish, S. A. *Developing paraprofessional manpower: Implications for training in community psychology.* Paper presented at the annual convention of the American Psychological Association, Chicago, 1975.
2. Aponte, J. A. *Training programs and internship settings in community psychology.* Paper presented at the National Training Conference in Community Psychology, Austin, Tex., April 1975.

3. Zolik, E., Sirbu, W., & Hopkinson, D. *Graduate student perspectives on training in community mental health-community psychology.* Paper presented at the National Training Conference in Community Psychology, Austin, Tex., April 1975.

REFERENCE

Kelly, J. G. Antidotes for arrogance: Training for community psychology. *American Psychologist*, 1970, *25*(6), 524–531.

19 From Noah to Babel

Relationships Between Conceptions, Values, Analysis Levels, and Social Intervention Strategies

Julian Rappaport

And the Lord saw that the wickedness of man was great in the earth, and that every imagination of the thoughts of his heart was only evil continually (Genesis 6:5).

And for three days and three nights the Austin Conference convened with all manner of beast (both clean and unclean). And they went forth from the conference that they may swarm in the earth, and be fruitful and multiply upon the earth (Austin 1:1).

And they said: "Come, let us build us a city, and a tower, with its top in heaven, and let us make us a name; lest we be scattered upon the face of the whole earth" (Genesis 11:4).

And the Lord said: ". . . and now nothing will be withholden from them that they propose to do. Come, let us go down, and there confound their language, that they may not understand one another's speech" (Genesis 11:7).

And were God willing they would now build the tower at Austin; but even as the descendants of Noah they speak in many languages (Austin 1:2).

In Genesis, so the story goes, after Noah and his sons left the ark the generations that followed wanted to build a city with a tower to heaven. But God refused to allow them to have heaven on earth, and so caused them to speak different languages and to be unable to communicate and to understand one another's directions. Despite the noble efforts of over 80 psychologists who emerged from the Ark of Austin, the tower to heaven is no more likely to be built today than it was at Babel. In the 10 years between Swampscott and Austin, community psychology may have discovered that humans must settle for something less than the heavenly city on earth (cf. Sarason, 1975). While people of religion have known this, people of science often disregard it.

This paper was prepared while the author was supported by a Sabbatical Award from the James McKeen Cattell Fund, to whom appreciation is extended.

In the words of Rene Dubos (1959):

The golden age means different things to different men, but the very belief in its existance implies the conviction that perfect health and happiness are birthrights of men. Yet, in reality, complete freedom from disease and from struggle is almost incompatible with the process of living. (p.13)

At Austin many different languages were spoken. Early in the conference multiple "models" were acknowledged, and it was deemed most productive to divide into smaller subgroups where those speaking the language of each model could best communicate. The models are those presented in other sections of this volume. One observer, Emory Cowen, toward the end of the conference noted that rather than distinct models, the participants might find that they were talking about a kind of continuum, and that it would be helpful to look at "representative points or slices" along it. One of the things that became clear was that the languages along the continuum are not separated by data so much as by different aims for our discipline. The values and goals of one community psychologist are not necessarily those of another, and to the extent that we seek to build that tower to heaven, where we presume that these values and goals will all blend into a happy perfection, we will be confounded, be it by nature or by divine plan. To the extent that we are willing to recognize that there are going to be many different brands of community psychology, each with its own values and goals, we may begin to understand not how to get to heaven, but that we require different levels of analysis, conceptions, strategies, and tactics, depending on our particular values and goals. In this sense community psychology, as well as perhaps all of social science, requires that social values not be hidden by the language of social science and that we actively pursue clarification of value differences, not as truths so much as what they really are: different beliefs about the kind of society toward which we wish to work.

When we hide behind the terminology and euphemisms of social science, we often sound as if we all speak a common tongue in which the logic of experimental design and empirical tests determine our actions. However, when we stop and look at ourselves nondefensively, we will see that most of our differences are really matters of faith. That means faith quite literally in the religious sense, despite the discomfort this may arouse among a group of scientists. When we choose a model or a paradigm to guide our work, we select it on the basis of faith that it will solve the puzzles we as community psychologists have selected as worthy of study. As Kuhn (1970) has made clear, paradigms allow some problems as legitimate for study and others as outside of their scope. It is reasonable to contend that, at least in the social sciences, both our selected problem areas and our faith in our different paradigms reflect our social values, rather than reflecting our scientific differences.

Much of community psychology, because of our desire to extend it to problem areas outside the historical scope of our traditions, has overstepped the bounds of psychological paradigms. By bringing this about, we have brought on ourselves a crisis in the Kuhnian sense of the term. The traditional paradigms of our discipline are not relevant to many of the puzzles we now seek to solve. While the older paradigms are partly workable for some of our purposes, they are inadequate for others, and we are led to a frantic search for new ones. Although logically our conceptions should lead to our actions, a good deal of the search is guided by our actions, which help us think about what we have already done and, in turn, lead to new conceptions. What guides much of this activity, but are often either implicit or forgotten in the quest to appear "scientific," are our values and goals. Table 1 is an attempt to clarify the often confusing relationships between values, level of analysis, conceptions, and actions.

To enhance an understanding of Table 1, several orienting ideas need to be introduced. Reiff has often suggested that society can be conceptualized in terms of multiple levels of organization (cf. Reiff, 1971; Seidman & Rappaport, 1974). In Table 1, four such levels are presented: the individual, the small group, the organization, and the institution.[1] Depending on an interventionist's values and goals, a different level of analysis will be required for the selection of conceptions to guide the strategies and tactics of social intervention. Some conceptions are going to be appropriate for one level and others are not. Only from the study of an appropriate level can we arrive at appropriate conceptions and, ultimately, appropriate strategies and tactics for action. The appropriate conceptions at one level are not necessarily the same as those at other levels. In short, things may not work the same at differing levels of society. Individuals function by principles different from those governing organizations, and so on.

Please note that in the preceding remarks the word *appropriate* was used. What makes a given level of analysis appropriate? At least in part it depends on the values and goals of the interventionist. Differing value/goals require differing analysis levels, and only then can conceptions, strategies, and tactics be selected. If one hides values and goals behind a mask of scientific terminology, confusion will result. A failure to recognize this leads to what Watzlawick, Weakland, and Fisch (1974) have termed an *error of logical typing*. By this they mean that so long as one tries to create change by means of solutions based on a level of analysis inappropriate to one's goals, genuine change cannot be accomplished. For example, to the extent that problems of severe "mental illness" are seen to be a function of social labeling and a social policy of isolation, efforts aimed only at changing identified patients will necessarily lead to what Watzlawick et al. (1974) term *first order change*. Genuine or second order change requires questioning the institutions of

---

[1] The distinction between organizations (specific facilities, usually but not necessarily contained within walls, e.g., a particular school) and institutions (sets of social values, goals, and abstractions that tell organizations how to function, e.g., the institution of public education) is crucial (see Rappaport, 1977).

TABLE 1 Relationships between value/goals, level of analysis, conceptions, and strategies and tactics of social intervention[a]

Value/goals	Level of Analysis[b]	Conceptions[b]	Strategies and tactics[c, d]
1. Social problems are a function of the inability of some people or even an entire subculture to fit into the structures of society, or to be comfortable being different. People have deficits. The place of applied behavioral science is to help as many people as possible adjust to the goals and norms of the small groups and organizations of which they are a part. The values of the institutions of society are basically benign, and the organizations developed to accomplish these values do as good a job as one can expect, given human fallibility. If an individual differs from society, the problem is to decrease discomfort to self and others by changing the person or helping him or her live with the difference in a nondestructive way.	*Individual level* of analysis is emphasized because understanding a human being as a person is the key to changing her or him to be more competent, adaptive, to fit in and be comfortable with himself or herself and the available structures of society.	Various individual conceptions ranging from behavioral through psychodynamic. Depending on the specific problem, this level of analysis may require, in Sabin's (1970) terms, helping the person find his or her place in the self-maintenance, transcendental, or normative ecology. Social change is implied to be a summation of individual changes.	Person-centered interventions. Community mental health oriented therapies such as brief treatment. Consultation to socialization agents. Crisis intervention. Training of new person power. Also includes employment training techniques for individuals as well as other educational programs for children and for parents. The specific content varies with the specific conception of individual behavior.
2. Social problems are created by interpersonal difficulties within primary groups such as the family, peer, and work groups. Deficits in the group rather than the individual members are emphasized. Sometimes the problem is an inability of	*Small group level* of analysis emphasized. Because the problems lie in interpersonal communication and conflict, understanding the dynamics of interpersonal relations and small group interaction is stressed.	Two primary sources of conceptions are the group dynamics literature of social psychology and the group and family treatment literature derived from clinical psychology. Ecological principles can be used to understand and adjust the functioning of the group.	Family therapy, interpersonal communications training, sensitivity groups, group therapy. May include retraining agents of socialization to communicate more effectively with themselves and with the target people.

people in different groups to communicate with each other, for example, policemen and members of a given community. When these groups are not functioning well internally or are in conflict with other groups, they not only have a negative impact on individual members, but also inhibit the ability of organizations to accomplish the necessary tasks of administering society's institutional values and goals.			
3. Social problems are created by the organizations of society that fail to implement as well as they might the desirable values and goals of our social institutions. Concrete organizations are imperfectly structured and administered such that they often fail to accomplish the values and goals of socialization as stipulated by work, education, health, and welfare institutions. The aim remains to enhance the likelihood that organizations will help individuals fit into society; but the problems are in the organizations themselves, rather than in the person. Less obvious emphasis on weakness and deficits of targets, but often implied.	*Organizational level* of analysis. Because a great deal of behavior is under the control of the social structures of organizations these structures, and techniques for changing them, are the key to solution of social problems.	Systems-centered conceptions from public health, social, and organizational psychology. May include conceptions of deviant subcultures and norms. Power and alienation are psychological rather than political variables. Principles of social systems analysis, ecological and environmental psychology applied to adjust the functioning of the organization.	Public health and organization development strategies. Systems-centered consultation. Development of new structures and communication channels and styles within existing organizations through use of various organization development techniques. Includes programs of early identification of "high risk" in various locations such as schools, the armed services, or in the general mental health system. The strategy of early identification may be combined with secondary prevention, which usually involves such tactics as development and introduction of new programs, including any of the person or small group level strategies identified above.
4. Social problems are created by our institutions rather than by persons or by our organizations. While there are many problems in organizations that may be solved by specific changes,	*Institutional and community level* of analysis is emphasized because the institutions of society support and determine relationships with- in and between organizations and	Systems-centered conceptions from various social sciences. Power is a political-economic as well as a psychological variable. Principles of social action, social policy, and com-	Two major classes of social intervention are the community organization- social advocacy model and the parallel institutions or creation of settings model. Tactics emphasize power and

TABLE 1 (*continued*) Relationships between value/goals, level of analysis, conceptions, and strategies and tactics of social intervention[a]

Value/Goals	Level of Analysis[b]	Conceptions[b]	Strategies and tactics[c, d]
the real key to social change is in the attitudes, values, goals, and political-economic ideology and social policy of which the institutions themselves are composed and on which the organizations are based. The distribution of power (political as well as psychological) among various communities is an important variable. Values supportive of diversity and the need for alternative pathways to success. Explicit emphasis on strengths of target people, cultural relativity, and the need for resources.	communities. These relationships limit the alternatives and the resources available to members and, therefore, hold the key to social change.	munity organization are emphasized. Because many people require new alternatives, ecological principles applied to this value system and level of analysis lead to a search for new environmental alternatives.	control of disenfranchised groups either within existing organizations or in newly created organizations. In either case, the aim is to build organizations based on institutional assumptions different from those currently dominant in society. Choice between changing existing or creating new settings is a function of the specifics of the situation, including the resources of the particular group and the belief that existing structures ultimately will or will not yield power and control. May also use any of the strategies of change at other levels of analysis as well as any available research methods for data collection leading to social policy recommendations.

[a] Adapted from Rappaport (1977). The social intervention strategies tabled here all assume a seeking rather than waiting mode and an emphasis on change through direct action. Ultimately, each requires research and evaluation, although this is not always emphasized by adherents.

[b] The level of analysis may be cumulative as one goes down the column. Willingness to engage in strategies at the institutional and community level does not necessarily preclude a willingness to engage in any others at other levels of analysis. Often levels and strategies are combined in practice.

[c] Examples presented include some of the major classes of strategies and tactics in which psychologists engage today. Other specific intervention forms are also logically possible. For example, urban planning programs of various kinds may be implemented at the organizational, institutional, or community level, the specifics of which will vary with the values of the planner as well as the perspective of the intervention as based on a strengths or a weaknesses view of community development.

[d] Public education and social policy recommendations, in various forms, aimed at spreading the values that underlie a particular strategy so as to make the tactics themselves more acceptable, is a technique to which most change agents ascribe, and appears to be nonspecific with regard to values or level of analysis.

society, or the very rules by which the mental health system operates, that is, the process of social labeling and isolation.

Another example can be found in many preschool education programs. To the extent that the children of the poor are forced to contend with an educational institution that ignores their culture, no amount of tutoring to repair their supposed individual "cognitive deficits" will be able to solve the social problem of educational failure. Tutoring is an intervention based on the study of individuals. If the aim of community psychology is to effect change in the institutions of society, conceptions, strategies, and tactics based on appropriate institutional assessment are required. These arguments have been pursued in detail elsewhere (Rappaport, 1977). The point here is that the only way one can know if one's level of analysis is appropriate is to step back and examine the values and goals that underlie one's efforts.

Each of the four sections of Table 1 details one set of value/goals and the analysis level, conceptions, strategies, and tactics that follow from each. One intention in presenting this summary is to encourage would-be interventionists to ask themselves which set of values they ascribe to before they become involved in their next community psychology project and to consider the possibility that their strategies and tactics should be consistent with their values.

The first section of the table presents, under the column *Value/goals*, a set of assumptions about society. In brief, these assumptions suggest that the values and goals of our current social institutions are basically benign, and that the problem for applied behavioral science is to help as many people as possible adjust to the norms of the small groups and organizations of which they are a part. An individual level of analysis is emphasized because that is the key to changing a person to be more "competent" or "adaptive" and to "fit in." Various individual conceptions of human behavior, ranging from behavioral through psychodynamic, are appropriate to this level of analysis, which views social change as a summation of individual changes. The strategies and tactics of person-centered interventions that follow from these value/goals include community mental health oriented therapies, consultation to the agents of socialization, crisis intervention, and so on. Exact content of the "treatments" varies with the specific conception of human behavior, but all are focused on changing people to fit into available environments.

The second section has a different emphasis because it has different value/goals. It is suggested that social problems are the result of interpersonal difficulties within primary groups, including family, peers, and work groups. Deficits in the group, rather than in its individual members, are emphasized. Communication skills are often implicated as problematic. Inability to communicate is said to adversely affect not only individuals but also the ability of organizations to accomplish the necessary tasks of administering society's institutional values and goals. A small-group level of analysis follows from this view of society. Because problems lie in interpersonal communication and conflict, the dynamics of interpersonal relations are stressed. Conceptually, one can draw from the group dynamics literature of social and clinical psychology. The aim is to adjust the functioning of the group to help its members get along better with one another and to fit into societal expectations. Family therapy, group therapy, interpersonal communications training, sensitivity groups, and consultation to the agents of socialization that enable them to communicate more effectively with themselves and the target people, are common strategies and tactics of such intervention.

The table's third section lists under the column *Value/goals* a somewhat different set of assumptions about society. Basically, it says that social problems are a function of the organizations of society that fail to implement, as well as they might, the desirable goals and values of our social institutions. Concrete organizations are imperfectly structured so that they often fail to accomplish the socialization tasks as stipulated by work, education, health, and welfare institutions. From this viewpoint the goals of community psychology are to enhance the likelihood that organizations will help individuals fit into society; and the problems are seen to be in the organizations themselves rather than in the person or the small group. This belief leads to a study of organizations rather than to a study of individuals or small groups as detailed in the first two sections of the table; it also leads to different concepts as well as different strategies and tactics of social intervention (for example, those who assist the agents of socialization, rather than the individual people who have problems in living). Organization development as well as other strategies of intervention are noted in the table.

To the extent that one ascribes to these beliefs but limits one's activities to a level of study and set of conceptions and strategies derived only from individual and small group psychology, one will commit an error of logical typing and find that genuine change as defined by one's own value/goals is impossible to attain. It is well known that organizations will not be changed by changing individual people within them (Reppucci, 1973; Walton, 1972); rather, the basic organizational processes must be changed. Please note that the error of logical typing, or selection of an inappropriate level of analysis, is a function of the value/goals one ascribes to. If one really believes that individual deficits are the cause of social problems, one properly seeks to ameliorate them. In that case conceptions and intervention strategies based on an individual psychology are called for. However, it is incumbent upon the community psychologist to tell the consumer what his or her values are. Indeed, it may be unethical to tell them you are working for social change when in fact you really intend to change them.

An organizational level of analysis is also quite different from the type described in the fourth section of the table. It is inadequate if one's value/goals suggest that social problems are created by our institutions rather than by persons or organizations. If one believes that the real key to social change lies in the values, goals, political-economic idiology, and social policy of which the institutions themselves are composed and of which organizations are but a specific manifestation, a different set of conceptions is necessary. If one's values suggest that a redistribution of power (both political and psychological) and of money and other resources is important for genuine social change; and if one believes in values supportive of diversity and alternative pathways to success based on autonomy, respect for differences among people, strengths, cultural relativity, and the right to resources; then to limit interventions to those enhancing the ability of organizations, small groups, or individuals to socialize others and to distribute resources on the basis of conformity to a single standard of "competence" would be to commit an error of logical typing—by the criteria of one's own value system.

The difference between an organizational and an institutional level of analysis was best described in cybernetic terms by Gregory Bateson (1972), using the commonly known example of a thermostat. A thermostat sets the temperature range within which a heating system fluctuates. Within the limits of the setting the heat will fluctuate around a given level. In a social system the "rules of the game," those social institutions that determine the bias of the system, are the thermostat. To the extent that these rules are unquestioned, there are clear limits to the kind of social change possible. It is only when one is willing to step outside the system and consider resetting the social thermostat that the possibility for change is realized. To the extent, then, that one's value/goals require institutional rather than individual, small group, or organizational change, different conceptions, strategies, and tactics must be considered. In the examples in Table 1, strategies and tactics of community organization-social advocacy and the creation of autonomous settings are included. These are strategies new to psychology. They require different sets of conceptions and a search for new paradigms.

At the bottom of Table 1 are several footnotes, the most important of which says that the level of analysis may be cumulative as one goes down the column. Willingness to engage in strategies at the institutional and community level does not necessarily preclude a willingness to engage in any others. Often levels and strategies are combined in practice. It should be emphasized that multiple levels of study and intervention are desirable. What we must keep in mind, however, is that unless each of us is willing to openly state our basic value/goals to ourselves, our professional colleagues, and our colleagues in the communities we serve, we will surely build a tower of Babel. We must recognize that there is no single community psychology, and that the basic distinctions between the variants may turn out to be more a matter of social values than of science.

REFERENCES

Bateson, G. *Steps to an ecology of the mind.* New York: Ballantine, 1972.

Dubos, R. *Mirage of health: Utopias, progress and biological change.* Garden City: Doubleday, 1959.

Kuhn, T. S. *The structure of scientific revolutions* (2nd ed.). Chicago: University of Chicago Press, 1970.

Rappaport, J. *Community Psychology: values, research, and action.* New York: Holt, 1977.

Reiff, R. R. From Swampscott to swamp. *Division of Community Psychology Newsletter,* 1971, *4,* 1–3.

Reppucci, N. D. The social psychology of institutional change: General principles for intervention. *American Journal of Community Psychology,* 1973, *1,* 330–341.

Sarason, S. B. Psychology "To the Finland station" in "The heavenly city of the eighteenth century philosophers." *American Psychology,* 1975, *30,* 1072–1080.

Sarbin, T. R. A role theory perspective for community psychology: The structure of social identity. In D. Adelson & B. L. Kalis (Eds.), *Community psychology and mental health: Perspectives and challenges.* Scranton, Pa.: Chandler, 1970.

Seidman, E., & Rappaport, J. The educational pyramid: A paradigm for training, research, and manpower utilization in community psychology. *American Journal of Community Psychology,* 1974, *2,* 119–130.

Walton, R. E. Frontiers beckoning the organizational psychologist. *Journal of Applied Behavioral Science,* 1972, *8,* 601–629.

Watzlawick, P., Weakland, J. H., & Fisch, R. *Change: Principles of problem formation and problem resolution.* New York: Norton, 1974.

20 Research, Knowledge, and Professional Growth

Edison J. Trickett and Nancy Meyer Lustman

As any field of inquiry and action evolves, it undertakes certain steps to clarify its progress and problems, consolidate its gains, and conceptualize its future. The Austin Conference was designed to serve this developmental goal in the area of community psychology, for there had been changes in both focus and clarity in the 10 years since the first conference at Swampscott. This chapter delineates issues of knowledge and research relevant to various areas of community psychology that surfaced at Austin. In relation to the question, what do we need to know and how might we learn about it, two complementary questions emerged: (1) What are some of the substantive areas of research and knowledge in community psychology? (2) What domains of research inform community psychologists about issues facing community psychology as a field?

RESEARCH ACTIVITIES AND KNOWLEDGE BASE

As Rappaport noted in his biblical metaphor, when the generations that followed Noah and sons wanted to build a tower to heaven, their problems transcended the inability to speak in a common language. Beyond the hope and the vision symbolized in the idea of a tower, a series of substantive questions remained, regardless of one's particular "tongue." How do you build a tower? What do you need to know about towers and what do you need to believe about heaven in order to proceed? What conceptions and actions are necessary to translate beautiful visions into deeds that work? Questions such as these—questions of method, design, appropriate knowledge, conceptual level of analysis, and epistemology—were pivotal in the small group meetings, improvised conversations, and invited addresses in Austin.

The diversity of hopes, cares, values, and aspirations expressed by conference participants dashed any possibility for an integrated synthesis of research strategies and knowledge base in community psychology. Rather, various metaphors were invoked as useful orienting stances, each with its own set of

An earlier draft of this chapter was presented at a symposium entitled "A Report on the Austin Conference: The Future of Community Psychology," American Psychological Association annual convention, Chicago, Illinois, September 1, 1975.

The authors wish to thank N. Dickon Reppucci for his helpful comments on this chapter.

heuristic implications for the substance, process, and methods of research. At one end of the spectrum, individually oriented clinical psychologists discussed strategies for stretching their understanding of individuals to include the relationship of persons to social settings. From this perspective the development of knowledge in several areas seemed timely. The question of how socializing institutions might be structured if based on implications of research in child development provided one example; how personal coping styles are expressed in natural environments, another. Evolving alternative models of psychological consultation and the use of group dynamics as intervention strategies also flowed from this predominantly clinical orientation. At a point near the other end of the spectrum, ecologically oriented psychologists framed a declaration of interdependence, emphasizing the development of research that would clarify the structure and function of institutions and neighborhoods. Alternative definitions of the term *community* and the psychosocial implications of social policies augmented this ecological orientation.

Beneath these differing metaphors, however, were some general ideas and stances about the process and content of research in community psychology. Three elements may serve as unifying themes: the dual substantive focus of understanding and intervening in naturally occurring social situations, institutions, and communities; the commitment to naturalistic research; and the concern about the nature of the research relationship with the locale where it occurs or the group it involves.

Substantive Research Orientation

The coequal status of seeking knowledge for understanding and using knowledge for effective action dominated the discussion on the substance of research in community psychology. The specific substantive emphases were as diverse as the backgrounds and professional roles of conference participants—backgrounds ranging from clinical and social psychology to epidemiology and public health, roles ranging from student and university faculty to agency supervisor and program developer. Therefore, rather than an outline of these many areas, a summary follows of the orientations and of select examples from the discussions. (See Cowen, 1973, and Zax & Specter, 1974, for more elaborate summaries of research in community psychology.)

Knowledge for understanding. A general orientation of the Austin conference that has specific research implications was promoting the positive development of individuals (see Sanford, 1972). In moving to what James Kelly has called a "psychology of healthiness," the life processes of communities, the enriching of the socialization institutions for children and youth, and the capability of settings and neighborhoods to recruit and develop resources all become research orientation, which provides an integrative force among several areas of psychology (for example, developmental, organizational, and clinical). They also form a working agenda for reaching out to other disciplines (such as urban planning, public health) concerned with the growth and quality of community life. The current lack of knowledge in these areas highlighted the importance of developing conceptual bases as a central intellectual agenda for community psychologists.

The multiple meanings of the term *human ecology* provided much of the substance of this general orientation. Conceptual stances and empirical research in groups and systems (e.g., Argyris, 1970), social ecology (Moos, 1974), the ecological analogy (e.g., Kelly, 1967; Trickett, Kelly, & Todd, 1972), and ecological psychology (e.g., Barker, 1968) were cited as helpful beginnings. In addition, an emphasis on individuals in settings united the psychology of individuals with the dynamics of social systems. This, in turn, yielded a concern with how people cope with different kinds of environments and how they are differentially affected by participation in social systems.

Yet the knowledge-relevant areas extended far beyond this kind of research and thinking. One particularly salient subset of the social system frame of reference, for example, involved the systematic analysis of social policies, especially in the broad area of human services. The psychological, social, and economic implications of such policies as deinstitutionalization of mental patients served as examples of areas in which community psychologists should study and then act. Racism, sexism, and the study of power emerged as important areas for understanding as well as change among conference participants. This led more immediately and forcefully into the second primary focus of research: intervention and social action for change.

Knowledge for action. In discussions of knowledge relevant to intervention activities or social change roles, the terms themselves were broadly defined to include such diverse activities as the training of nonprofessionals for helping roles, the development of new services for select populations, and community organization and advocacy approaches. Crosscutting many of the specific approaches was the concept of evaluation (for example, Suchman, 1967; Weiss, 1972). The development of evaluation skills and methodology was broadly supported as having both scientific and political importance.

In addition to evaluation, more theoretical propositions about the nature of change and the development of models of intervention were stressed. Statements of value and political ideology tied many participants to propositions about change, while various existing research programs highlighted propositions about models of intervention. Mental health consultation, in socialization settings or with various groups (such as police), was described as extending a predominantly clinical role to include social system implications (e.g., Mannino, Maclennen, & Shore, 1975). Early intervention programs for children (e.g., Zax & Cowen, 1967) provided models for preventing more serious psychological maladaptation in later years. Research in organizational development (e.g., Schmuck & Miles, 1971) and systems theory-oriented interventions added to the multiple models of change discussed in Austin.

Methods Befitting the Substance

The varied content discussed by participants underscored the importance of "taking psychology out of the laboratory" and orienting research toward a more naturalistic approach. The tone of this orientation toward psychological research was by no means new. Lightner Witmer, whose psychoeducational clinic began over 75 years ago in Philadelphia and foreshadowed with greater specificity the ideology and strategies of the recent Community Mental Health Movement, wrote in 1906 (in Levine & Levine, 1970):

> Although clinical psychology is closely related to medicine, it is quite closely related to sociology and pedagogy. The school room, the Juvenile Court, and the streets are a larger laboratory of psychology. An abundance of material for scientific study fails to be utilized because the interests of psychologists are elsewhere engaged, and those in constant touch with the actual phenomena do not possess the training necessary to make their experiences and observations of scientific value.

In reaffirming the timeliness of these words, conference participants accepted the yet unfulfilled challenge to work toward developing and refining methodologies that facilitate the conceptualization, execution, and interpretation of data gathered in naturally occurring situations. The scope of naturalistic research was both qualitative and quantitative, encompassing a broad range of methodologies and spanning many epistemological traditions (e.g., Becker & Geer, 1960; Campbell & Stanley, 1963). Thus, the understanding of multivariate analysis coexisted with the importance of developing the interviewing skills of a Studs Terkel. Issues of sampling and questionnaire development in survey research found their qualitative counterpart in discussions of the internal logic of descriptive case studies. The search for naturally occurring "real life" experiments was mentioned as an underutilized approach to hypothesis testing in nonlaboratory situations, while researching the social history of programs or places provided a means for gathering data on the creation of settings in general (Sarason, 1972).

Both the problem-centered focus and the diverse roles of psychologists attending the conference led to an examination of the methods of disciplines other than psychology. From sociology, for example, both the qualitative method of participant observation and the statistical techniques of regression, cross-lag correlation, and the use of panel data to make causal inferences were considered promising (Borgatta & Bohrnstedt, 1970). From journalism, the validation and inference process of investigative reporting were discussed.

In sum, the conference emphasized the importance of attending to issues of method in naturalistic research, in both qualitative and quantitative domains. The traditional strength of psychology in the areas of design and measurement were seen as providing a solid foundation for enriching the emerging research methods in community psychology.

The Research Relationship

Mediating the issues of substance and method is the research process itself, which determines how something is carried out and what values it embodies. Many Austin participants were vocal in their worry about how research has been implemented in various communities. If the naturalistic research stance is taken seriously, they suggested, then attention must be given to the process by which such research is developed and executed. The search for alternative forms for the research relationship raised many questions. For example, what plausible roles can citizens play not only in doing research but also in defining the research problem? What kind of reciprocal relationships might universities develop with their communities? As one conference participant put it, "Are there any community training programs where local citizens help determine the curriculum?" Is it possible to develop collaborative research relationships that endure, that are perceived by both scholar and citizen as worthwhile, and that, over time, generate trust and support rather than suspicion and antagonism? Can we develop antidotes to the implications of Tom Cottle's article "Show me a scientist who's helped poor folks and I'll kiss her hand" (Cottle, 1974)?

A number of participants shared the belief that the very act of community research is a direct and visible intervention that can yield enduring effects not only on the validity of the data gathered, but also on the willingness of both researcher and community to meet again over a real problem. Several areas of the community research process were specified as deserving immediate and sustained attention. These included (a) the process by which the goals of research are defined, (b) the nature of the accountability of the research to the various groups involved, and (c) the process for defining issues of power and decision making at various stages of the research. While local circumstances would affect the resolution of these areas in their specifics, the conference did underscore the importance of viewing research itself as an intervention involving all the considerations of ethics, values, and priorities with which more direct action-oriented interventions must cope.

Various models were cited as current efforts for coping with these issues. From the community perspective, such structures as citizen review boards were seen as protective responses to past experience in the research process. From the university perspective, the current legal and ethical debate over the use of human subjects in research reinforced the importance of these issues.

Collaborative efforts between university personnel and citizens were also cited as models for working with citizens, not only in decision making about whether or not research should proceed, but also in what should be studied. To cite one example: Citizens in a town in the Northeast developed—in collaboration with academicians—an information-gathering action research project that gave them information about community opinion on an important community issue. Community residents were involved in selection of citizen-interviewers, decisions about the content of the interview, the process for contacting respondents, and the dissemination of results.

Regardless of whether this concern about the implications of the conduct of research took the form of control mechanisms or the articulation of various models for collaborating with citizens, it was agreed that a more reciprocal and collaborative *process* was one antidote to the stereotype of research as an aloof, if not insidious, activity, far removed from the everyday cares of citizens, and done to, rather than with, fellow human beings.

THE EVOLUTION OF COMMUNITY PSYCHOLOGY AS A FIELD

The varied approaches at Austin to the substance of research and the research relationship with citizens evoked many discussions about the evolution of the field in general—what Jack Chinsky calls "the community psychology of community psychology." That the field has been growing is certain: During the past decade Division 27 has been added to the APA and two community psychology journals have been started. While an assessment of the issues accompanying this evolution is beyond the scope of this chapter, two recurring themes at Austin affirm the need to study the growth of community psychology: (1) the issues of professional identity raised when new social roles are emerging and old roles are shifting, and (2) the issues of collaboration with other disciplines.

A review of the natural history of one profession can serve as a general background to both these issues, especially if one notes the social conditions affecting its creation and the developmental stages it passed through (see Wilensky, 1964, for a more general statement). The field of social work, described in detail in the Levines' book, *A Social History of the Helping Professions* (Levine & Levine, 1970), provides a provocative and informative source.

The origins of the field are found in the settlement house movement at the end of the last century. The settlement houses originally were founded as a means of coping with social disorganization induced by rapid industrialization, urbanization, and immigration after the Civil War. University affiliated social scientists, both men and women, felt the need to become involved with the problems of the "real world"—to make themselves useful. Innovative approaches such as school lunch programs, the concept of the visiting teacher and the school nurse, and college extension programs evolved as individuals, living in the community, improvised their way through periods of social turmoil to provide new services embodying new concepts for developing neighborhoods. The ethic was one of mutual assistance and self-help, of concern and caring between people, and an appreciation of the naturally occurring systems of personal support, which neighbor provides neighbor and which exist independent of professional helpers. "It is terrible," said Stanton Coit in 1891, "when men draw together only in suffering; whereas those who have laughed and thought together, and joined in ideal aims, can so enter into one another's sorrow as to steal much of its bitterness away" (Levine & Levine, 1970).

Over time, the settlement house took hold as a community institution and with this change came an increased thrust toward professionalism on the part of those involved in running these establishments. By the 1920s forces within the field were pushing toward the development of specified training curricula, standards of professional accountability, and a power of selection into the fields that rested with the faculties of professional schools. The concept of the original settlement house worker who had lived in and contributed to the local neighborhood had evolved into one emphasizing training in professional schools with scientific expertise in casework.

This example is not intended to overgeneralize the specifics of the rise of the profession of social work, though some parallels may seem plausible. And if it is seen as a cautionary tale about the constraints of professionalization, let the caution be mild. The central point is to underscore the dual propositions that new areas of endeavor—even if they do not reach the status of professions—must change over time, and that, as they change, they must go through stages where choice points exist to help determine the future of the field. Two such issues emerged at the Austin Conference as a direct result of the growth of the field of community psychology.

Professional Identity and Changing Social Roles

During the past 15 years an increasing number of psychologists have, through their professional activities, taken on new tasks, attempted to develop new roles, and experienced the need to gain new competencies. In particular, many psychologists in Austin have been involved in the effort to create new forms of professional activity. Anecdotes of frustrations and successes in attempting to implement new ideas were abundant and revolved primarily around two related questions: How might existing social roles, predominantly clinical, be redefined to increase the probability of social systems impact? And how can new social roles for community psychologists be created?

The questions about building on existing social roles came primarily from psychologists with clinical backgrounds who were functioning in clinical settings. Psychological consultation served as one important aspect of the discussions, and various examples were offered to demonstrate the potential for community-oriented clinical psychologists in this role. One psychologist, for example, described how an initial consultative relationship involving psychological assessment of problem adolescents led over time to programs of inservice training, increased staffing for mental health-related areas, and the creation in town of a youth center.

Some psychologists, on the other hand, expressed concern about how to create roles that do not currently exist, or that exist only in select places. Program evaluation was cited as an area in which psychologists have specific expertise to contribute, and agencies or institutions need valid data to improve their functioning with clients. Still, many agencies were perceived as having neither the resources nor the will to make a commitment to program evaluation. How might such allegiances be formed? Can one "prepare the environment" for a role that does not currently exist? These substantive intellectual issues go hand in hand with the development of community psychology as a field.

Underlying both these questions was the issue of the professional identify of the community psychologist. As roles emerge and gain clarity, the task of defining and redefining areas of competence continues. The diversity of opinions about the specific nature of certain roles did not alter the shared perception that the ongoing task of defining one's professional identity has profound implications for the future of the field. The plea was not for premature closure on a still-expanding area; rather, it was for a self-consciousness about the relation of various aspects of community psychology to other disciplines or areas of study and action.

Problem Solving and Interdisciplinary Collaboration

The issue of professional identity is crosscut and in some ways complicated by a central orientation toward substantive problems that often transcend disciplinary boundaries. The dual concern with developing unique skills and knowledge yet maintaining a problem-solving orientation led many to conclude that a critical task for the field involved the ability to collaborate across disciplines. However, two factors mentioned at the conference suggest that interdisciplinary collaboration is a complex and difficult task: (1) its relation to the socialization practices of established fields, and (2) its relation to the institutional structures that support disciplines.

Sociologists of professions see the professionalization of a field as a necessary task for its survival (Elliot, 1972; Wilensky, 1964). The carving out of an exclusive domain of expertise and the creation of specific training facilities and curricula perpetuate the profession. Indeed, the 19th century guilds in England were considered less important as structures for organizing work tasks than as means of insuring status and minimizing external competition (Elliot, 1972). These same forces, however, have understandably socialized allegiance to disciplines and discipline-bounded areas of study.

In addition to socialization practices, the institutional structures that confer legitimacy on disciplines reinforce disciplinary allegiance. The organization of universities by departments exemplifies the general rule. However, institutional structure may constrain even in those settings within which collaboration was intended to occur. For example, Yale's Institute for Human Relations (IHR) was created 50 years ago to encourage people from different academic backgrounds to "cross-fertilize." However, the budget and review boards, in terms of promotion and tenure, were controlled by each individual department whose members were part of IHR. This structural situation was a recurrent reminder of the disciplinary orientation and became one of several factors hampering the potential for interdisciplinary collaboration (Ellis, Note 1).

To the degree to which the foregoing is valid, it suggests serious tensions between the growth and institutionalization of disciplines and the viability of interdisciplinary collaboration. Currently, however, new institutional structures are being created and new breeds of professionals are emerging that may alter the balance. In this regard, it will be instructive to understand the creation and current functioning of multidisciplinary ventures such as the College of Human Development at Pennsylvania State University, the Wallace School of Community Service and Public Affairs at the University of Oregon, and the Social Ecology Program at the University of California at Irvine. Each stands as a different kind of approach toward overcoming the institutional constraints on collaborative work.

These two areas—the evolving of new forms of professional activity and the importance of interdisciplinary collaboration—highlight the need to think as hard about "the community psychology of community psychology" as about its substantive knowledge base and research methods. The Austin Conference can serve no better purpose than to act as a catalyst for clarifying, framing, and confronting these issues as the field of community psychology progresses.

REFERENCE NOTE

1. Ellis, P. *A study in the prehistory and creation of a setting.* Unpublished predissertation, Yale University, 1974.

REFERENCES

Argyris, C. *Intervention theory and methods.* Reading, Mass.: Addison-Wesley, 1970.

Barker, R. *Ecological psychology.* Stanford, Calif.: Stanford University Press, 1968.

Becker, H. S., & Geer, B. Participant observation: The analysis of qualitative field data. In R. N. Adams & J. J. Preiss, *Human organization research.* Homewood, Ill.: The Dorsey Press, 1960.

Borgatta, E. F., & Bohrnstedt, G. W. (Eds.). *Sociological methodology 1970.* San Francisco: Jossey-Bass, 1970.

Campbell, D. T., & Stanley, J. C. *Experimental and quasi-experimental designs for research.* Chicago: Rand McNally, 1963.

Cottle, T. J. Show me a scientist who's helped poor folks and I'll kiss her hand. *Social Policy,* 1974, *4,* 33–37.

Cowen, E. L. Social and community interventions. *Annual Review of Psychology,* 1973, *24,* 423–472.

Elliot, P. *The sociology professions.* New York: Hurder & Hurder, 1972.

Kelly, J. G. Naturalistic observations and theory confirmation: An example. *Human Development,* 1967, *10,* 212–222.

Levine, A., & Levine, M. *A social history of the helping professions.* New York: Appleton-Century-Crofts, 1970.

Mannino, F. V., Maclennen, B. W., & Shore, M. F. (Eds.). *The practice of mental health consultation.* New York: Gardner Press, 1975.

Moos, R. H. *A social ecological approach: Evaluating treatment environments.* New York: Wiley, 1974.

Sanford, N. Is the concept of prevention necessary or useful? In S. Golann & C. Eisendorfer (Eds.), *Handbook of community mental health.* New York: Appleton-Century-Crofts, 1972.

Sarason, S. B. *The creation of settings and the future societies.* San Francisco: Jossey-Bass, 1972.

Schmuck, R. A., & Miles, M. B. (Eds.). *Organization development in schools.* Palo Alto, Calif.: National Press Books, 1971.

Suchman, E. A. *Evaluative research.* New York: Russell Sage Foundation, 1967.

Trickett, E. J., Kelly, J. G., & Todd, D. M. The social environment of the high school: Guidelines for individual changes and organizational development. In S. Golann & C. Eisendorfer (Eds.), *Handbook of community mental health.* New York: Appleton-Century-Crofts, 1972.

Weiss, C. H. *Evaluation research.* Englewood Cliffs, N.J.: Prentice-Hall, 1972.

Wilensky, H. The professionalization of everybody. *American Journal of Sociology,* 1964, *25,* 132–158.

Zax, M., & Cowen, E. L. Early identification and prevention of emotional disturbance in a public school. In E. L. Cowen, E. A. Gardner, & M. Zax (Eds.), *Emergent approaches to mental health problems.* New York: Appleton-Century-Crofts, 1967.

Zax, M., & Specter, G. *An introduction to community psychology.* New York: Wiley, 1974.

21 Nine Coalescing Themes

Jack M. Chinsky

INTRODUCTORY NOTE

To better understand this report, it is important to consider the process and context of its preparation. The report was written and presented at the Austin Conference and reflects my efforts as a participant-conceptualizer there. I spent a good deal of time visiting and listening to as many task groups as I could. I tried to drop my own notions of needed conceptual directions in community psychology and, instead, concentrated on obtaining the essential themes generated at the conference itself. The procedure was enhanced by audio taping, and a good deal of the paper consists of the thoughts and complete statements made by a variety of participants at the conference. These were extracted from the tapes and woven into an organized form. In an important sense, then, this is not a singularly authored report, but one that reflects, at least in part, the issues and concerns of many people at the conference.

CHANGE

The first major theme I heard repeatedly at the conference was that of change. Change this, change that, everybody was into changing something. More specifically, a variety of questions were asked: How do we implement change? How do we change individuals? How do we change groups? How do we change organizations? How do we change social systems? How do we assess this change? How do we know we have made a change? Of particular concern was: What are the total effects of a change—both the intended and the unintended consequences? Other questions centered on different issues: How do we maintain change? How do we build change into permanence?

Although there was considerable talk about promoting positive change, there was some discussion of reducing negative change. The notion of

Portions of this chapter were presented under the title "Experiencing Community Psychology: Reflections of a Participant-Conceptualizer at the Austin Conference" in I. Iscoe (chair) *Report on the Austin Conference: The Future of Community Psychology.* Symposium presented at the meeting of the American Psychological Association, Chicago, September 1975.

Cary Cherniss, Gerry Goodman, Judy Kramer, Steve Larcen, Stanley Sue, Dave Todd, Forrest Tyler, and members of the Special Interest Group on Conceptual Directions provided special help and suggestions for the final form of this report.

preservation—the preservation of adaptive aspects of individuals, groups, and systems that seems to be receding in our culture today—was also considered. Change is a concept that links us because we are all dealing with this process. Understanding, implementing, and evaluating change is one of the central themes of community psychology.

POWER

The second issue of significance was power. There were several ramifications of the theme of power across groups, each relating to community psychology's own sense of power vis-a-vis individuals, groups, and institutions. A frequent question was: Who are we to suggest things to people? This issue dichotomizes somewhat into others: Are we going to be leaders? Are we going to tell individuals and groups what to do? Are we going to develop collaborative interactions where we work together? Another issue concerned power in relation to the field's institutional base. What can community psychologists do within, without, and outside of particular institutions? The concept of power has implications for individuals, particularly their power to make choices and to control their own destiny. It also includes institutional power over individuals and the power dynamics in the community.

We talk about power, and it is interesting. But there will be some people who misunderstand. "There you go," they might say. "That is what community psychologists were after all along—their own power." This misunderstanding, if it does occur, reflects the issue just highlighted, for power generally is not understood.

Power is also effectiveness. Traditionally, it has been associated with hoarding, greed, and self-aggrandizement. Alternative conceptions of power should be promoted—the power of rationality, of patience, of empathy, of consensus; the power of effective change. Helplessness, in today's culture, is becoming as dated as the concept of motherhood and apple pie.

INTERDEPENDENCE

The third theme addressed across groups was interdependence. Essentially, the questions concerned: What goes with what? What are the ecological relationships? This is reflected in terms of multiple inputs, coordinating entry and perhaps more important, multiple outcomes, leading to multiple changes as a result of interventions. This leads, in turn, to other expressed concerns: Do we know enough to make interventions? If we promote change in one area, are we preventing change in another? Community psychologists must explore the concepts of intended and unintended consequences. We are accustomed to thinking in a linear fashion—input-output, side effects, dropouts. Now we must begin to discover relationships—in individuals, between values, attitudes, and behavior; between groups; within systems; and between institutions.

RELATIONSHIPS

The fourth common concern noted was the need to discover the relationships between the person and the environment, or "person and environment fit," as it is often called. It is clear that this is a reciprocal relationship: environments affect people, but people also affect environments. It is also fairly clear that the relationship between person and environment is not isomorphic. That is, if you change environments in one way, you don't directly and proportionally change individuals in the same way. Understanding this relationship is one of the field's most difficult challenges.

HISTORY

The fifth theme explored was an appreciation of history. Within this general area are many conceptual issues that need to be addressed. These include the history of the individual, that is, developmental notions. Simplified concepts like immaturity to maturity once were adequate, but now it is time to consider more complex developmental notions. It is time to address, in terms of history, how social systems evolve. What is the developmental sequence of organizational growth? What changes can we expect to occur in institutions as they grow? In the context of history, it is also time to talk about the future and the creation of future settings (e.g., Sarason, 1972).

CRITERIA FOR OPTIMAL FUNCTIONING

The sixth general area that reflects many common concerns deals with the criteria for optimal functioning. There were many questions: What is and how do we define optimal functioning in individuals, in systems, and in societies? For example, when institutions are optimally functioning do they hum? What do they do? The answers are as yet unknown. We may be left with relative levels of optimal functioning. This whole area needs to be explored, and short- and long-term goals need to be made more explicit.

The topic of optimal functioning in individuals leads into the concept of competence. We talk about ecological matches on another level. On the societal level, using Glidewell's (Note 1) framework, we talk about the cultural concerns of reducing pain and social conflict, as well as increasing enhancement and the equitable distribution of justice.

Related to the criteria for optimal functioning is a concern to avoid being caught in the clinical trap, to not get wrapped up only in social problems but to look at creative and positive alternatives. We should look at what we find to be optimally functioning systems in order to create alternatives. Projects such as intentional communities (Rhodes, as quoted by Bloom, Note 2) from which to draw resources for ideas, to input into less well functioning systems, are important and need to be supported.

EVALUATION

The seventh area concerned the need for new conceptions of evaluation, including such process issues as developing new methodologies appropriate to our interventions. There are common concerns related to such a question as: What is the effect of current evaluation strategies on limiting what we can evaluate? It seems clear that current psychological methodologies may not be able to handle the questions that we are trying to address. In fact, they may curtail knowledge rather than enhance it. Most of the statistical methodologies found in community psychology curriculum apparently are based on the linear agricultural model. They may be good for raising tomatoes, but how applicable they are to people is not yet clear. We have to develop new methodologies while being careful to maintain our critical perspective. To paraphrase Trickett (1975), our concern with traditional psychology is that it has lost its heart and soul, and our potential concern is that community psychology may lose its mind.

Other questions commonly addressed were: What is the effect of data? What is the effect of our evaluations on change? Research on the critical edge can be called "research to know versus research to change." The pioneering work of Fairweather (e.g., 1967, 1972) is especially important to consider here.

Let me give an example of research to know and research to change. I did some research in a state training school setting. We spent almost a year on the wards observing upward of 13,000 interactions between aides and children. We found that the average child in the state training school on this particular ward received a total of 4.5 minutes of formal training a day (Chinsky, 1975), and this training was distributed inequitably. We also have data to show that if the child is more attractive, he/she gets far more positive interactions than if he/she is not attractive; and the number of positive interactions is relatively independent of objective mental level (Dailey, Allen, Chinsky, & Veit, 1974).

I have those data, but what do I do with them? How do we affect change on the basis of those kinds of data? I could cite, as we all could, numerous examples of acquiring data. We do have some understanding of data but are only beginning to determine how to use it as a basis for action. The question is, "How do we turn that data into action?" And that was a common concern at the Austin Conference.

COMMUNITY PSYCHOLOGY OF COMMUNITY PSYCHOLOGY

The next issue concerns the "wheelbarrow" area, to borrow from an anecdote that Glidewell related at the conference. Can we push the wheelbarrow while we sit in it? Another way of conceptualizing this is the "community psychology of community psychology." This has several ramifications and introduces a lot of tension areas. The issues of social values caused some conflict at the conference, and it is clear why they did. Many participants are members of particular groups and classes that, as can be seen in our data and by our observations, give us benefits at the same time that they oppress and exploit others. How do we deal with that irreconciliation?

The issue to be faced is twofold: How much change do we really want to see; and are we potentially, covertly preventing change? We have to pursue this issue, and we have to put our values on the line. We want to preserve parts of the system, for some parts are beneficial and need to be strengthened. Some of us moved up through the educational system and now we want to help others use its positive aspects. We need alternatives here.

Another implication of the community psychology of community psychology concerns how to build intra- and interprofessional networks. Who are the allies? Where and how do we go for help and ideas? We need to lay out the interrelationships between community psychology and other disciplines. In the same light, possibly one of the best things to come out of this conference is a sense of community of our community, a sense of community of Division 27. After all else is said and done, this may be the most powerful outcome of the conference.

A related issue to address is who our constituencies are. Who are we conceptualizing and writing for—each other, the people in the community, or both? Who is giving us the credit? Who is promoting us? Whose reinforcement schema are we really working under? Caplan and Nelson (1973) have noted that people who please those above them move up in the system. We might add that those who please people below them are frequently considered charlatans and freaks and not "professionals." Again, this has to be addressed.

DEVELOPING AN EXPERIENCE BASE

The last theme, and an important one, was, How do we develop or redevelop our experience base? How do our experiences catch up with our conceptualizations? How do we make contact with, understand, experience, and observe diverse groups, individuals, settings—the community? These are complex questions because they concern interacting with people who don't necessarily share our ideologies; they probably mean working with people who don't think "psychology." This is so important that it seems appropriate to conclude with a personal anecdote that in a sense reflects the history of many others of my age and level.

I grew up in a candy store. My father owned the candy store, and I worked in it through adolescence, through college, up to the time I went to graduate school at Rochester. I noticed as I went to school—I got a state scholarship so I went to school and I learned about psychology—that the more I learned about psychology and the more I went up the educational ladder, the less that learning and experience related to the people in the candy store.

I could not talk to them anymore; I was moving away from them. I went into psychology because I wanted to help people. I was 17 and naive, and I thought I would learn how in clinical psychology. I found out, however, that clinical psychology didn't really help the people in the store. They didn't understand it ... it was too expensive ... it was on a different conceptual level ... it wasn't relevant to them. Community, it seems to me, has the opportunity to relate to those people.

To understand what is now going on in community psychology, we can, if we combine our own biographies with history, conceptualize as a group of people who came up from the working class, entered academics, looked around and found that it wasn't relevant, and decided that now we want to change it. Now we have to bring psychology back and consider what the real issues are.

We talked a lot about Barker at the conference, and it is rather ironic that one thing that was mentioned was the fact that Barker (1968) made some detailed observations in the fountain of a corner drug store much like the candy store in which I grew up. It seems that now people are saying that that's where the action was all the time. I think we all have to remember our own "candy stores." We can do this in two ways. The first is to remember our personal ties to the community. The second is to continuously integrate our work with the "real" world. We must understand the community, relate to the community, and bring our conceptions to bear in the community, if we are truly to have a psychology of the community.

REFERENCE NOTES

1. Glidewell, J. S. *Critique of the models presented in the preconference material.* Paper presented at the National Training Conference in Community Psychology, Austin, April 1975.
2. B. L. Bloom (Ed.), *Preconference materials of the National Training Conference in Community Psychology.* Unpublished manuscript, University of Colorado, 1975.

REFERENCES

Barker, R. G. *Ecological psychology: Concepts and methods for studying the environment of human behavior.* Stanford, Calif.: Stanford University Press, 1968.

Caplan, N., & Nelson, S. D. On being useful: The nature and consequences of psychological research on social problems. *American Psychologist,* 1973, *28,* 199–211.

Chinsky, J. M. Collaborative interventions in community mental health: A personal perspective. In S. E. Golann & J. Baker (Eds.), *Current and future trends in community psychology.* New York: Human Sciences Press, 1975.

Dailey, W. F., Allen, G. J., Chinsky, J. M., & Veit, S. W. Attendant behavior and attitudes toward institutionalized retarded children. *American Journal of Mental Deficiency*, 1974, *78*, 586–591.

Fairweather, G. W. *Methods for experimental social innovation*. New York: Wiley, 1967.

Fairweather, G. W. *Social change: The challenge to survival*. Morristown, N.J.: General Learning Press, 1972.

Sarason, S. B. *The creation of settings and the future societies*. San Francisco: Jossey-Bass, 1972.

Trickett, E. J. Review of *Community mental health: Social action and reaction* by B. Denner & R. H. Price (Eds.). *American Journal of Community Psychology*, 1975, *3*, 77–79.

V CURRENT TRENDS IN TRAINING AND THE PRACTICE OF COMMUNITY PSYCHOLOGY

INTRODUCTION

Bernard L. Bloom

The chapters in this section provide the empirical base necessary for any reality-oriented discussion of training issues in community psychology. The first three chapters report the major results of studies commissioned and partially subsidized by the Division of Community Psychology of the American Psychological Association. Preliminary results of these studies were presented at the annual meetings of the APA in 1974. The fourth chapter is based on data collected as part of a larger project funded by the Mental Health Services Development Branch of the National Institute of Mental Health, Grant no. MH 24428, Howard J. Parad, Principal Investigator. The authors acknowledge, with thanks, these sources of support.

These four studies have a special coherence and a synergistic impact. Each sought to assess activities and attitudes pertinent to community psychology training, obtaining data from (a) directors of university and field-based training programs in community psychology, (b) Division of Community Psychology members, (c) current doctoral-level graduate students in clinical and community psychology, and (d) staff members in community mental health centers. Following their presentation is a brief analysis of their themes and the significance of their results.

22 Training Programs in the Mid-1970s

A. Keith Barton, Dennis P. Andrulis,
William P. Grove, and Joseph F. Aponte

Prior to 1965, when the Boston Conference on The Education of Psychologists for Community Mental Health (Bennett, 1965) was held, and 1966, when the formation of the APA Division of Community Psychology took place, university community psychologists had not established credibility as members of a recognized subspecialty within departments of psychology. In the 10 years since the Boston Conference a variety of changes have occurred in the education and training of community psychologists as a consequence of changing concepts about their roles and functions. But while position statements have been prepared to define what community psychology is and what community psychologists do, the field itself has not yet achieved a clear identity. The discipline is characterized by a range of orientations and activities, including (a) extension of clinical psychology into the community, (b) organization of community services and personnel around primary prevention, (c) development of conceptual issues pertinent to planning and implementing interventions, and (d) viewing the community from an ecological perspective (Aponte, 1974).

There is little doubt that university and internship settings have become more responsive to community needs in the past decade and that they are undertaking serious reexamination aimed at the reconceptualization of training goals (Bloom, 1969b). From past studies (Bloom, 1969a; Golann, 1970; Golann, Wurm, & Magoon, 1964), it appears that a small number of ideologies are being identified. At the same time, special community psychology and community mental health vocabularies are developing. The authors concur with Bloom (1969b), however, that unless these ideologies are transformed into clearer and more rigorous concepts and methodologies within training programs, community psychology may forfeit the opportunity to influence change in academic and nonacademic communities. It seemed crucial, therefore, to examine the extent to which community psychology concepts and methodologies are being taught and practiced in university and internship

From "A Look at Community Psychology Training Programs in the Seventies" by A. K. Barton, D. P. Andrulis, W. P. Grove, and J. F. Aponte, *American Journal of Community Psychology,* 1976, *4*(1):1–11. Copyright 1976 by Plenum Publishing Corporation. Reprinted by permission.

Thanks are extended to Drs. Bernard L. Bloom, F. T. Miller, and Charles D. Spielberger for their constructive comments on earlier drafts of this chapter.

settings, and to compare more recent trends in community psychology offerings with those of earlier studies. By ascertaining the characteristics and similarities of community-related university programs and internships, psychologists should be better able to integrate research, theory, and practice. Implicit in this comparison is the recognition of the need for varied training experiences and the realization that training must take place in a variety of settings, using a variety of individuals, strategies, and program linkages.

SURVEY DESIGN AND METHOD

The survey design paralleled the earlier survey by Bloom (1969a). No distinction was made between the terms *community psychology* and *community mental health*. Of specific interest were (a) the degree to which community psychology training was offered as a distinguishable curriculum or specialization involving course requirements and sequencing, (b) course format and contents, (c) rankings by order of importance of community training experiences in preparing students for community work, (d) number of community-identified psychology faculty and their interest areas, and (e) student field-training experiences.[1]

The survey form was mailed in April 1974 to directors and heads of 341 master's and doctoral (university) programs, and 114 internship settings, representing all graduate programs in psychology (APA, 1973b) and all APA-approved internships (APA, 1973a). Follow-up letters and survey forms were mailed in July and November of that year to programs that had failed to respond.

RESULTS

Response rates were 69% (237 returns) from university programs and 53% (60 returns) from internships. The first question asked whether *any* community psychology or community mental health academic or field training was provided within their curricula. Findings from the returned surveys indicate that 141 university programs (59%) and 47 internship settings (78%) include some community psychology or community mental health content in their programs.

Program Format and Content Areas

Table 1 contains information on the characteristics of the training being provided by university programs and internships offering community psychology academic or field-training experiences. Approximately 15% of

---

[1] The survey was also concerned with program and student support, current student enrollments, and training programs in community colleges at the associate of arts degree level. These results are not reported in the present article but may be obtained from the authors upon request.

TABLE 1   Programs offering community psychology academic
or field-training experiences

	Type of program setting			
	University (N = 141)		Internship (N = 47)	
Program format	N	%	N	%
Community mental health fieldwork experiences	107	76 (84)[a]	45	96
Sequence of courses within the psychology department	79	56 (44)	2	4
Portions of one or more courses within the psychology department	75	53 (62)	6	13
Interdepartmental collaborative program	32	23 (16)	11	23
Portions of one or more courses within a behavioral science area	25	18	7	15
Distinguishable curriculum or specialization in community psychology	21	15	1	2
Other	14	10	7	15

[a]The percentages in parentheses are taken from Bloom's (1969a) survey which indicated 50 program offerings in community psychology.

university programs provide a distinguishable curriculum or specialization in community psychology, a finding identical to the figure reported in Golann's 1967 survey (Golann, 1970). Approximately one out of two reporting university programs offer community psychology coursework, primarily within psychology departments. At least three out of four university programs and nine out of ten internships offer fieldwork experiences in community mental health settings. Academic opportunities are becoming more elaborate, with the trend going from portions of one or more courses to course sequence and interdisciplinary programs.

Course and experience content areas of university and internship programs, as checked by survey respondents, are shown in Table 2. While the relationship is far from perfect, there is a general similarity between universities and field settings in program content. The areas most frequently offered tend to be in the relatively traditional mental health service domain or in activities associated with community mental health as distinguished from the community psychology movement. Compared to university programs, internships offer significantly more content coverage in mental health service delivery issues, program planning and evaluation, staff development, and case consultation, and significantly less content in basic community mental health

TABLE 2 Percentage of programs indicating various course content offerings

Course content	Type of program setting	
	University (N = 141)	Internship (N = 47)
Comparison of intervention strategies	85	81
Crisis intervention	79	89
Case consultation	77 (50)[a]	85
Community mental health center, neighborhood health center organization	74	83
Urban community-based action programs	74	79
Mental health program planning and evaluation	72	85
Prevention of mental disorders	67 (62)	43
Group process	66 (73)	68
Mental health program evaluation	64	66
Consultee-centered consultation	64 (50)	68
Federal, state, and local mental health activities	63	72
Brief psychotherapy	61	70
Applied community mental health research	60	53
Community organization	59 (25)	55
Issues in the delivery and financing of mental health services	56 (46)	81
Public health concepts	54 (13)	44
Administrative or system consultation to program or agency	53 (50)	62
Growth-enhancing counseling	50	40
Social milieu and their relationships to emotional disorders	49 (62)	36
Aftercare and other rehabilitation programs	48	64
Intervention programs for high-risk groups	48	66
Health and welfare agency structure and function	45	62
Mental health legislation at national and state levels	45	53
Mental health education	45 (35)	57
Screening and early detection programs	44	53

TABLE 2   (*continued*) Percentage of programs indicating
various course content offerings

| | Type of program setting | |
Course content	University (*N* = 141)	Internship (*N* = 47)
Mental health manpower issues	42 (44)	38
Basic community mental health research	40 (40)	25
Behavioral-science-oriented instructional programs	39	43
Identification of high-risk groups	39	40
Staff development	38	77
Rural community-based action programs	35	19
Identification of etiological factors in emotional disorders	35	28
Epidemiology of emotional disorder	33 (21)	28
Mental health program administration, e.g. financing, personnel, grantsmanship	27	40
Community small-area analysis	26	25
Industrial mental health	9	11

[a]The numbers in parentheses refer to the percentages obtained by Golann et al. (1964) in a 1962 survey, which indicated 46 psychology departments providing from 1 to 18 community mental health topics, with a median of 10.4 topics.

research. Such findings are congruent with the research emphasis of university programs and with agency administrative and consultative service emphases of internship settings.

Academic Training Experience Rankings

Academic training experiences were ranked according to their importance in preparing students for future employment in community psychology and/or mental health. The results of this analysis appear in Table 3. It was found that both university and internship settings emphasize consultation skills, community field placements, therapeutic skills, and program development and evaluation. Administrative skills, research in the community, and community organization are consistently ranked as least important. University programs value research in the community more than do internships, while internship facilities place greater emphasis on administrative skills.

TABLE 3 Rankings in importance of academic training
experiences preparing students for community work[a]

	Type of program setting	
Academic training experiences	University ($N = 141$)	Internship ($N = 47$)
Consultation skills	3.17	2.68
Community field placement	3.28	3.41
Therapeutic skills	3.50	3.14
Program development and evaluation	3.60	4.10
Research in community	4.42	5.61
Community organization	4.45	4.33
Administrative skills	5.71	4.85

[a]Rankings range from 1 = important to 7 = unimportant.

Community-Identified Faculty and Interest Areas

There is no significant difference in the mean number of community
psychology faculty for university (3.7) and internship (3.6) settings.[2] Within
each program setting, approximately 80% of the faculty express an interest in
specialized community mental health activities such as consultation and
education, crisis intervention, organizational development, program planning,
and evaluation, as contrasted to approximately 20% who express an ecological
or community psychology perspective.

Field-Training Experiences

The locations of field-training experiences are shown in Table 4. For
university and internship students, the most likely field settings are with
schools, mental health outpatient clinics, community mental health centers,
mental health inpatient facilities, and law enforcement agencies. Overall,
field-training experiences are minimal in city planning and public health
agencies, church settings, and mental retardation facilities.

A student-faculty coconsultation question was asked to determine the
extent to which students may obtain firsthand community psychology field-
training experience from direct observation and interaction with faculty

---

[2]Although numbers of faculty with substantial community interest were specifically
requested, some university and internship programs included larger listings of their
psychology departmental faculty, thereby inflating these values by some unknown degree.

TABLE 4   Percentage of program settings providing field-training experiences preparing students for community work

Field-training experiences	Type of program setting	
	University (N = 141)	Internship (N = 47)
Schools	68	85
Mental health outpatient setting	65	87
Community mental health center	65	74
Mental health inpatient setting	56	66
Law enforcement, prisons, courts	56	74
Mental retardation outpatient setting	37	45
Social service agency	35	51
Mental retardation inpatient setting	29	45
Church setting	18	40
Public health agency	14	28
City planning	7	17
Other	21	8

serving in a consultation function: 67% of university programs and 70% of the internships indicate that the coconsultation model of training is in use.

DISCUSSION

These data are useful for comparing recent trends in community psychology in university and internship settings with those of earlier studies (Bloom, 1969a; Golann, 1970; Golann et al., 1964). Identifiable course content relevant to community psychology and community mental health has increased from less than 20% in 1962, to 44% in 1967, to the 69% reported in this study. Furthermore, in comparison with the 50 programs reported in 1970, 141 university psychology departments now report course coverage in community psychology and community mental health topics. University programs offering a sequence of self-contained courses in community psychology have increased, while university psychology departments offering community psychology concepts as portions of one or more other psychology courses have decreased. Another important trend is the doubling of university PhD programs with a specialized community psychology curriculum, from the 10 departments reported in Golann's (1970) survey of academic departments of psychology to 20 today.

With respect to community psychology program content areas for university and internship programs, present results parallel findings of similar surveys conducted in the past. Emphasis continues to be placed on program planning and community mental health center administration, crisis intervention, and case consultation. Brief individual psychotherapy training is still important, but is more likely to be crisis oriented, short term, and community focused.

Thus, in university programs and internships, substantial gains (in absolute numbers) have been made in establishing community psychology and mental health experiences as relevant and identifiable training components within psychology departments and field settings. The data indicate that graduate psychology programs are providing students with increasing opportunities to learn about communities as social systems. The extent of this community involvement must be qualified, however, in that the data suggest a concentration of university involvement in the traditional mental health settings. The choice of more traditional practicum agencies has apparently determined the psychological techniques to be learned (Spielberger & Iscoe, 1972).

University programs and internships provide experiences defined more in terms of community mental health activities than in terms of community psychology activities. Within each program setting, program emphasis is primarily service oriented. Practicum experiences are obtained mainly from traditional mental health agencies, in part because most faculty members maintain greatest involvement in these agencies.

These results support Spielberger and Iscoe (1972) in their assertion that university psychology departments and internships are likely to make their most important contributions in the areas of social planning, conceptual analysis, program evaluation, and research on community problems. More psychology departments and internships are developing specialized, distinguishable curricula in community psychology with course sequencing today than they were five years ago, when community psychology concepts and methodology were less defined and were more often offered as portions of other psychology coursework. The data also suggest a conservative unfolding of the field with regard to student and faculty field-training experiences. The bridging of community psychology theory, research, and practice remains incomplete, in part because the knowledge and skill base for the practice of community psychology remains unresolved.

REFERENCES

American Psychological Association. APA-approved internships for doctoral training in clinical and counseling psychology: 1973. *American Psychologist*, 1973, *28*, 846–848. (a)

American Psychological Association. *Graduate study in psychology for 1973-74*. Washington, D.C.: Author, 1973. (b)

Aponte, J. F. In search of an educational model for community psychology. *The Journal of Community Psychology*, 1974, *2*, 301–305.

Bennett, C. C. Community psychology: Impressions of the Boston Conference on the education of psychologists for community mental health. *American Psychologist*, 1965, *20*, 832–835.

Bloom, B. L. Training opportunities in community psychology and mental health: 1969-70. Washington, D.C.: Committee on Manpower and Training, Division of Community Psychology, American Psychological Association, 1969. (Mimeo) (a)

Bloom, B. L. Training the psychologist for a role in community change. *APA Division of Community Psychology Newsletter*, 1969, *3*, 1–7. (b)

Golann, S. E. Community psychology and mental health: An analysis of strategies and a survey of training. In I. Iscoe & C. D. Spielberger (eds.), *Community psychology: Perspectives in training and research*. New York: Appleton-Century-Crofts, 1970.

Golann, S. E., Wurm, C. A., & Magoon, T. M. Community mental health content of graduate programs in departments of psychology. *Journal of Clinical Psychology*, 1964, *20* 518–522.

Spielberger, C. D., & Iscoe, I. Graduate education in community psychology. In S. E. Golann & C. Eisdorfer (Eds.), *Handbook of community mental health*. New York: Appleton-Century-Crofts, 1972.

23 Training Programs from the Perspective of Graduate Students

Edwin Zolik, William Sirbu, and David Hopkinson

As the general framework of community psychology has developed, increasing attention has been given to identifying the basic elements of effective training programs in community psychology and community mental health. This attention has taken the form of conceptual commentaries and critiques (Kalis, 1973; Powell & Riley, 1970; Rosenblum, 1973), as well as surveys on the status of graduate psychology programs (Golann, Wurm, & Magoon, 1964; Jacob, 1971). Spielberger and Iscoe (1970) have emphasized that graduate programs in psychology must be modified in order to meet community needs for a variety of psychological services.

Based on the perspectives of graduate students, however, no information is available concerning the training experiences and needs of graduate students interested in community psychology and community mental health. This study, conducted under the auspices of Division 27, was directed toward providing a comprehensive evaluation of training in community psychology and community mental health from the viewpoint of the consumers of training, i.e., graduate students.

Students were asked to evaluate their exposure to each of 30 specially selected topical areas related to community psychology and community mental health, as well as the adequacy of coverage of the topic in relation to their needs. Similarly, the availability and adequacy of field experiences in each of the 30 areas was assessed. To delineate student views about the concepts and practices subsumed under community psychology and community mental health, graduate students were also asked to rate each of the 30 topical areas in terms of its perceived importance. The focus of this report is the analysis of the evaluation by advanced clinical students of the adequacy of their training experiences in relation to their perceived needs.

From "Perspectives of Clinical Students on Training in Community Mental Health and Community Psychology" by E. Zolik, W. Sirbu, and D. Hopkinson, *American Journal of Community Psychology*, 1976, *4*(4):339-349. Copyright 1976 by Plenum Publishing Corporation. Reprinted by permission.

Thanks are extended to the graduate students and training directors who have participated in this survey. Acknowledgements and thanks for critiquing the preliminary survey forms and recommending modifications are extended to Dennis Andrulis, Joe Aponte, Keith Barton, Bernie Bloom, Emory Cowen, Barbara Dohrenwend, Ira Iscoe, Len Haas, and Bob Newbrough. The efforts and dedication of Marguerite Pozzi and Linda McHugh in assisting the authors is gratefully acknowledged.

PROCEDURE

Subjects

To obtain broad survey participation by graduate students, graduate training program directors were requested to distribute survey forms to students in their programs. Since community psychology/community mental health (CP/CMH) topics are covered in a variety of programs, a mailing list was compiled of all doctoral programs in clinical, community, counseling, school, social, and ecological-environment psychology. This list was based on program descriptions published by the APA (1973). If a university offered both the master's and doctoral degree, only the doctoral program was included.

A letter, information form, and six sets of the survey form were sent to the training directors of every identified doctoral program and the department chairmen of every identified master's program in clinical, community, counseling, social, ecological-environmental, and school psychology. Receiving survey packets were 128 clinical and community, 41 counseling, 106 social, 29 school, and 110 master's programs. Community psychology programs were classified as primarily clinical or social on the basis of their program description. This paper deals only with respondents from doctoral programs in clinical and community psychology.

The directors were asked to request a maximum of six of their advanced doctoral students who were in their last year of academic work or at the dissertation stage, and who had demonstrated interest in CP/CMH, to complete the survey forms. Advanced students were selected as the subject group on the presumption that information they provided would be based on broader experience as consumers of graduate education. Training directors were requested to complete a form indicating the number of students participating in the survey and the number of courses in community mental health and community psychology offered in their programs. Accompanying each survey form was a letter addressed to the graduate student explaining the purpose of the survey and requesting his or her participation. An addressed, postage-paid return envelope was included with each survey form. Three months later a second mailing was sent to programs from which survey returns had not been received.

Survey Instrument

The survey instrument consisted of three forms. The first was a questionnaire designed to obtain: (a) background data on the respondents, (b) information about the student's graduate program, and (c) information about the relation between the student's career goals and the fields of community mental health or community psychology. The second survey form consisted of a checklist of the availability and adequacy of academic and practicum training experiences in 30 topical areas associated with CP/CMH. These areas were selected to span the wide spectrum of the CP/CMH field and to allow for variations in emphasis among graduate programs. To keep the list within manageable limits for respondents, topics relating to basic and typical clinical areas, such as psychotherapy, and community areas, such as case consultation to mental health agencies, were excluded in view of their high frequency of coverage in training programs. The third survey form consisted of a five-point rating scale that assessed the student's opinions of the importance of the same 30 topical areas that were included in the second form.

RESULTS

The initial mailing resulted in 302 completed surveys, received from students representing 84 doctoral programs in clinical, clinical-community, and community psychology. The second mailing increased the sample to 385 respondents representing 102 programs. In addition, four program directors responded that their programs did not offer any coursework in CP/CMH. Accordingly, 80% of the identified programs are represented in the survey sample. In the design of the survey it was considered that by requesting the participation of up to six students from each program, an assumed adequate return rate of 50% would be obtained; it was further considered that the number of programs included in the sample would be maximized by the provision for flexibility necessary for programs that had only one or two advanced students interested in CP/CMH. The mean number of respondents from the 102 programs was 3.7 students.

Characteristics of Respondents

The 385 subjects were predominantly white (90%), male (69%), advanced (3.7 years of graduate study) students, three-quarters of whom indicated that psychology was their undergraduate major. In this sample, 5% of the respondents were black and 3% were Chicanos or of other Spanish descent. Prior to enrollment in graduate school, 58% of the subjects had had no psychological experience; 11% had had less than one year; and 26% had had between one and four years experience. Community mental health or community psychology was reported by 14% of the respondents as their major area of concentration, and of the 86% who indicated clinical psychology as their major, 70% reported that they would consider CP/CMH as being a minor or subarea in their personal academic program. The remaining 14% of the respondents either did not consider CP/CMH to be their major or minor area or as yet had not selected a minor area.

In this sample, 64% of the subjects had not yet completed an internship; 45% had not had a CP/CMH practicum that carried academic credit; 24% had had one practicum; and 17% reported having had two such practica. The remainder of the sample (15%) had had three to five such practica for credit. The range of CP/CMH courses taken by the respondents was zero to eight courses; 26% reported no course, 30% reported having taken one course, 18% having taken two courses, 12% having taken three courses, and 14% reported having taken between four and eight courses.

Program Characteristics

Whereas only 28% of the respondents reported that there was a specific CP/CMH sequence at their university, 68% expressed the opinion that a special or separate curriculum in the theory and practice of CP/CMH should be available as one of the programs offered in graduate education in psychology. Of the subjects, 21% reported that CP/CMH was available as a major area of specialization, and 44% indicated that it was available on a departmental or interdepartmental basis as a minor or subarea of concentration. Although few (28%) students could avail themselves of a specific CP/CMH sequence, more students (44%) could develop a minor through appropriate course selection. However, 60% of the students reported that they considered CP/CMH as a minor or subarea in their personal academic program. These data suggest that student interest and demands for training in CP/CMH are greater than what is available to them in their academic program.

The departmental orientation toward CP/CMH programs was reported by 46% of the subjects as being general or eclectic in nature, thereby allowing each student to develop her or his own conceptual framework. Only 6% described the orientation as having been developed around a central organizing theory.

Faculty attitude toward the allocation of curriculum time and space to CP/CMH was reported by 18% of the respondents as very accepting and by 39% as moderately accepting. The remaining 43% of the group reported that the allocation of curriculum time or space to the field was only slightly accepted or was not accepted at all by the faculty. When asked to rate the adequacy of the training in CP/CMH available in their program in relation to their career goals, only 4% of the subjects considered it as more than adequate; 31% considered it adequate, 46% less than adequate, and 19% inadequate or simply not available.

CP/CMH Orientation of Respondents

The majority of the subjects are highly oriented to CP/CMH, as indicated by their responses to several questions: (a) 60% of the respondents believe that their future professional duties will be strongly related to CP/CMH, (b) 66% consider training in CP/CMH as "very helpful" to their career goals, and (c) 54% are "very much interested" in obtaining further training in CP/CMH after completing their degree programs.

Academic and Practicum Training in CP/CMH

Students were requested to indicate whether the 30 CP/CMH topics (listed in Table 1) had been covered in "any formal course or seminar that you have taken," and, if the topic had been covered, whether "the coverage was sufficient or adequate for your needs." Table 1 presents the specific analyses for each item; some of the major highlights follow. The percent of subjects reporting coverage of topics ranged from 12% to 70%. Only four topics, however, were reported as having been covered by 50% or more of the respondents: (1) primary prevention, (2) ethics of community intervention and research, (3) research and program evaluation, and (4) crisis intervention. At the other extreme, five topics were reported as being covered by 25% or less of the respondents.

With respect to assessed adequacy or sufficiency of the coverage, the percent of respondents who considered the coverage of any topic to be adequate ranged from 40% to 67%. Since adequacy of coverage was assessed in terms of each subject's perceived needs, adequacy could be the result of either comprehensive coverage of the topic or of minimal coverage coupled with minimally perceived need for additional knowledge on the specific topic. Some of the topics reported as adequately covered by 60% or more of the respondents included: ethics of community intervention and research; normative stresses (i.e., adjustment problems following retirement, forced relocation, etc.); mental health-related epidemiology; public health philosophy and concepts; case- and consultee-centered consultation to service (nonmental health) organizations; and primary intervention.

The marked variability in the coverage of the topics is indicative of wide variations among graduate programs in providing students with exposure to areas related to the fields of community mental health-community psychology. The data also suggest that CP/CMH as a content area is in various stages of development in the departments represented in the survey. The topics related to clinical community mental health, as contrasted to those more closely associated with community psychology, are reported by a higher percentage of respondents as being covered in their academic coursework and also as being adequately covered. With the continued conceptual development of community psychology-community mental health, it can be anticipated that both the extent of coverage and student-perceived adequacy of coverage will increase in both components of the field.

Table 1 also presents data on the availability and adequacy of field experience or practicum in each of the 30 topical areas. Survey comments by some of the respondents indicated that, in many cases, availability meant that obtaining experiences was possible only through the student's initiative, rather than a planned field placement as part of the training program. Between 10% and 64% of the respondents indicated that field experience was available in the various areas, and between 64% and 91% of the respondents who had had

TABLE 1 Academic coverage and field experience: Availability and adequacy

Topic	Topic covered academically (N = 385)	Academic coverage adequate[a]	Field experience available (N = 385)	Field experience adequate[b]
	Percent of respondents indicating			
Alcoholism and drug abuse	43	40	61	76
Crisis intervention	51	55	64	70
Early screening and identification	48	59	46	75
Primary prevention	70	60	44	78
Follow-up and aftercare services	27	54	39	68
Normative stresses, e.g., retirement	13	67	21	73
Case consultation to service deliverers	49	60	52	80
System consultation to service deliverers	38	52	40	77
System consultation to mental health agencies	40	55	38	79
Interagency coordination issues	32	53	29	70
Paraprofessional training	41	57	38	73
Community structure and analysis of political organization	37	59	24	77
City and regional planning	12	51	10	79
Social system analysis and change	40	49	21	71
Advocacy and social action	33	51	19	71
Citizen participation issues	32	47	18	71
Public health concepts and philosophy	30	62	10	84
Social policy	28	52	15	74
Developmental disabilities	33	59	33	78

TABLE 1 (*continued*) Academic coverage and field experience: Availability and adequacy

	Percent of respondents indicating			
Topic	Topic covered academically (N = 385)	Academic coverage adequate[a]	Field experience available (N = 385)	Field experience adequate[b]
Preschool and daycare issues	36	56	41	70
School mental health programs	45	60	54	78
Mental health program planning	37	45	31	77
General human service program planning	18	44	16	64
Research and program evaluation	63	59	48	74
Mental health-related epidemiology	41	65	15	83
Uses of social indicators for program development	28	51	18	80
Management information system utilization	12	52	10	91
Assessment of consumer attitudes	28	56	20	80
Ethics of community intervention and research	64	67	22	85
Research on quality of life	21	53	14	86

[a]Percent reporting adequate academic coverage is based on number reporting that the topic had been covered.
[b]Percent reporting field experience as adequate is based on number who had field experience available less the number who had not taken a practicum in the particular area.

field or practicum experiences in the different areas reported the field experience as being adequate for their needs. The data in Table 1 indicate that community mental health field experiences were more readily available than community psychology experiences. Further, a greater percentage of students reported field experiences adequate than reported academic coverage adequate for the same topical area.

Student Comments

Many students availed themselves of the opportunity to make comments on the different sections of the survey. Although a number of comments were positive, especially in relation to recent or planned program changes providing for greater exposure CP/CMH, many others expressed concern about the lack, or limited availability, of both academic training and field experience. While CP/CMH field experiences are more readily available than are appropriate and relevant academic training experiences, many students have to seek them out on their own, for they are not formally available through the training program. Others described their programs as traditional and clinical-community in name only. Concern was expressed over the need for academic courses to provide an integration of field experiences at the conceptual level. The lack of faculty support of student interests in CP/CMH was frequently noted.

The following comments express some of the student reactions and concerns. "Students often find outside work in particular areas, but this is not connected to coursework. I have, unfortunately, gotten almost no support from the faculty." "There are no specific practica available. Students find them on their own." "You could seek out experiences in most of these areas on your own, but they are not formally available through the program." "I've gained experience in several agencies doing CMH, none of which were connected to or sanctioned by the university." "The only CMH training occurs in placement settings." "Our program is flexible, and students can conceivably have any experience they wish and the faculty would do their best to find them this experience or help them obtain it." "Training is inadequate; however, I have the freedom to do my own learning." "While there is no formal community program either in a major or a minor way, there are a number of good practicums with strong community mental health focus. It would be most helpful to have related or concurrent courses that could stimulate greater integration of experience and conceptual approaches." "Although my department sometimes advertises its graduate program as community oriented, it is, in fact, a traditional clinical program with one course in community psychology." "The program has changed considerably ... many of these areas are now covered either through seminars or practicum." "This (survey) list makes one aware of how few areas we've covered, and most are important." "Reading through this (survey) list, I am shocked to find how deficient my training has been." "I like this form very much ... but perhaps we must consider what limitations exist in training within universities and decide whether that system can or should be changed to meet defined needs, or if, instead, we should focus on the development and utilization of other training systems."

DISCUSSION

In the last decade there has been a steady increase in course content relevant to community psychology and/or community mental health. Student comments in this study confirm this increase. However the data also indicate wide variations in CP/CMH-related course content and courses. In many academic departments CP/CMH training is still in an early developmental stage. Such variability is not atypical of a newly emerging area of specialization and is related, in part, to the degree of faculty acceptance of the area as being important enough to necessitate curriculum modification and change.

While acknowledging the incremental growth that has occurred and is planned in many departments, students have many concerns about the growth rate and present state of training in CP/CMH. A major concern is for greater integration between conceptualization and application. The action orientation in applied settings has resulted in many advances, which are beginning to percolate back to academic programs for integration with the growing body of CP/CMH theory.

The strong underlying foundation of clinical psychology is still in evidence. Much contemporary training is characterized by an extension of clinical psychology into the community, as both academic exposure and practicum training are more readily available in the community mental health dimensions of the CP/CMH continuum than in community psychology dimensions. This development is not unexpected in view of the clinical background of the majority of community psychologists, the demands for improving service delivery, and the knowledge base available to the field over the last decade. The results also indicate that the community psychology dimensions are receiving varying degrees of attention in some academic programs and that some nontraditional field experiences are becoming available to students. The present state of training indicates that the greatest amount of development in the near future may occur in the community psychology dimension of the CP/CMH continuum. With such a development the variety of roles available to the community psychologist of the 1980s will be much greater, and the recommendation of Spielberger and Iscoe (1972) that psychology can make its most important contributions in the areas of social planning, conceptual analysis, program evaluation, and research on community problems will be closer to realization.

The 1975 Austin Conference promulgated a number of training models based on contemporary trends and directions envisioned for the future development of community psychology. The implementation of these models will most often require academic departments to make choices, based on the expertise and interests of available faculty, on both a departmental and an interdisciplinary basis. The unevenness in the availability and adequacy of academic and field experiences depicted in the survey data is partially the result of the lack of clearly defined training models in many departments. The breadth of the field is such that the specification of the training model underlying each program should be available for informed decision making by prospective students.

The potential contributions from the field of community psychology can only be realized through periodic evaluations of its programs. The ease of placing graduates is a popular and convenient evaluation, but while it contributes to the self-enhancement of trainers it does not result in meaningful program evaluation. For effective evaluation, departments need to develop conceptual models of their training programs, including the definition of program goals and objectives, the values involved in the program, and the expected outcomes. The models developed at the 1975 Austin Conference present an opportunity for initiating such an undertaking, for only through internal, systematic evaluations of its programs can community psychology most effectively meet the needs of students and society.

REFERENCES

American Psychological Association. *Graduate study in psychology for 1973-74.* Washington, D.C.: Author, 1973.

Golann, S. E., Wurm, C. A., & Magoon, T. M. Community mental health content of graduate programs in departments of psychology. *Journal of Clinical Psychology,* 1964, *20,* 518–522.

Jacob, T. A survey of graduate education in community psychology. *American Psychologist,* 1971, *26,* 940–944.

Kalis, B. L. Orientation to community mental health for clinicians in training. *Community Mental Health Journal,* 1973, *9,* 316–324.

Powell, T. J., & Riley, J. M. The basic elements of community mental health education. *Community Mental Health Journal,* 1970, *6,* 196–202.

Rosenblum, G. Advanced training in community psychology: The role of training in community systems. *Community Mental Health Journal,* 1973, *9,* 63–67.

Spielberger, C. D., & Iscoe, I. The current status of training in community psychology. In I. Iscoe & C. D. Spielberger (Eds.), *Community psychology: Perspectives in training and research.* New York: Appleton-Century-Crofts, 1970.

Spielberger, C. D., & Iscoe, I. Graduate education in community psychology. In S. E. Golann & C. Eisdorfer (Eds.), *Handbook of community mental health.* New York: Appleton-Century-Crofts, 1972.

24 Training Experiences from the Perspectives of Community Psychologists

Dennis P. Andrulis, A. Keith Barton,
and Joseph F. Aponte

This study focuses on the Division 27 (Community Psychology) membership of APA to determine their (a) demographic and educational characteristics, (b) employment status, (c) attitudes toward training issues, and (d) ideas about professional activities deemed essential to the field of community psychology. Division 27 members are assumed to be closely identified ideologically and methodologically with community psychology theory, research, and practice; and understanding their perspectives on issues related to community psychology can assist materially in planning training programs.

METHODS AND RESULTS

A list of current members of Division 27 (about 1,200) was obtained from the American Psychological Association, and survey questionnaires with a self-addressed stamped envelope and cover letter were mailed in April 1974. The survey questionnaire focused on (a) background and demographic data, (b) past and present employment settings, (c) relevance of community psychology training to current employment, and (d) roles and functions considered essential to community psychology.

There were 460 (38%) surveys completed and returned. The respondents were predominantly white (95%), male (85%), with PhD or EdD degrees (90%). The group was relatively young, with 30% between 25 and 34 years of age, 36% between 35 and 44 years, 25% between 44 and 54 years, and only 8% 55 years or older. More than half of the respondents received doctorates within the past ten years.

Academic and Employment Characteristics

The vast majority of respondents were psychology majors as undergraduates, and, of course, psychology graduate students. About 5% of the members who

From "Training Experiences from the Perspective of Community Psychologists" by D. P. Andrulis, A. K. Barton, and J. F. Aponte, *American Journal of Community Psychology*, in press. Reprinted by permission of Plenum Publishing Corporation.

Thanks are extended to Drs. Bernard L. Bloom, F. T. Miller, J. Robert Newbrough, Charles D. Spielberger, and Ed Zolik for their constructive comments on earlier drafts of this chapter.

completed graduate school in an area other than clinical psychology became involved with clinical psychology after graduate school. A very small portion of the sample graduated from a community psychology program in graduate school (3%), 20% had one or two courses in community psychology, and 67% had never taken a community psychology course.

With regard to present employment status, as can be seen in Table 1, at least 64% of the respondents are employed in positions partially related to community psychology. Their principal work settings are in community mental health centers (24%) and in colleges or universities other than community psychology programs (23%).

Of the respondents who belong to other APA divisions, nearly half of Division 27 members also belong to Division 12 (Clinical Psychology). Other membership includes 18% in Division 8 (Personality/Social), 18% in Division 9 (The Society for the Psychological Study of Social Issues), and 14% in Division 29 (Psychotherapy).

Most respondents (55%) perceive their present position of employment to be strongly related to community psychology, 58% indicate that their interest

TABLE 1   Employment characteristics of division 27 respondents

Present employment status	N	%
Full time in community psychology	202	44
Part time in community psychology	91	20
Full time not in community psychology	115	25
Other	52	11

Principal work setting	N	%
Community mental health center	109	24
College or university, other than community psychology program	106	23
Psychiatric inpatient facility	45	10
College or university community psychology program	42	9
Health agency other than inpatient facility	37	8
Private practice	32	7
Medical or other health professional school	22	5
Social agency	15	3
Public school system	10	2
Other	42	9

TABLE 2 Competences judged as essential to the field of
community psychology

Professional activity	N	%
Consultation	158	34
Community change and social planning	129	28
Program evaluation	124	27
Education and training	108	23
Program development in the human services	107	23
Clinical mental health skills	98	21
Research	85	18
Community organization	85	18
Health and mental health education	82	18
Mental health and general health program administration	74	16
Interagency coordination	67	15
Staff development and inservice training	67	15
Political aspects of community planning	59	13
Theory building	58	13
Preventive services	57	12
Need assessment and epidemiological studies	54	12
Systems analysis	52	11

in community psychology was enhanced by their academic training, and 61%
report substantial interest in further training.

Roles and Functions Perceived as Essential to Community Psychology

In an open-ended question, respondents were asked to name five activities
essential to the field of community psychology. Table 2 presents the areas
that are listed as essential to the field by more than 10% of the respondents.
Because the question was open-ended, it was sometimes difficult to evaluate
the replies. But the list of essential competencies is long and broad and clearly
includes areas well removed from traditional clinical training program content.

DISCUSSION

Clinical psychologists dominate the Division 27 membership in terms of both
area of graduate study and employment setting. Yet, although a majority of

the membership is involved with patient care, most perceive indirect services and nonclinical activities to be at least as essential to community psychology as direct service skills. Active participation in community change through multilevel programming and a general human services framework are frequently seen as essential by the membership. The need for an inter-disciplinary approach is partially supported, as is the need for evaluation and consultation training (Golann, 1970). Like Reiff (1970), the membership perceives the necessity of training in social systems interventions through design and development of human service programs and community organizations.

Community psychology, in theory, is moving away from individual issues and toward broader social system concerns. This is especially noteworthy when one considers that clinical psychology is the predominant field in which the present membership trained. At present, such nonclinical activities as community change and social planning and the design and development of human service programs are increasingly seen as alternative areas of training that should be considered as core elements of community psychology.

REFERENCES

Golann, S. E. Community psychology and mental health: An analysis of strategies and a survey of training. In I. Iscoe & C. D. Spielberger (Eds.), *Community psychology: Perspectives in training and research.* New York: Appleton-Centruy-Crofts, 1970.

Reiff, R. The need for a body of knowledge in community psychology. In I. Iscoe & C. D. Spielberger (Eds.), *Community psychology: Perspectives in training and research.* New York: Appleton-Century-Crofts, 1970.

25 Professional Activities and Training Needs of Community Mental Health Center Staff

Bernard L. Bloom and Howard J. Parad

The community mental health literature of the past decade has presented in detail the ideological position of the mental health movement and the implications of this position for how mental health center staff might best distribute their professional activities (e.g., Bloom, 1973). The special emphases of the community mental health movement have been on preventive programming, crisis and emergency services, consultation and education, interagency coordination and collaboration, and community involvement in program planning. One would like to assume that community mental health center staff would spend significant portions of their time in these activities. The National Institute of Mental Health (Bass, 1974) reported that between 5 and 6% of community mental health center staff time is devoted to consultation and education. But there have been no staff surveys to which one might turn in an effort to examine professional staff activities comprehensively in relation to the ideological positions that mental health centers are designed to represent.

This chapter provides information on community mental health center staff activities and expressed training needs, based on data collected as part of a larger project studying knowledge and skill needs of such staffs.[1] The larger study focused on 13 western states and included an examination of how mental health centers describe their activities and define their training needs and how they view interdisciplinary team functioning and collaborative practice. The special emphasis in this report is on the activities and training needs of psychologists.

METHOD

Letters describing the project were sent to the directors of all federally-assisted community mental health centers in the 13 western states. Directors were invited to appoint a staff member to serve as the local study coordinator

[1] Supported by Mental Health Services Development Branch, NIMH (Grant No. MH24428), Howard J. Parad, Principal Investigator.

who would be responsible for distributing, collecting, and returning completed questionnaires. Of the 87 federally assisted centers in the West, 77 appointed a local study coordinator. The others indicated that they would be unable to participate in the project. Draft copies of the questionnaire were distributed to these local study coordinators with the request that they share their comments and suggestions for revision and, in a subsequent communication, that they indicate how many copies of the final questionnaire they would need so that there would be a copy for every clinical staff member.

The questionnaire was divided into seven sections: (a) demographic and occupational information (15 items), (b) time spent per week in various professional activities (33 items), (c) patterns of interaction with other professional groups both within the mental health center and with other organizations in the community (35 items), (d) major sources of knowledge for professional activities (19 items), (e) nature of training needs pertinent to professional activities (19 items), (f) attitudes toward interdisciplinary practice (49 items), and (g) a professional value orientation scale (68 items).

A total of 10 local study coordinators indicated either that their mental health centers would be unable to participate in the project, usually because the questionnaire was too time-consuming, or that they would only be able to sample the staff. A total of 3,850 questionnaires was distributed on request to the 67 remaining mental health centers during early 1975, and replies were received from 55 of these centers by June. Along with returning the completed questionnaires, each local study coordinator also reported the number of clinical staff in each professional category employed at the center. In sum, 3,448 staff were identified and 1,503 completed questionnaires (43.6%) returned.

In interpreting the data to be presented, two cautions should be kept in mind. The first is that counting numbers of staff in a community mental health center is a complex and somewhat unreliable task, particularly when the center consists of a consortium of collaborating agencies. Thus, the questionnaire return rate estimates shown in Table 1 should be interpreted as maximum estimates. Second, it is not possible to assess the representativeness of the questionnaire replies. It is not known whether or how those mental health centers that participated in the project differ significantly from those that did not, nor is the extent known to which participating staff members may differ from nonparticipants.

STUDY RESULTS

Demographic and Occupational Information

Assignment of respondents to one of six occupational categories was based on reported highest level of education and field of specialization. All psychiatrists had, of course, completed medical school. The master's degree or above was required for assignment to the psychologist category; in fact, however, more than 60% of psychologists held the PhD. Attainment of the master's degree was also required for the social worker designation. Educational background of nurses varied, with 52% having diploma-level training, 30% bachelor's-level training, and the remaining 18% master's degrees. The category called "other mental health professionals included counselors, physicians other than psychiatrists, and rehabilitation specialists and social scientists, all with masters' degrees or higher. Nearly one-quarter of this group had completed doctoral-level training. The mental health worker category included paraprofessionals and licensed vocational and practical nurses. Nearly half of the respondents in this occupational category were college graduates, 47% were high school graduates, and only 3% had not completed high school.

Table 1 shows the number of staff and number and percent of questionnaires completed by profession. A somewhat larger proportion of psychologists than other groups completed the questionnaire, but the differences are not great.

The six professional groups differ dramatically in sex and age distribution and also in marital status and racial or ethnic identification. While 50% of the total sample is female, 81% white, 64% married, and 48% between ages 25 and 34, the more highly trained staff tend to be older, more often male, married, and white. The only significant representation of minority group members is found in the mental health worker category (36% nonwhite). A large proportion of the most highly trained staff was educated in the East—three quarters of all psychiatrists, more than one-third of psychologists and social workers, and more than one-quarter of nurses and other mental health professionals. The older mental health staff tend to have been in the mental health field longer, but length of time employed by the present agency or in the present position within that agency is not age related. Virtually all

TABLE 1 Number of clinical staff and questionnaire completions by profession: 55 western c mmunity mental health centers

Profession	Clinical staff	Questionnaire (N)	Completions (%)
Psychiatrists	278	116	41.7
Psychologists	401	211	52.6
Social workers	676	327	48.4
Nurses	525	227	43.2
Other mental health professionals	445	138	31.0
Mental health workers	1123	484	43.1
Total	3448	1503	43.6

respondents are fulltime employees, and there is no significant difference among professional groups in the length of the normal work week. With regard to the position held prior to joining the present agency, psychiatrists and nurses often came from general medical settings, and one-third or more of the four core mental health disciplines came from other mental health settings. Concerning current primary job responsibility, two-thirds of all respondents list direct clinical service, with the balance divided more or less equally among supervision, administration, and other activities.

Distribution of Professional Activities

In order to ascertain how community mental health center staff distributed their time among various professional activities, the questionnaire instructions read as follows:

The following section asks you something about how you distribute your time in your current job. We are interested in obtaining an estimate of how much time our respondents devote to selected activities. In order to do this we are asking each respondent to estimate the total time devoted to these activities for the *five full working days immediately prior to the day in which this item is completed.* The listing below is not meant to be exhaustive, and it is recognized that some respondents may spend considerable portions of their time in activities not included. There is a space for you to indicate activities you performed last week which are not on this list, and to indicate whether or not these last five days were typical for you. You may find that it is useful to examine your appointment book to refresh your memory. When you are all done, the total number of hours listed should be the same as the hours you work per week.

A total of 19 different activities were listed, divided into three major categories: diagnostic and treatment services; community activities; and administration, supervision, and research. If the respondent indicated that the previous five full working days were not typical, he or she could list which activities typically took more time and which typically took less time. Of all respondents, 87% indicated that the previous five full working days were typical for them in terms of how they spent their time. Respondents, on the average, reported spending less than five minutes per week in activities other than the 19 listed on the questionnaire. Thus, the 19 listed activities apparently identified virtually all of the functions typically performed by community mental health center staff. Diagnostic and treatment services took up just over 18 hours each week, on the average; community activities required 7 hours (of which slightly more than 2 hours were devoted to mental health consultation and education); and administrative, supervisory, and research activities used 13.5 hours.

The distribution of professional activities by profession is found in Table 2. One-way ANOVA results are shown in the last two columns—significant F

TABLE 2 Mean hours per week allocated to professional activities: Staff in 55 community mental health centers

Professional activity	Psychiatry	Psychology	Social work	Nursing	Other mental health profession	Mental health worker	Total	F	p
Clinical diagnosis and assessment	4.91	3.18	2.64	1.80	2.50	1.63	2.43	22.90	<.001
Individual treatment	5.36	8.12	7.65	5.31	6.37	6.30	6.63	7.83	<.001
Family and group treatment	1.25	3.45	4.36	2.83	3.44	5.31	3.98	15.08	<.001
Crisis/emergency services	1.95	1.23	1.75	3.17	1.10	1.51	1.77	8.04	<.001
Deciding on hospitalization	0.70	0.22	0.32	0.58	0.19	0.31	0.36	3.07	ns
Prescribing medication	3.03	0.00	0.01	0.12	0.09	0.01	0.27	95.62	<.001
Administering medication	0.28	0.01	0.03	2.96	0.07	0.46	0.63	52.97	<.001
Patient and ward management	2.46	0.81	0.80	5.13	0.50	2.73	2.18	22.74	<.001
Total clinical activities	19.94	17.02	17.56	21.90	14.26	18.26	18.25	12.21	<.001
Mental health consultation	1.32	2.81	1.93	1.02	1.65	1.03	1.55	14.88	<.001
Working with citizens	0.73	0.99	1.20	0.67	2.01	1.84	1.33	8.82	<.001
Mental health education	0.41	0.82	0.79	0.87	0.86	0.94	0.83	1.08	ns
Aftercare	0.34	0.18	0.58	1.17	1.26	1.62	0.99	9.86	<.001
Home visiting	0.22	0.30	0.47	1.11	0.64	1.41	0.84	16.36	<.001
Interagency collaboration	0.82	1.19	1.86	1.21	1.68	1.44	1.44	6.03	<.001
Total community activities	3.84	6.29	6.83	6.05	8.10	8.28	6.98	9.95	<.001
Research and evaluation	0.89	1.90	0.62	0.33	2.06	0.69	0.93	10.97	<.001
Training and supervision	3.89	2.85	3.07	2.55	3.82	2.17	2.81	5.62	<.001
Administration and program development	2.34	3.31	3.38	1.61	3.28	1.77	2.49	11.56	<.001
Report writing, correspondence	2.97	3.52	3.83	3.70	3.69	4.25	3.82	3.47	ns
Staff conferences	3.11	3.30	3.77	3.17	3.07	3.43	3.39	2.02	ns
Total administration	13.20	14.88	14.67	11.36	15.92	12.31	13.44	8.75	<.001
Other	0.07	0.05	0.03	0.09	0.15	0.09	0.08	0.69	ns
Grand total	37.05	38.24	39.09	39.40	38.43	38.94	38.75	1.75	ns

values indicate that the six professional groups devote different amounts of time to the activity in question. Psychiatrists and nurses spend significantly more time in the provision of diagnostic and treatment services than do all other mental health professionals. The four core mental health disciplines spend less time in community activities than do other mental health professionals and mental health workers. Psychologists and the group of mental health professionals other than the core disciplines spend most time in administrative, supervisory, and research activities, largely because of their somewhat greater time spent in research.

As for distinguishing features of each professional group, the following findings should be stressed. Psychiatrists spend significantly more time than any other group in clinical diagnosis and assessment and in prescribing medication, and significantly less time than any other group in family and group treatment and in community activities in general. Psychologists spend significantly more time than any other group in mental health consultation. Nurses spend significantly more time than any other group in crisis and emergency services, dispensing and administering medication, and patient and ward management. Mental health professionals other than the core disciplines spend significantly less time than any other group in clinical activities. Mental health workers spend significantly more time than any other group in providing family and group treatment (which is perhaps best explained by the fact that time spent in day treatment and partial hospitalization services are included in this category, and mental health workers are frequently involved in these programs).

In the case of respondents –13% in all–who indicated that the previous five working days were not typical of their normal work week, analysis of their responses to the questions regarding those activities normally more or less common are consistent with the general findings reported. Respondents whose work week was atypical ordinarily spend more time in clinical activities, notably individual treatment, and less time in a variety of activities in which community services and supervisory and administrative activities are conspicuous.

Mental Health Center Staff Training Needs

Expressions of training needs were solicited in another section of the questionnaire by means of the following instructions:

Listed below are the same 19 community mental health functions as in previous sections. We are now interested in the extent to which you feel you need additional training in these functions. First, place ONE check mark after each function where you feel you need additional training and place TWO check marks next to those functions where you feel you have the *greatest needs* for additional training. Second, after each function you have checked, indicate, again by checking, whether you feel you need further theoretical knowledge (check column A), or skill learning (check column B), or both (check column C).

Only data regarding felt need (single or double checked) for additional training are presented. The latter part of the instructions did not yield remarkable results, since about two-thirds of all people expressing a need for training consistently acknowledged needs in both theory and skill building. The analysis of expressed needs for additional training by profession is presented in Table 3.

Examination of Table 3 shows substantial differences in felt needs for additional training by profession and by function. First, greatest needs for additional training are expressed in clinical areas, particularly family and group treatment, clinical diagnosis and assessment, and individual treatment. It will be remembered that these were among the most common activities of mental health center staff. In fact, the correlation of average hours spent per week on each activity and felt need for additional training in the case of all respondents combined is significantly positive, $r(17) = +.53; p < .01$. Second, the need for additional training is inversely related to education, with mental health workers expressing greatest need and psychiatrists and psychologists least need. Of the 15 functional areas where significant interprofessional differences in training needs were found, mental health workers express greatest need for training in 10. As a consequence, there is a variable relationship between how much time a particular professional group spends in a specific function and the felt need for training in that function. In the case of clinical services, for example, psychiatrists, who spend more time than any other profession in clinical diagnosis and assessment, have lowest expressed need for additional training in that function. Similar findings are seen in the case of psychologists and individual treatment. But in the cases where staff members other than psychiatrists or psychologists allocate most time to that activity, the negative relationship does not hold. Mental health workers, for example, express greatest need for training in family and group treatment and in report writing, two activities in which they spend more time than any other occupational category. A notable exception to this second finding is seen in the case of research and evaluation activities, where greatest need for additional training is expressed by psychiatrists, possibly because of the current emphasis on cost benefit analysis and on the evaluation of program effectiveness. Third, a moderately high level of need for additional training is found regarding activities commonly associated with community mental health practice—crisis and emergency services, mental health consultation, working with citizen groups, mental health education, and interagency collaboration.

TABLE 3 Percentages of staff expressing need for additional training: 55 western community mental health centers

Function	Psychiatry	Psychology	Social work	Nursing	Other mental health profession	Mental health worker	Total	F	p
Clinical diagnosis and assessment	33	48	69	67	65	67	62	18.26	<.001
Individual treatment	34	47	57	65	46	69	58	18.31	<.001
Family and group treatment	54	67	76	75	64	74	71	5.67	<.001
Crisis/emergency services	39	48	42	52	44	52	47	6.68	<.001
Deciding on hospitalization	13	26	23	19	27	31	25	5.36	<.001
Prescribing medication	24	8	8	10	13	10	11	2.72	ns
Administering medication	5	4	5	13	7	12	8	3.97	ns
Patient and ward management	22	12	12	29	17	21	19	6.19	<.001
Mental health consultation	41	44	58	47	43	43	47	6.67	<.001
Working with citizens	43	39	45	42	36	41	41	1.06	ns
Mental health education	28	26	32	39	29	46	36	8.99	<.001
Aftercare	15	14	16	28	20	34	24	13.47	<.001
Home visiting	9	10	7	15	16	24	15	11.99	<.001
Interagency collaboration	45	33	31	36	33	36	35	1.08	ns
Research and evaluation	56	31	39	34	38	38	38	4.12	ns
Training and supervision	33	29	43	42	32	38	37	3.42	ns
Administration and program development	52	46	50	41	39	39	44	4.45	ns
Report writing, correspondence	11	12	16	32	17	39	25	21.85	<.001
Staff conferences	11	12	15	30	22	26	21	9.32	<.001

Professional Activities and Training Needs of Psychologists

It is appropriate to examine in greater detail the reported professional activities and training needs of the 211 psychologists in the sample. At least one reply from a psychologist was received from 51 of the 55 participating mental health centers, and the average number of replies by psychologists from each of these 51 centers was slightly over four. Of these replies 85% indicated that they were describing a typical work week. Mean number of hours spent in each of the 19 professional activities for psychologists has been shown in Table 2. In Table 4, additional information concerning how psychologists spend their time is provided. As can be seen, Table 4 contains information for each of the 19 professional activities as to modal, median, minimum, and maximum hours per week, and gives the 20th and 80th percentile on each distribution. That is, in the case of total clinical activities, for example, the median number of hours per week spent in this activity by psychologists is 17. Responses range from a minimum of zero hours to a maximum of 40, with 14 the most frequently reported number of hours per week. The bottom 20% of the respondents report 10 or less hours per week in total clinical activities; the top 20% report 24 or more hours per week in total clinical activities.

The positively skewed nature of the distribution of psychologists' activities can be seen in the fact that mean scores are almost always higher than median scores. In the case of total community activities, the mean number of hours per week reported by psychologists is 6.29; the median is 4.56. That is, the mean value is influenced by the relatively small number of psychologists who spend unusually large amounts of time in community activities. As can be seen in Table 4, the maximum number of hours per week reported by any psychologist in all community activities combined is 28, and the top 20% of psychologists spend only 11 hours or more per week in all community activities combined. In the case of crisis or emergency services, to cite another community mental health activity, the maximum number of hours reported by any psychologist is nine and the top 20% of respondents spend only two or more hours per week in this activity.

For people who look to the psychologist as the major contributor to research and program evaluation, the data are not reassuring. While the mean number of hours spent each week in research and evaluation activities is nearly two hours (itself not a very striking commitment), this figure is heavily influenced by the six responding psychologists who report spending 20 or more hours each week in these endeavors. The median figure is a mere 18 minutes per week! Of all psychologists responding, 63% report spending less than one hour each week in research and program evaluation activities. The data in Table 4 regarding psychologists serve to reinforce data presented in Table 2, which indicate that psychologists' activities in community mental health centers are not dramatically different from those reported by any other

TABLE 4 Professional activities of community mental health center psychologists in hours per week ($N = 211$)

Professional activity	Mini-mum	Maxi-mum	20th per-centile	Median	80th per-centile	Mode
Clinical diagnosis and assessment	0	20	0	2.42	5	0
Individual treatment	0	25	3	7.88	12	10
Family and group treatment	0	23	0	2.76	6	0
Crisis/emergency services	0	9	0	0.68	2	0
Deciding on hospitalization	0	4	0	0.10	0	0
Prescribing medication	0	0	0	0.00	0	0
Administering medication	0	1	0	0.01	0	0
Patient and ward management	0	40	0	0.05	0	0
Total clinical activities	0	40	10	17.00	24	14
Mental health consultation	0	22	0	1.63	4	0
Working with citizens	0	20	0	0.25	2	0
Mental health education	0	10	0	0.23	2	0
Aftercare	0	11	0	0.03	0	0
Home visiting	0	6	0	0.09	0	0
Interagency collaboration	0	10	0	0.42	2	0
Total community activities	0	28	1	4.56	11	0
Research and evaluation	0	32	0	0.30	2	0
Training and supervision	0	21	0	1.77	4	0
Administrative and program development	0	23	0	1.58	5	0
Report writing, correspondence	0	20	1	3.08	5	4
Staff conferences	0	16	1	2.89	5	2
Total administration	0	46	8	12.88	23	10
Other	0	4	0	0.01	0	0
Grand Total	3	59	38	39.98	41	40

professional group. Most of their time is spent in direct clinical service and in those activities associated with clinical services, e.g., report writing, staff conferences, and supervision.

More detailed examination of psychologists' expressed needs for additional training parallels the findings regarding their professional activities. The six topical areas that all respondents indicate as their areas of greatest need for additional training are identical to the top six areas identified by psychologists. The most commonly expressed needs are for the improvement of clinical skills, notably family and group therapy (67% of psychologists indicate some need for additional training in this area and 18% list it as among their greatest needs). Nearly half of psychologists mention the need for additional training in crisis and emergency services and in mental health consultation, and 8% indicate these needs to be among their most important. Expressed training needs consistently include skill building more often than theoretical understanding. Finally, psychologists are clearly interested in additional training in mental health administration and program planning. Nearly half of the respondents mention this need; 15% identify it as one of the areas of greatest need for additional training.

DISCUSSION

While a large number of significant differences have been found among occupational categories in how time is allocated in community mental health centers and in expressed needs for additional training, it would be well to note that these differences are often remarkably small in actual time units. That is, the differences are often statistically significant but programmatically unimportant, and they should not obscure what seem to be the two most important findings of this data analysis—the relatively small differences between how all of the six professional groups allocate their time during a typical week; and the fact that activities of community mental health center staff are similar to the generally held view of how mental health professionals spent their time before the advent of the community mental health movement. To illustrate the assertion that the obtained significant one-way ANOVA findings are of limited importance, calculation of omega squared for clinical diagnosis and assessment reveals that, in spite of the highly significant difference in time spent in this activity by profession, less than 7% of the variance is accounted for by professional identification. Traditional direct diagnosis and treatment services occupy nearly half of the work week. If one adds the activities indirectly associated with treatment activities, e.g., supervision, staff conferences, report writing, and correspondence, the amount of time spent on activities related to clinical work approaches 75% of the work week. Activities thought to be associated with the special emphases of the community mental health ideologies, such as crisis and emergency treatment, mental health consultation and education, working with community and citizen groups, and interagency collaboration, occupy less than seven hours each week in total, or less than 18% of the working week.

Three findings, however, document the impact of the community mental health movement on mental health center staff. First, the seven hours allocated each week to the activities associated with community mental health ideologies, while modest to many observers, undoubtedly represent far more time devoted to these activities than was the case a decade ago. Second, there is a substantial general interest in additional training both in theory and in skill building regarding community mental health-oriented activities, an interest that may be the harbinger of increased allocation of resources to these activities in the future. While more traditional areas of clinical service are associated with the highest levels of expressed needs for additional training (i.e., clinical diagnosis and assessment, individual treatment, and family and group treatment), the second echelon of topical areas for which additional training needs are recognized includes the two technologies most directly associated with the community mental health orientation, namely, crisis and emergency services and mental health consultation. Third, mental health centers have achieved one important objective, the utilization of community workers and other personnel outside of the traditional mental health disciplines. Staff with diverse skills are being afforded greater opportunities to address themselves to community needs.

The relatively modest differences in the professional activities being performed by psychiatrists, psychologists, nurses, and social workers confirm the observations of other investigators concerning the overlapping roles of mental health professionals (see, for example, Henry, 1971). As expected, only one function is unique, namely, prescribing medication, which is still the exclusive responsibility of the psychiatrist. Since all other functions are widely shared, perhaps it is again time to ask whether the present disciplinary boundaries are artificial and even dysfunctional. It may be time to reconsider the need for further experimentation with training programs for a generic mental health professional with diverse skills.

REFERENCES

Bass, R. D. *Consultation and education services: Federally funded community mental health centers, 1973* (Statistical Note 108, U.S. Department of Health, Education and Welfare Publication No. (ADM) 75-108). Washington, D.C.: U.S. Government Printing Office, 1974.

Bloom, B. L. *Community mental health: A historical and critical analysis.* Morristown, N.J.: General Learning Press, 1973.

Henry, W. *The fifth profession: Becoming a psychotherapist.* San Francisco: Jossey-Bass, 1971.

26 The Rhetoric and Some Views of Reality

Bernard L. Bloom

It is a rare opportunity to be able to step back and examine a number of independent studies whose findings converge on a single general question, in this case, the question of how training and practice in the fields of community psychology and community mental health mesh with its articulated ideologies. As this volume attests, the ideologies are fairly clear. They include a focus on the building of community competence as well as individual competence, on prevention rather than remediation, on less expensive and thus broadly available short-term crisis-oriented services rather than more expensive and less readily available long-term therapy, on enhancing the skills and effectiveness of social caregiving systems by the processes of consultation and education, and on an interest in community well-being in its least restrictive sense, including but by no means limited to mental health and mental illness. So much for the rhetoric.

These four studies describe the convergence of training and practice as of 1974–1975 in a cross-section of people identified in greater or lesser degree with the field of community psychology and community mental health. The primary conclusion that seems inescapable is that the orientation is generally toward the mental health end of the community psychology-community mental health continuum, and that the extent of this orientation is highly associated with seniority. While the ideologies of community psychology are most actively espoused by some of the senior leaders in the field, the group that appears to have been most influenced by these ideologies are graduate students. And perhaps this is as it should be.

Staff members in community mental health centers, including psychologists, continue to spend the bulk of their time in activities directly or indirectly related to clinical practice, and their interests in the development of additional skills are concentrated in clinical topics. Directors of graduate training programs in community psychology and community mental health continue to place major emphasis on the development of clinical skills and the use of clinical field settings. Members of the Division of Community Psychology of the American Psychological Association, while more involved in community psychology than are training program directors, work in mental health settings, come from clinical psychology training programs, identify very strongly with clinical practice and clinical concerns, and even though most describe themselves as involved in the field of community psychology, few have had any training in the area.

The clear exception is the graduate student. The students' views of the faculty are a reasonably accurate reflection of the faculty's self-description, namely, that they are often not greatly interested in significant departures from fairly traditional clinical training, and when they are, they are far more interested in community mental health than in community psychology. The graduate students see their future careers closely linked to community psychology and accordingly often find themselves dissatisfied with their academic training. They feel far better about the adequacy of their field experiences, even though it is often difficult to arrange for them.

It is clear, however, that the opportunities for graduate training in community psychology and mental health have increased dramatically in the past five years, but the primary emphases in this training are on the technologies of community mental health. Whether one discusses academically-based or field-based training, the concentration of effort is on the mental health service function; that is, on the development of consultation and crisis intervention skills and on strategies of program evaluation. Interest in conceptualization, theory building, and more basic empirical research appears to be lagging far behind. The obviously growing interest in mental health program evaluation raises the important problem of identifying the optimal degree of training necessary to carry out various community psychology-related tasks. It would not be difficult to argue, for example, that far less than PhD-level training is required to carry out technical program evaluations, however important such evaluations might be.

The emerging field of community psychology has not made a qualitative break with community mental health, with which it is still very strongly identified. The findings in these four studies provide converging evidence for this general conclusion. In the profession of psychology at large there is a growing interest in how environmental characteristics influence and are influenced by behavior. But there is little evidence that those people interested in what is often called environmental psychology or human ecology gravitate to those clusters of people already identified with community psychology. Rather, as a recent article in the *APA Monitor* suggests (1976), psychological researchers interested in environment and behavior see their intellectual home bases within the fields of engineering or population psychology. The continued identification of community psychology with community mental health and the relatively weak role of empirical research and conceptualization in the training and functioning of the community psychologist are at least partially responsible for the failure of the field of community psychology thus far to attract a broader constituency.

REFERENCES

"New breed" of psychologists study environment and behavior. *APA Monitor*, February 1976, p. 15.

VI PROBLEMS OF CONCERN TO THE COMMUNITY PSYCHOLOGISTS

INTRODUCTION

Charles D. Spielberger and Ira Iscoe

Early in the planning for the national conference it was recognized that it would not be possible to schedule time for discussion of all the important issues and topics that had been suggested from various sources. Therefore, to at least minimally accommodate as many of these topics as possible, the conference format included a general discussion session on issues and topics not otherwise considered. At this session, participants were given an opportunity to brainstorm, voice concerns, and offer suggestions. In the first part of Chapter 27, Bernard Lubin summarizes the main themes expressed in this free-wheeling session.

In convening the conference, the Executive Committee of Division 27 charged its Education and Training Committee with the primary responsibility for follow-up activities and implementation of conference recommendations. Immediately after the conference representatives of the Education and Training Committee met in Austin with the Conference Planning Committee to initiate follow-up activities. In the second part of Chapter 27, J. Robert Newbrough, chairman of the Education and Training Committee, reports on the organization of five task forces given responsibilities to follow up on a number of recommendations growing out of the conference.

The decision to report the proceedings of the Austin Conference in book form permitted the editors to invite participants to contribute brief position papers dealing with topics of special interest to them that were informally discussed but not considered in depth at the conference. These papers, reported in Chapters 28–32, reflect a variety of concerns. Some of the invited papers are central to community psychology, while others are germaine to the entire discipline of psychology because of their contemporary social significance. Several papers suggest new directions or approaches to training, research, and practice in community psychology, and provide a potential focus for future meetings and conferences.

Collectively, the papers in Part IV represent an inventory of issues and topics of concern to conference participants that were discussed only briefly and informally at the Austin Conference. Many of these issues are of central importance to American society and require thoughtful consideration by all psychologists working in community settings.

27 Unresolved Conference Issues and Future Plans

A. Issues Briefly Considered at the Conference

Bernard Lubin

As is the case at most conferences, time restraints limited the number of issues that could be discussed at the Austin meetings. To at least partially overcome the omission of potentially important areas of discussion, a session was held on "Issues Not Discussed at the Conference." The session was based on the fact that almost no psychological role requires as varied a set of skills as that of the community psychologist. The community psychologist has many opportunities, and is often expected, to convene various-sized groups for purposes of training, information sharing, data collection, organization, etc. Designing meetings in a way that will provide for participant needs, such as demonstration of competence, security, belonging, ownership, and impact, is important. Providing opportunities for participant input, in keeping with the value placed on client involvement in decision making by many community psychologists, also is important.

The session was designed to meet several objectives:

1. To discover unmet learning needs of the participants
2. To provide opportunities for all participants to make additional contributions to the total conference
3. To maximize the opportunity for participants to work with others whom they had not yet met
4. To provide a change of pace in the conference format
5. To begin to collect ideas about conference follow-up activities

To form discussion groups, participants were asked to count off by three from left to right in each row. Beginning on the left in the first row, the first three people were asked to turn and form a sextet with their counterparts in the second row; continuing left to right, the next three were asked to do the

I want to thank Ms. Bertha Shanblum for retrieving the items, Lynette Smith and William Rooney for assistance in categorizing the items, and all the participants who contributed their ideas.

same. The arrangement was repeated with each pair of rows so that the total group was quickly restructured into a large number of sextets.

For the first 10 minutes, the sextets were asked to get acquainted, then to (a) discuss how they felt about the conference at this point, (b) list the learning needs that had not yet been met, and (c) make suggestions they considered important to the conference or for the follow-up period. Each sextet was asked to appoint a reporter who, at the end of the period, came forward to read that group's list and write it on the slate board that extended across the large room. These opening activities were accompanied by intensive and sustained interest of all participants.

Participant comments were given in a large number of areas, which have been categorized under 11 headings. A summary of the comments, by category, follows.

CONFERENCE IN GENERAL

In this area comments were largely individual. There was concern about lack of closure, namely, "Where are we going?" There was concern that more participants had not done their preconference homework. And there was discussion of what had been gained and lost by not including community psychology workers (the "doers") and representatives of constituent communities at the conference.

OPENING INFORMAL COMMUNICATION

While most agreed that there was a need for more avenues of communication, the suggestions for achieving this were varied. They included: (1) an informal newsletter that would be distributed not only to Division 27 members but also to public concern groups; (2) workshops and other meetings to deal with ongoing problems close to home, rather than with long-range issues; (3) more time at conferences for airing conflicts and confronting concrete issues; (4) the development of informal communication networks through Division 27 channels; (5) continuing education, use of experts as resources, and other methods of transmitting experiential knowledge from established community psychologists to newcomers; and (6) research on dissemination and utilization processes to help the field reach more people.

SELF-ASSESSMENT OF COMMUNITY PSYCHOLOGY

Participants were in accord that there was a need for an assessment of community psychology—accomplishments, failures, lessons learned, and implications of these lessons. Such an assessment would include minority issues, short- and long-term planning and goals, and the move from a reactive to a proactive stance. Individual concerns centered on the lack of studies of the middle class, the focus on the lower class, the need to become more political, and the development of a rural community psychology to address the needs of a large percentage of Americans.

ROLES OF THE COMMUNITY PSYCHOLOGIST AND RELATIONSHIP OF COMMUNITY PSYCHOLOGY TO OTHER FIELDS

Apparently there is still some confusion about the difference between clinical and community psychology. Some participants noted a need to clarify the relationship of Division 27 to APA as a whole, of community to clinical psychology, and of Division 27 to SPSSI. Others were concerned that community psychologists are being spread too thin, which increases their lack of identity, and that they often do not model the ideals of community psychology. A need was expressed for parameters of the field as an occupation.

FINANCIAL AND POLITICAL SUPPORT BASES

As federal resources are becoming more limited, there is need to find new sources of financial support. More questions were asked than answers provided: Can we free people from embeddedness in systems by offering independent outside funds? How can we break out of the locked-in system we are now in? How can we increase NIMH support? There was debate over the idea of developing new models, in contrast to belief in continual monies that could be reallocated.

FORMAL TRAINING ISSUES AND SKILLS

There is a need to identify skills, to focus more on concrete skills than conceptual issues, to make effective use of traditional clinical skills as a means of entry into community settings and intervention processes, and to develop more political "savvy." There was some discussion about devoting more attention to the teaching process of community psychology itself.

UNIVERSITY TRAINING PROGRAMS

There was some concern that training programs should more accurately describe their orientations, and that PhD programs should deliver what they promise when attracting applicants. One way to assure meeting these concerns is for each department to provide honest information and direction to its own undergraduates. Need also was noted for improving the dissemination of information to undergraduates about graduate training programs in community psychology. From another aspect, participants discussed dealing with resistance to the evolution of community psychology programs by clinical programs, increasing faculty acceptance of community training so that students will not have to play dual roles, and providing mechanisms for the exchange of trainees between programs.

SPECIFIC TRAINING SUGGESTIONS

Suggestions focused on improving communications, with specific reference to a West Coast, a Northeast, and a Texas-Texas Tech consortium. There was a suggestion to implement reciprocal visits by students and faculty to nearby universities for a week or two during the summer, and one to develop a self-planning internship program.

UNIVERSITY/FORMAL TRAINING SUGGESTIONS

Needs were expressed for establishing interdisciplinary institutes, changing training policies, and taking a stand on the extent and types of nonuniversity involvement for trainees. Participants from the Connecticut area had already planned to implement an idea for a postconference activity that would capitalize on the conference experience. The plan involves an informal, student oriented, interuniversity conference consisting of a day-long workshop focusing on student presentations of their work. Faculty and advanced graduate students would serve as consultants. Informal and inexpensive, the conference is seen as a way of enriching individual training programs and a start to building crossuniversity collaboration.

VALUES AND ETHICS; OPENNESS
TO THE VALUES OF OTHERS

Values deemed important included the accountability of community psychologists for their research and experimentation in community settings, their responsibility for critically analyzing psychology's own testing movement, their relevance to minority concerns, and their awareness of women's roles in the field.

CROSSCULTURAL APPROACH

The differences in values across cultures should be recognized and respected. These differences include race, ethnic background, socioeconomic status, and geographic region.

PROFESSIONAL ISSUES

Issues on the minds of many community psychologists and graduate students include entry levels, defining competencies at each degree level, licensure and certification, and continuing education.

B. Preliminary Plans for the Implementation of Conference Recommendations

J. R. Newbrough

Implementation of the results of conferences does not usually happen in a very organized or systematic way. Training conferences have been for the purpose of mediating and consolidating forces within the discipline, and not for charting new directions (Lloyd & Newbrough, 1965). The Austin Conference is unique in the history of those sponsored by the American Psychological Association; it was developed by a division. This placed the deliberations closer to a membership group, and within an organization that could see to the follow-up. The Education and Training Committee of the division was assigned the responsibility for continuing work on issues deriving from the conference.

ALTERNATIVES FOR DIVISION 27

The APA Division of Community Psychology has functioned as a profession-oriented organization since its formation in 1966. Its concerns have been with knowledge, practice, and standards for training. In the establishment of any new speciality, it is understandable that the orientation will be inward (Newbrough, 1970). The Austin Conference gave one the sense that the discipline, now ten years old, does not have to continue the process of self-definition. It began to attend to matters that go beyond psychology, that take us into the larger society, and that concern themselves with future possibilities.

IMPLEMENTATION STRATEGIES

Following the conference, a day-long meeting of the Education and Training Committee was held just prior to the 1975 APA Meeting in Chicago. The committee proposed five task forces and a working group. These were approved by the Executive Committee and set to work in September 1975.

Task Force on Graduate Programs in Community Psychology

Conference participants recognized the long-standing problems that an applicant faces in knowing just what the graduate program offers and whether it actually provides the training that the person desires. This task force was created to address the matter of "truth in advertising" and to come up with a program description that will help the applicant properly evaluate programs.

A survey of programs was planned for 1976 that would provide a report for people applying for 1977. The task force was chaired by Meg Gerrard (University of Texas).

Task Force on Market Conditions and Production of Community Psychologists

It was noted at the conference by an NIMH psychologist that approximately 35,000 people were engaged in graduate study in psychology in the U.S.–far more than there would be jobs. While there was considerable interest in this, no data were available to help understand the situation. This task force was formed to gather information from the National Register on Scientific and Technical Personnel and as many other sources as possible to answer questions about how and whether the job markets would be saturated over the next 10-15 years. They were also to explore alternative jobs that might be done by psychologists but are not now classified as such. The task force was chaired by Suzanne Bachman (University of South Carolina). It was expected to take two to three years to report since the matter is complex and may need a special data collection.

Task Force on Continuing Education

Continuing education has become a requirement for continued licensing in a few states and appears to be a national trend affecting all the helping professions. The conference discussions noted the importance of this area and explored the possibilities of holding some workshops prior to the next APA convention. The task force was charged with organizing professional workshops for the regional and national conventions, and working with the larger APA in establishing record-keeping systems for giving participants documented credit when they request it. The task force was chaired by F. T. Miller (University of North Carolina).

Task Force Entry Levels: Masters Level Training

While the conference was oriented to doctoral training, there was a special interest topic group directed specifically at masters level training. The task force was established to explore the curricula and competencies available and to develop the rationale and details for an exemplary masters level training program. The importance that the Vail Conference gave to the masters holder as the "journeyman" was to be taken seriously and considered in detail.

The issue of master's level training attained major status when the Division of Clinical Psychology (12) and American Board of Professional Psychology issued a joint statement calling for a cessation of masters level training (*APA Monitor*, March 9, 1976). The task force met in the summer of

1976 with the Southern Region Education Board in Atlanta to begin the development of a position in support of such training. It was to be made public later that year, after processing through the division at the APA meetings. The task force was chaired by Steven Danish (Pennsylvania State University).

Task Force on Internships and Field Training

The conferees were very interested in field-based training and wished to explore this area in great detail. Many students were interested in alternatives to APA-approved clinical internships and wished to explore how some students had created their own. The task force put out a report on internships during late 1975. It was to be revised and improved for winter, 1976. Further, the task force was to begin discussing a national conference on field training—possibly to be the next APA-sponsored training conference. This task force was the largest and attracted the most member interest. It was cochaired by Judith Kramer (Red Bank Community Mental Health Center, New Jersey) and Edison Trickett (Yale University).

Working Group on the Development of a Notebook on Teaching Materials

A small group at the conference was very interested in sharing teaching and training resources that were found to be useful. A notebook was suggested as something to which new materials could be added easily and quickly. A working group was encouraged to develop this and to see if it could be informally distributed in the division. Martha Katheryn Key (Tennessee Department of Mental Health/Mental Retardation) was the chairperson.

These six efforts were expected to provide the structure for pursuing many of the immediate concerns in the division. At the same time, it was recognized that there were social processes that might be considered in formulating longer term goals for community psychology.

LONG-TERM MATTERS

Several areas of social change were identified at the Austin Conference, and at the APA meetings in Chicago, that could provide opportunities for the division.

1. The local community was recognized as a social structure that badly needs study, support, and development in America. Many social policies are destructive to citizen participation and sense of community. Future alternatives for the locality and for service delivery to the residents need to be generated so that planful development can take place. Research and development into alternative futures might be a fruitful avenue for community psychology to pursue.

2. The impacts of federal legislation and programs on the locality—the family, the neighborhood, the municipality—need sustained research. Further, a legislative reference service on "community impacts" could be very important in influencing future legislation at local, county, and state levels. This is an area where the social indicators movement becomes very relevant in emphasizing a long-term monitoring approach to community change research.

3. Community psychology has often seemed to identify with the needs and welfare of the general community citizen—the "interest" in the local political process that does not seem to be very well represented. Citizen advocacy and ombudsman programs have exemplified the interest in this area. At the conference, it was suggested that the division develop a Ralph Nader-like organization that would be consumer-oriented and concerned with producing responsive government. One idea was to do research for groups like Common Cause, at the national level.

4. Some conferees noted that community psychologists are usually not very knowledgeable about theories of community and are usually concerned with service delivery in the context of the local community. Alternative theories, including radical analyses, might become the topic of a task force trying to generate theories that build human resources, hold down real costs, and conserve nonrenewable energy.

Community psychology was described at the conference as a problem-oriented profession that was not particularly concerned with disciplinary boundaries. While this may be generally true, the division has not been very active in promoting the interdisciplinary character of it. On the basis of this, the division was urged to provide participation for nonpsychologists and to establish direct working relationships with such fields as sociology, community development, political science, education, divinity, and law.

OCCUPATIONAL IMPLICATIONS

As social needs change and new forms of service delivery are developed, community psychologists may have an opportunity to take on new types of jobs. The following jobs are some examples.

1. *Technical assistance.* The Bureau of Education to the Handicapped funded several years ago a technical assistance center to help local programs get organized, relate appropriately to the local community and state developmental disabilities councils, and evaluate their programs.

2. *Technology transfer.* The National Science Foundation has a program, through Public Technology, Inc., that assigns an Urban Technology Agent to the mayor's office in 27 cities. The agent's job is to identify problems in the city for which new technology and technical resources are needed.

3. *Worker retraining.* The President's Council on Productivity has estimated that a substantial proportion of the work force will soon be displaced by industrial modernization and will need to be retrained (and perhaps relocated).

4. *Service delivery improvement.* Project Re-Ed found it necessary to invent a new professional role, Liaison-Teacher-Counselor. The job involved work with families, schools, and local agencies to ensure that services were properly delivered to families who found it impossible to obtain comprehensive services for their children (Hobbs, 1975). Liaison work is an indirect (secondary) service role familiar to many community psychologists.

5. *Community development.* The Housing and Community Development Act of 1974 provides for substantial citizen involvement in housing and community problem-solving programs. Planning, participation, and evaluation are needs that many localities must face if they wish to participate in the federal revenue sharing programs. The community school movement is becoming a means for participation of community psychologists (Newbrough, 1976). It represents a social form that is familiar to many Americans and should be especially useful in rural settings (Minsey & LeTarte, 1972). The community school can serve as a focus of neighborhood activity and an organized way of obtaining broad-scale citizen involvement. There are training grant funds provided in both the Housing and Community Development Act and the Community Education Act. These might enable community psychologists to get into this area in substantial ways.

These examples initiate speculation about the types of positions that could be trained for. Community psychologists have techniques and theories that could be applicable to these developing areas. Training programs might do well to try some new experimental training approaches.

The general implication of this chapter is that the Division of Community Psychology has the possibility of a wide and varied agenda of activities for its work for the next five years. It could become a nationally important group should it choose to grapple with basic issues concerning local communities and local families. By being attentive to social trends, it can transform itself internally, and perhaps, through this, the whole of psychology (Murphy, 1969).

REFERENCES

Hobbs, N. *The futures of children.* San Francisco: Jossey-Bass, 1975.

Lloyd, D. N., & Newbrough, J. R. Previous conferences on graduate education in psychology: A summary and review. In B. Lubin, & E. E. Levitt (Eds.), *The clinical psychologist: Readings on background, roles and functions.* Chicago: Aldine, 1965.

Minsey, J. D., & LeTarte, C. *Community education: From program to process.* Midland, Mich.: Pendell Press, 1972.

Murphy, G. Psychology in the year 2000. *American Psychologist,* 1969, *24,* 523–530.

Newbrough, J. R. Community psychology: A new specialty in psychology? In D. Adelson & B. L. Kalis (Eds.). *Community psychology: Perspectives on community mental health.* San Francisco: Chandler, 1970.

Newbrough, J. R. Editorial opinion: The community school and community education. *Journal of Community Psychology,* 1976, *4,* 209–210.

28 Social Change and Community Psychology

Thom Moore

"And why beholdest thou the mote that is in thy brother's eye, but considerest not the beam that is in thine own eye?" (Matthew 7:3)

In April 1975, Division 27 of APA sponsored a National Training Conference on Community Psychology at the University of Texas in Austin. On official and unofficial levels, the conferees reaffirmed a commitment, as community psychologists, to devote themselves to the enchancement of life through the study of and intervention in communities. The spirit of this commitment recognized both the demands of the professional standards of psychology and the responsibility that professionals have to the society. The model that most nearly represents this spirit is Fairweather's Experimental Social Innovations, in which the professional (either practitioner or researcher) employs an empirical approach to the conception and implementation of changes in social system (Fairweather, 1967; Fairweather, 1972; Fairweather, Sanders, & Tornatzky, 1974). Thus, data-based theories are developed, and application of psychological principles is accomplished.

CONCERNS OF BLACK PSYCHOLOGISTS

Few of those present disagreed with the fundamental definition of community psychology, although several had some concern regarding the actual implementation of the concept. More specifically, a contingent of black psychologists expressed concerns about certain communities, to the exclusion of others, targeted for intervention. From conversations with white community psychologists particularly, it became clear that there exists a misunderstanding between them and black community psychologists as to the functional concept of communities.

Black psychologists concluded from references made and examples given at the conference that communities were being defined along socioeconomic and racial lines, and that the focus of the community psychologist's intervention was on poor and black geographic locations. Black community psychologists voiced strong opposition to this position, claiming that

The author would like to acknowledge the contributions of Ernest R. Myers, K. E. Renner, Dalmas Taylor, David Terrell, and Henry Tomes. Without their continued support and guidance this paper would not have been completed.

considerable interest should be directed toward affluent white communities. White community psychologists at the same training conference interpreted the definition of communities to refer to small, self-contained units such as various social and institutional settings. However, socioeconomic and racial variables were viewed as subclasses. Furthermore, they stressed the social structure and its impact on service recipients in schools, hospitals, industrial organizations, social service systems, etc.

These two interpretations exemplify the serious problems that persist between blacks and whites in general and contribute to the ambivalence that blacks have about the goals and effectiveness of community psychology. The uppermost concern in the minds of black psychologists is white researchers in Afro-American communities. For obvious reasons the outcome of such an effort is at best questionable. The most glaring examples of destructive social science research and its relationship to blacks are those of Arthur Jensen (1969) and Daniel P. Moynihan (1965). Each has succeeded in portraying black America in a negative light. Herzog (1971) says, "It is time to shift our research light away from the poor and the black, who have begun to resent and resist unremitting service as study targets. More appropriate research subjects are groups and institutions that are in a position to obstruct or to tolerate needed change" (p. 4). While research has had its detrimental effects on black and other minority Americans, it is also clear that it can be useful. Given the level of technological development in today's society, survival and progress depend on research sophistication and equal access to information. Minority groups must begin an active critical review of research as it affects them.

While the basic commitment of community psychologists clearly referred to "communities" without categorizing them, it was apparent that black, minority, and poor communities would serve as primary targets for a substantial proportion of the envisioned work. The constant referral to these settings as a place for "us" (community psychologists) to do "our thing" implied that there is something wrong with these communities and that our involvement in them will facilitate constructive and positive changes. Although a systematic study of communities may in fact be beneficial to community residents, as proposed it represented an attitude of intervention by the expert professional directing change strategies for others. It is just this attitude against which black community psychologists react. Much of the opposition is supported by the results of the Joint Commission report (1961), the Community Mental Health movement, and various social action involvements by psychologists. Each one of these events supported, among other things, the notion that in many cases the long-term community residents could better deliver human services than could the nonresident professional.

Since that time there has been a proliferation of nonprofessional/ indigenous worker programs. Reiff and Riessman (1965) describe the unique aspects of the indigenous nonprofessional in a poverty program. They claim that such nonprofessionals have their own methods for dealing with poverty and that they are often of more concrete assistance than middle-class professionals. There is a growing recognition that research and program development must be a joint effort. Those who are objects of the intervention must participate in its design and operation. Furthermore, instead of being the overseer, the social scientist must become a participant-observer (Sommer, 1973; Gaulet, 1971; Gordon, 1973).

The fact that the discipline of community psychology is still young and pliable is encouraging. Inherent in community psychology is the absence of data-based theories, for it has primarily been an applied force reacting to social issues. Although there have been 10 years of knowledge building, the field has witnessed only minimal attempts to solidify the material (Cowen, 1973; Murrell, 1973; Zax & Specter, 1974). During this time the role of values has received considerable mention, and it continued to be a focal point at the conference. Community psychologists have recognized that the form and content of a particular science are greatly determined by a set of personal, professional, and scholarly values. In the world of scientific research, empirical data are treated as though they maintain a value-free position. Gergen (1973), in describing research in social psychology as a reflection of history, states,

We are well aware of the biasing effects of strong value commitments. On the other hand, as socialized human beings, we harbor numerous values about the reaction of social relations. It is the rare social psychologist whose values do not influence the subject of his research, his methods of observation, or the terms of his descriptions. (p. 311)

Robert Williams (Note 1), in a recent presentation to black students, specified that personal and professional values are significant in the selection of a research topic throughout the many disciplines of psychology. This realization is of particular importance for black Americans. More specifically, Williams noted that researchers cannot help but be influenced by their own sets of values.

Williams' and Gergens' comments have been preceded by comments from black leaders for years. They have implied that values held by whites directly influence their behavior toward blacks. Carmichael and Hamilton (1967), therefore, in describing Black Power, indicate that change in the black community must follow directions identified by blacks. Change identified by whites will be based on their perception of what *they* want for blacks, which over time will not serve a black interest. An example of this phenomenon more relevant for psychologists is given by White (1970) as he makes a case for a black psychology. Explaining the process occurring in an encounter group between blacks and whites, he says, "One of the primary reasons why interracial group sensitivity encounters often fail to make adequate progress may be due to the fact that black people and white people have different priorities, expectations, and ways of viewing the world and life styles." His implications here are that people hold values that affect their perception of things around them, and because of this it is difficult for those in conflict to be sensitive to each others' needs.

Thus, the philosophies of social psychology, Black Power, and black psychology hold special insight for black psychologists. In particular, they suggest that blacks must be acutely aware of the role that human values play in the social sciences. Wherever the goal is to effect changes within the lives of Afro-Americans, a demand must be made that the motivations and values underlying the proposed change be articulated. One need not look or think hard about psychology to understand the reasons for this position.

It is not uncommon for Afro-Americans to be the audience for high sounding moral and human-oriented ideas, but rarely have they been the recipients of the proposed outcomes. In the larger society there have been promises of freedom from slavery, resources (economic and natural) to begin an independent self-supporting life, and repeated reassurances that equality in American life was soon to be achieved.

Likewise, throughout the history of psychology in America numerous concepts and techniques have been developed and couched in humanistic statements that point the way to equality, democracy, and a better life for all. For some reason the mechanisms developed never quite reached the stated goals. For example, the development of IQ tests to insure that children would receive appropriate education led to the establishment of sophisticated classification systems and corresponding educational methods (Kamin, 1974). By and large these have proven detrimental to Afro-Americans (Hobbs, 1975). On the government scene, scores of psychologists during the Lyndon B. Johnson War on Poverty, each with his or her speciality, promised to contribute to the eradication of poverty. Many of today's community psychologists were among this group. Clark and Hopkins (1968) stated that after six years of operation, programs initiated under this philosophy did little, if anything, to alleviate the social problem of poverty. In retrospect, these and other programs have been presented as mechanisms for individual and social improvement; they held out promises to millions of minority people, and at their overall best they have had only token effect.

As black psychologists hear the community psychology struggle to "do something different and be more relevant," they see old patterns developing and know that if these patterns are allowed to go unchecked, they will result in questionable futures for their brothers and sisters. Herein lies the dual responsibility of black professional psychologists. They must strive to develop concepts and add knowledge to the field of psychology that more accurately describes human behavior, while at the same time they must ensure that concepts do not become obstacles to the growth of black Americans. At times this requires them to be watchdogs of science while actively bringing new perspectives to the field. In the case of community psychology, the black participant feels that the goals of social change and the techniques of social action are much too distant and vague.

The zest and zeal of the Austin Conference carried the participants' thoughts and designs into areas that offered more glamour for applied psychologists than did other, more traditional areas. They began to envision themselves in the larger social system (government, law, economics, education, etc.), able to direct changes for masses of people. They failed to see that these were areas in which they presently have little control. To better understand the problem created by their vision, a definition of a *system* is in order. Buckley (1967) describes a system

generally as a complex of elements or components directly or indirectly related to a causal network, such that each component is related to at least some others in a more or less stable way within a particular period of time.

In other words, larger systems are collections of interrelated components. Change efforts would result in more effective outcomes if initial intervention steps included an extensive description of the system. The rationale for this procedure is related to the need to build a knowledge base. Community psychology must reason its intervention methods and understand that systems will not be changed in their totality unless each component is likewise changed.

Ira Goldenberg's (1974) address concerning the relationship of the university to the community is pertinent to the present discussion. He suggested: It is time we (community psychologists) begin to make some crucial decisions about ourselves, our own setting, our own aspirations, and our own willingness to reorder what have already become traditional community psychology and community mental health programs. He believes that this has specific implications for community psychology; one is "that we commit ourselves to studying, understanding and changing our own settings (i.e., the University) and to accepting the risks that will invariably follow all such attempts" (p. 173).

This is exactly the position that we as black psychologists take. Community psychology must change community psychology.

A PROPOSED PLAN FOR REDIRECTING COMMUNITY PSYCHOLOGY

The above-stated goal does not place the broader goals of community change in a secondary role, but it does say that a double focus is needed. Following a long tradition of requests (Meyers, Note 2) and proposals (Smith, 1973; Williams, 1974) to APA, it is proposed that Division 27 adopt as a project the following plan, which is geared to developing community psychology into a study area that will enhance life through study of and intervention within its own community.

The proposed plan grew out of black psychologists' concern about research innovation and change designed by whites for blacks and minorities. This is an old issue and one that appears in various disciplines including psychology. As black people view the sciences, they see their value weighing heavily as a political tool to be used against them (Gordon, 1973). Therefore, the objection to the position of community psychology was that concepts about all minorities and strategies to change their lives were developed without ever consulting them. Given this, it seemed only logical to request that minority representation[1] be built into Division 27 at all levels. On further consideration it became clear that this was only part of the problem. The appointment of a minority member as the solution represents secondary prevention. Therefore, consideration was given to a plan that would have a long-term effect and could be viewed as primary prevention. The key to the following plan is minority student recruitment.

Proposed Plan

I. Minority recruitments and admissions
   A. Undergraduate
   B. Graduate

II. Program development
   A. Creation of minority-oriented training within minority institutions
   B. Establishment of field settings
      1. Practicum
      2. Internship

III. Minority representation
   A. APA
   B. Division 27
   C. Faculty
   D. Practicum

Following considerable discussion, the issue of minority representation in Division 27 gave way to the more pressing problem of minority representation among graduate students. This was targeted as an area of concern because a sustained involvement on the part of minority psychologists is related to the number of potential participants, and an increase in the student population would increase the availability pool. In a recent survey of black PhDs in America, Mommsen (1974) identified 166 living blacks holding PhDs in psychology and reported that "Blacks hold less than 1% of America's earned

---

[1] *Representation* in this sense has two components. Minorities would represent the viewpoint of their own communities, and this will be based more on political principles than on psychological principles. On a different level minorities, will deal with the psychology behind programs, intervention, and decisions.

doctoral degrees" (p. 253). Further, he projected that the future does not appear much brighter. He based this belief on data presented by Crossland (1968), who found that the proportion of blacks in America's graduate schools of arts and sciences was only 1.7%. He estimated that at best this would add 200 new black PhDs to the existing pool. Remember, this 200 is in all the arts and sciences fields. More specific to minorities and psychology, Padilla, Boxley, and Wagner (1973) report that although minorities (American Indian, Black, Chicano, Filipino, Japanese, Puerto Rican) represented 16.2% of the United States' population in 1972, they represented only 7.3% (348) of the total student population in doctoral-level clinical programs. The situation was even more glaring for faculty members. Minorities represented 3.3% (41) of faculties of doctoral-level clinical psychology programs. Regardless of which set of data one accepts, the overall picture of minority members currently holding or seeking PhDs is gloomy.

At the same time, we must not lose sight of the fact that minority students offer more to a program than just their presence. By virtue of life experiences, minority students bring a different perspective to the research and applied sciences. They bring with them a challenge to long-standing theories of human behavior. For community psychology, new thoughts and techniques are needed. Therefore, sound reasons for developing a strong minority recruitment program exist.

The second step in the plan is to encourage the development of graduate training programs at minority universities and community facilities. In the case of black people, there is no better place to begin such a process than at predominately black universities and colleges. At this time a black student wanting experience at the graduate level is limited to two such institutions. The primary problem is the identification and acquisition of financial, physical, and human resources. In addition to the establishment of new programs at predominately black institutions, training experience in existing predominately white insitutions needs modification. Rappaport, Davidson, Wilson, and Mitchell (1975) have described a concept and the process for creating a new setting to which minority students can relate. These settings can then serve as practicum and internship placements. Successful development of such a plan will demonstrate that community psychology is willing to accept challenges and that it possesses the knowledge and resources to bring about a change in its own operation.

The final step in the plan comes back to the original concern of minority representation in Division 27. The immediate solution to this problem is, in fact, the inclusion of minority members in the general operations of the division. But this is clearly a stop-gap measure and not an acceptable response to the present request. A better intermediate step involves some procedure that will insure that minority representatives will always be included. The proposed plan presents a more natural way of dealing with the problem by providing for a large pool of individuals who will, because of their own professional interest and actual functional roles, become part of Division 27.

Once admitted to various community programs, and having the opportunity to select relevant training experiences, they will be willing to invest themselves in the maintenance and growth of the division, and in this way they also will contribute representation in the sense of the psychological validity of the enterprise.

EFFECTING THE PLAN

In this manner the field of community psychology is more apt to realize its goals of devotion to the enhancement of life "through study of and intervention in communities." First of all, the present university system would require a structural change if more minority students were to be recruited and admitted to psychology programs. The same is true of developing minority-oriented training programs. For example, establishing PhD psychology programs at minority universities entails a financial commitment from current funding agencies. Success in these two areas would be a substantial social change. Second, minority students are likely to have an expansive effect on concepts and intervention in communities and other areas of psychology. Even if these students are molded to think and act like the present group of educators, once left to pursue their own interests the interaction between their training and years of life experiences will influence their professional activity. Finally, these students become cultural carriers. In other words, they begin to teach and spread the concepts and practices of community psychology. In this fashion, it can be expected that the radiating effects would be observed in various institutions.

Advocates of community psychology can take small concrete steps toward the realization of the goal of enhancing life through the study of and intervention in communities. Success cannot be judged only on the minority student as a product. In other words, just being a minority student with an advanced degree will not result in the creation of appropriate theories, methods, and intervention. The true test is in the willingness of training programs to change. If the values and expectations of the training faculty prevent them from incorporating the expected differences of minority students, then there will be little, if any, difference in the kind of student coming from such a program. On the other hand, faculty eager to challenge their own ideas and engage students and each other in honest rigorous exchange are likely to train students who think more creatively. Still further, those faculty who not only challenge their theories but also are willing to do things differently will clearly produce nontraditional students. It is important that the lines of socialization influence both participants.

Frankly, the concentration of effort in this limited area holds as much promise for community psychology as does involvement in the big arena.

REFERENCE NOTES

1. Williams, R. Personal communication, November 13, 1975.
2. Myers, E. R. *Black perspectives of community psychology.* Paper presented at the convention of the American Psychological Association, Washington, D.C., September 1971.

REFERENCES

Buckley, W. *Sociology and modern systems theory.* Englewood Cliffs, N.J.: Prentice-Hall, 1967.

Carmichael, S., & Hamilton, C. V. *Black power: The politics of liberation in America.* New York: Vintage Books, 1967.

Clark, K. B., & Hopkins, J. *A relevant war against poverty: A study of community action program and observable social change.* New York: Harper & Row, 1968.

Cowen, E. L. Social and community interventions. *Annual Review of Psychology,* 1973, *24*, 423–472.

Crossland, F. E. *Graduate education and black Americans.* New York: Ford Foundation, 1968.

Fairweather, G. W. *Methods for experimental social innovations.* New York: Wiley, 1957.

Fairweather, G. W. *Social change: The challenge to survival.* Morristown, N.J.: 1972.

Fairweather, G. W., Sanders, D. H., & Tornatzky, L. G. *Creating change in mental health organizations.* New York: Permagon, 1974.

Gaulet, D. An ethical model for the study of values. *Harvard Educational Review,* 1971, *41*, 205–227.

Gergen, K. J. Social psychology as history. *Journal of Personality and Social Psychology,* 1973, *26*, 309–320.

Goldenberg, I. The relationship of the university to the community: Implication for community mental health programs. In H. E. Mitchell (Ed.), *The university and the urban crisis.* New York: Behavioral Publications, 1974.

Gordon, T. Notes on white and black psychology. *Journal of Social Issues,* 1973, *29*, 87–95.

Herzog, E. Who should be studied. *American Journal of Orthopsychiatry,* 1971, *41*, 4–12.

Hobbs, N. *The futures of children.* San Francisco: Jossey-Bass, 1975.

Jensen, A. R. How much can we boast IQ and scholastic achievement? *Harvard Educational Review,* 1969, *39*, 1–123.

Kamin, L. J. *The science and politics of I.Q.* New York: Wiley, 1974.

Mommsen, K. G. Black Ph.D.s in the academic marketplace. *Journal of Higher Education,* 1974, *45*, 253–267.

Moynihan, D. P. The negro family: The case for national action. Washington, D.C.: U.S. Department of Labor, 1965.

Murrell, S. A. *Community psychology and social systems: A conceptual framework and intervention guide.* New York: Behavioral Publications, 1973.

Padilla, E. R., Boxley, R., & Wagner, N. L. The desegregation of clinical psychology training. *Professional Psychology,* 1973, *4,* 259–264.

Rappaport, J., Davidson, W. S., Wilson, M. N., & Mitchell, A. Alternatives to blaming the victim or the environment. *American Psychologist,* 1975, *30,* 525–528.

Reiff, R., & Riessman, F. The indigenous nonprofessional: A strategy of change in community action and community mental health programs. *Community Mental Health Journal,* Monograph No. 1, 1965.

Smith, P. M., Jr. Black psychologist as a change agent in the black community. *Journal of Black Studies,* 1973, *4,* 41–51.

Sommer, R. Evaluation yes; Research maybe. *Representative Research in Social Psychology,* 1973, *4,* 127–133.

White, J. Toward a black psychology. *Ebony,* September 1970, *25,* 44–45; 48–50; 52.

Williams, R. A history of the association of black psychologists: Early formation and development. *The Journal of Black Psychology,* 1974, *1,* 9–24.

Zax, M., & Specter, G. A. *An introduction to community psychology.* New York: Wiley, 1974.

29 Minority Groups, Women, and Students

A. Community Psychology and Racism

Ernest R. Myers and Henry Pitts

Some of the white participants at the National Training Conference on Community Psychology held in Austin, Texas, in April 1975, expressed "discomfort" in their involvements in the black community in spite of a sense of being effective. Clearly, outsiders must be both consciously aware of their feelings and motives and honest with the community clientele as to the intent of their actions. Yet, these issues arise: What is the nature of this discomfort? Do such feelings have a negative impact on the effectiveness of service? Can one feel uneasy in body and mind and not express this in ways that influence effective service delivery?

Today the missionary mind-set of yesterday's white "savior" in the American black ghetto is as obsolete as colonial rule in the black independent nations of Africa. A more individual kind of social change confronts the field of community psychology in terms of social and professional values and psychological readiness of its members.

HISTORICAL IMPACTS

Unfortunately, a great number of community psychology's younger "new guard" entered this evoling field at a time when the aura of law and order was surpassed only by the "benign neglect" mentality monopolizing national policies and priorities following the 1968 presidential election (several years after Division 27 arose in the American Psychological Association). The marketability of social change is influenced by the status of the appeal of innovation or new ideas for action. Consider the status of the "New Frontier" or the "Great Society" versus the "Watergate Administration."

Massacres at colleges like Jackson State and Kent State by the National Guard conveyed a compelling message to blacks and whites alike, while the "silent majority" theme spread to reinforce the notion that such action was in the public interest. Significantly, these events exemplified the new law and order edict and confronted radical liberalism. The Swampscott Conference, out of which community psychology emerged, came on the heels of the liberal administrations of JFK and LBJ, the March on Washington, and so on.

Division 27's membership, then, since 1968, has come about without the psychological and moral support of the progressive national mood characteristic of the pre-Nixon, or Great Society, era. Hence, these aspiring "agents of change" have necessarily been influenced by historical and political developments that have infused an apathetic spirit into many would-be change agent converts. Ambivalence has since appeared to characterize both APA's and community psychology's stances relative to social change and social action in urban America.

SOCIAL CHANGE WITHIN

Many of the conferees at Austin expressed difficulties with and incomprehension of the social change process and its diverse nature and methodology. To some extent it appears that this difficulty is because we are prone to deny that "we" are an essential part of the very system in need of change. The "we" and "they" dichotomy has introduced a blind spot. We, in fact, may be the primary target for the system's intervention rhetoric professed in community psychology circles. Reiff's model of intervention provides some clarity to the scope of the social change process. However, for community psychology to embrace a paradigm that institutional change is possible in the stark absence of individual (dispositional) behavioral changes, is to deny the organismic reality of the systems concept. Individuals make up the situational (group and environmental) context, and the situational variables are the basis for institutional arrangements. Thus, to change the system is to change its elements or parts, even though this does not necessarily guarantee changes in the whole system.

Bill Moyers, a former aide to the late President Johnson, notes that since 1971 the national mood has changed from antagonism to resignation. "I vacillate between the determination to change society and the desire to retreat into the snuggeries of myself and my family," he has said (p. 12). According to Moyers, Americans must be aware of their tendency toward defeatism or the nothing-can-be-done mind-set (as reported in the May 11, 1975 *Parade* magazine).

A CHALLENGE WITHIN

It was conspicuously observed by black participants at the Austin Conference that the topic of racism was not addressed. Further, this issue was not programmed into the agenda of conference topics even though clearly it remains a major mental health problem in America. Was not racism a target recommended by the late Rev. Martin Luther King, Jr. in 1968 when he addressed the American Psychological Association's conference? Again, was not that the era when community psychology became a division in APA? And the question must be raised: How far has the field of psychology come since then to attack this problem in human behavior? Does community psychology have a unique responsibility to address itself to such issues, or are such issues considered academic and outside the purview of this new thrust in the profession by its leadership?

The absence of discussion on racism at the Austin Conference in great part resulted from extremely abstract levels at which vital topics were generally discussed, that is: community, social structure, ideology, values, goals, and objectives. Thus, the community psychology training models formulated prior to the conference as part of the preconference materials for the conferees suffered from many overlapping abstractions that continue to beg the questions: What communities (laboratories?) are we talking about? What social structures are in need of change? What should or do we as community psychologists really believe in? What are appropriate goals for community psychology thrusts in the 1970s and beyond? These questions cannot be dealt with in the abstract. We must call it as we see it. Indeed, we must see it first and be courageous enough to acknowledge this vision: Racial antipathy and racism remain among America's most complex problems. And it has been observed that racism is perhaps the nation's greatest challenge as we emerge from the Bicentennial year.

The conference participants were repeatedly exhorted by the leadership to avoid getting "mired down in concrete problems," and instead to focus on the level of "general directions of growth of the profession." We were directed to concentrate on models for community psychology training and discouraged from explorations into concrete problems of training. Such an approach to model building is somewhat analogous to a construction procedure in which the builder chooses to focus on the roof and neglects detailed design specifications for the foundation requirements.

It is our view that appropriate, effective dialogue about a problem is advanced by concrete articulation of the natural causes and incidence of the phenomena. While *community* and *psychology* are somewhat abstract concepts, the study of these concepts at the conference would have gained focus by fuller examination of concrete issues relevant to the quality of life of various community populations in political, economical, and sociopsychological terms. This "roots" oriented approach to model development, based on problem definition, may have found the conference participants acknowledging that the typical community in America is essentially an urban-suburban contrast. Consequently, certain fundamental realities about community population characteristics come in to view: the continued exodus of white homeowners from the deteriorating urban areas, and critical "urban crisis" issues such as inadequate revenues, health services, and public education, to name a few.

The evolving practice of community psychology has developed within an urban framework, the "turf" of 80% of the nation's black population. Hence, not only should we concern ourselves with this reality but also with its implications for training and practice of the "art."

SUGGESTED CHANGES

A significant perspective of community psychology training should include a focus on institutionalized exploitation and oppression. At the Austin Conference, Reiff made a strong point of stressing the need for community psychology to face up to the realities of the "exploitive society" element in the character of America.

Following are some suggested areas of content for training.

1. The use and abuse of power in political, economic, and psychological terms. Racism and sexism are targets in this regard.
2. The methodology and techniques in therapy and counseling that support or combat racism and oppression, particularly as these conditions are perceived as community problems.
3. The development of social policies affecting community health, such as the methadone maintenance movement and its implications for the health of black urban areas. Other areas would be housing and education.
4. The influence of mass communications media in the institutionalization of racism, especially television and the movie industry.
5. The abuse of psychological research in support of racist notions about human intelligence, a notorious reputation of the psychology profession promulgated by some select "experts" of genetic deterministic persuasion.
6. The dynamics of power in terms of social system structures, both public and private.

A primary commitment of community psychology should also be the development of interaction strategies contributing to the eradication of racist attitudes, practices, and policies pertaining to the cited issues.

Community psychology is "out of touch" if its definition of goals, training content, recruitment and selection of trainees, and techniques and levels of interventions are not predicated on an acceptance of the realities of the colonized nature of the "black community" and its struggle against institutional racism. This struggle is essentially a social change process. The development of social change agents should, therefore, be a major emphasis for community psychology training.

REFERENCE

Special intelligence report. *Parade,* May 11, 1975, p. 12.

B. Community Psychology for Hispanos

Manuel Ramirez III

The concepts, theories, and testing instruments of traditional psychology have contributed to the view of Hispanos as having a culture inferior to that of the mainstream American middle-class, one that interferes with the psychological development of children. The community psychology movement offers the hope that psychology will view cultural differences as legitimate, give greater opportunity for Hispanos to become members of the profession, and in general help make cultural democracy a reality. This chapter reviews some of the problems fostered by the orientations and approaches of traditional psychology and indicates how changes are being attempted through opportunities offered by community psychology.

TRADITIONAL PSYCHOLOGY: ANGLO CONFORMITY

Traditional psychology reflects the Anglo-Western European world view. The theories, concepts, and instruments developed by traditional psychology have been used to devise and evaluate educational and mental health programs that have as a primary goal, explicitly or otherwise, forcing Hispanos to accept the values and life styles of the mainstream American middle-class. For example, standardized intelligence and achievement tests have been used to place Hispanos most closely identified with their culture in classes for the mentally retarded or in "tracks" that are unlikely to prepare students for a college education. Concepts such as locus of control, delay of gratification, and achievement motivation have been used to construct educational programs to acculturate Hispano children. Psychoanalytic theory, Piagetian theory, and concepts of behavior modification also have been used to explain the psychodynamics of Hispanos, usually in terms of what is considered to be pathology, and to develop treatment and educational programs that attempt to correct this pathology. Again, Hispano culture is viewed as a source of conflict and as a block to development.

Traditional psychology has encouraged the Anglo conformity view of acculturation and has provided the conceptual frameworks and techniques to develop educational and mental health programs to make this acculturation more effective and more rapid. Traditional psychology also has led to the assumption that since the culture of Hispanos is inferior and is potentially pathological, there is no need to train people to understand the sociocultural system or to offer services to Hispanos from the perspective of the world view that emanates from their sociocultural system. Hispanos, then, have been forced to accept the particular approaches, techniques, and instruments that have been developed by traditional psychology, and to accommodate themselves to the particular perspectives of the psychologists and the paraprofessionals trained in these concepts. Little attempt has been made to respond and be sensitive to the particular orientation and perspective of the Hispano who seeks treatment or serves as the subject for psychological research. Similarly, those Hispanos who have sought to become members of the psychological profession have had to accept the mainstream American middle-class orientation reflected in many graduate and undergraduate training programs in psychology and programs to train paraprofessionals. Traditional psychology has reached the conclusion that what is good for the Anglo mainstream is good for people of all cultural groups.

From another perspective, the only "problem" with Hispanos and members of other cultural groups is their unfamilarity with mainstream American culture. The object of so-called compensatory and intervention programs is to acquaint culturally "disadvantaged" persons with the sociocultural system of the mainstream American middle-class as quickly and as effectively as possible.

COMMUNITY PSYCHOLOGY: CULTURAL DEMOCRACY IN PRACTICE

The community psychology movement has encouraged sensitivity to cultural differences and recognizes that programs developed to serve the community must take into account the particular world view—the perspectives, values, and needs—of the community. This supports the philosophy of cultural democracy. Community psychology recognizes the importance of having individuals maintain their identity and identification with their ethnic group while at the same time becoming acquainted with the values and behaviors of the mainstream American middle-class. The importance and advantages of biculturalism, the ability to function in two cultures, are recognized. Community psychology values the important contributions that can be made by different cultures to life in the United States as well as to the understanding of the psychodynamics of individuals. The point of view fostered by community psychology allows a better understanding of the diversity among cultures as well as the diversity within any one cultural group. Community psychology calls into question the myopic view, engendered by traditional psychological approaches, of what is considered to be normal or adequate personality development. It has encouraged contributions made by community members born and reared in the Hispano sociocultural system, providing opportunities for them to enter the profession of psychology and more effectively serve their community. Community psychology provides an opportunity for Hispanos to develop the "competent community" described by

Iscoe (1974), to obtain training in psychology, and to help develop mental health and educational programs consonant with the world view unique to the Hispano sociocultural system.

All of this implies, then, that community psychology is encouraging replacement of the conflict model supported by traditional psychology with a model in which biculturalism or multiculturalism is viewed as an advantage, as encouraging flexibility of psychological functioning and development of self-actualization. The sociocultural systems of minority ethnic groups such as Hispanos are seen as the foundation on which the research and service programs in the community must be based.

A MESTIZO WORLD VIEW

To develop conceptual frameworks and programs consonant with the psychodynamics of Hispanos, it is necessary for psychology to be responsive to the Mestizo world view, a product of the amalgamation of Hispanic and Native American cultures. This point of view emphasizes identification with the family and ethnic group, personalization of relationships, humanism, cooperation, and unity and harmony with the environment. The first organized efforts to involve strategies for incorporating the Mestizo world view in psychology were made at a conference held at the University of California, Riverside. Participants at this conference included Hispano and other psychologists committed to the community psychology movement, as well as graduate and undergraduate psychology students from universities throughout the country. An attempt was made to define training, recruitment, and research and service programs from the perspective of a Mestizo world view. Recommendations were made to the American Psychological Association and to the National Institute of Mental Health for their participation in the attempts to achieve some of these goals and in support of the efforts of community psychology to promote cultural democracy for Hispanos.

The goals discussed at Riverside were presented at Austin to participants at the National Training Conference in Community Psychology. It was evident at Austin that the new wave of interest represented by community psychology is indeed providing a favorable climate for cultural democracy in America. Furthermore, the Austin Conference reaffirmed the belief that the approaches and instruments of traditional psychology are inadequate in light of the diversity now evident to psychologists everywhere. Community psychologists consider that one of their important goals is to help people who have been disenfranchised in the past develop a voice in the design and implementation of the programs that affect their lives. This commitment must be extended to others; it must become active reality through efforts of future conferences, research, training, and the dedication of those working to achieve the goals of cultural democracy and community mental health.

REFERENCE

Iscoe, I. Community psychology and the competent community. *American Psychologist*, 1974, 29, 607–613.

C. Women in Community Psychology: A Feminist Perspective

Margie Whittaker Leidig

From the start, the Austin Conference on Training in Community Psychology was different from other psychological meetings. Strong, concerted, and successful efforts were made to insure the attendance of women graduate students and young PhDs. Conference planners went out of their way to invite and subsidize women's participation. This was an important step in community psychology's attempts to insure full equality between the sexes and to invest a heretofore powerless group with broader participation.

Despite these efforts, however, women experienced a lack of validation during the conference. There were few role models, and with rare exceptions, women could not look up to the power structure of the organization and see their own sex represented. Many of the women present expressed "feeling grateful" at being invited to the conference—a feeling often expressed when a minority group begins to note inclusionary attempts. We sat in an audience and heard numerous jokes at our expense (e.g., "community psychology needing new girlfriends"), and when we expressed disdain at these kinds of comments, some of us were told to "not take things so seriously." Paternalistic hugs and pats were also evident. Bem and Bem (1971) call these subtle behaviors the expressions of a "non-conscious ideology" designed to help a woman learn her place.

Many of us felt powerless and overcome by a bit of the "Catch-22" confusion on hearing discussions of the psychology of power and powerlessness in our own model groups as well as in the special interest groups.

An experience comes to mind that may make these points clearer. As a former school psychologist concerned about the powerlessness of low-income groups, I once set up a meeting with Head Start mothers and fathers, principals, and teachers. The purpose of the meeting was to encourage participation of these parents in the planning of programs for their children. I thought I was being extremely sensitive when I arranged pick-up transportation, food, and baby-sitting services in order to facilitate their inclusion and participation. At the meeting the parents were asked for input in every possible way. They did not give any. After the meeting, the principals, teachers, and I sat around debriefing what had just happened (or not happened, as it turned out), surprised that our efforts seemed so unproductive. Why hadn't they spoken? Why hadn't they helped us in our planning?

The implications of this anecdote are obvious to any student of social action and the psychology of powerlessness. We, in this meeting, were asking a powerless group to counter a lifetime of conditioning experiences, experiences that had taught them to be nonverbal, nonassertive, inarticulate, and to feel that school authorities make decisions for them, not with them.

Many women are currently at this stage. We are trying to counter the conditioning of a lifetime that, for the most part, has taught us that we are subjective, irrational, poor leaders, unscientific, and emotional (Broverman, Vogel, Broverman, Clarkson, & Rosenkrantz, 1972).

There appeared, then, to be a discrepancy between community psychology ideology and what we experienced as participants. It was never expressed overtly, but the feeling was as if we were permitted to listen and learn but were placed in a passive, powerless, leaderless role. When these observations were shared with some of the men at the conference, the reactions were generally "Well, speak up, you don't have to feel powerless. That's your own fault if you don't feel competent."

A double bind occurs when a subordinate group internalizes the guilt for issues that have been socialized and conditioned. Women look inward and blame themselves for their lack of initiative in speaking out and for their fear of taking assertive roles. They know it is irrational, but their socialization teaches them what is right and wrong for women and their functioning, particularly with competent males. We know these facts about racial and ethnic prejudices—group self-hatred and the acceptance of the dominant group's conception of them (Hacker, 1951). Yet we appear short-sighted when the same issues revolve around women.

Community psychology theories about working with oppressed and exploited groups illustrate sensitivity for the double binds that minority groups feel. Yet, these very theories do not work well when it comes to male-female relationships. Could it be there is minimal application of our technology when we attempt to relate to each other in tolerant, non-discriminatory ways?

Why is this the case? I can offer three hypotheses. The first might be called the "benign" hypothesis. The assumption here is that the conference planners and people in the power structure were well motivated but less than optimally informed about the issues women face in their emergence as competent community psychologists. Psychologists in general, and community psychologists in particular, are supposed to be committed to civil rights. They make valiant efforts to show their commitments by their actions. When they fail, the "ingrates aren't grateful for their efforts." If this particular hypothesis is operating, supplying information should prove to be the key.

The second would be a "don't-rock-the-boat" hypothesis. A commitment to equal rights would produce a redistribution of power. Iscoe (1974) has correctly pointed out that redistributing power is often frightening and threatening, particularly for those in the power positions. However, knowledge of power distribution, effects of shifts in power, and a sincere attitude toward change would remedy this alternative.

The third might be called the "malevolent" hypothesis. This refers to the poorly intentioned and poorly informed superordinate group that really doesn't want to change. Group members enjoy the benefits of discrimination and oppression and aren't about to give them up.

This last hypothesis was not and is not viable with community psychology pre- and post-Austin, because there has been a clear and open commitment to change. (Indeed, inviting a feminist to express her views as a conference participant is an affirmation of this.)

I would like to assume the "benign" hypothesis is operating. I would like to assume the goodwill and commitment to the redistribution of power, both in this organization and in those organizations and institutions we study. Assuming this to be the case, what can we do to change the position for women in community psychology and in the institutions that employ us?

From social psychology, we know that it is often the younger, least experienced of the species who will first experience new or radical ideas. Then the older ones will change as a result of modeling after the young (Itani, 1961). Numerous recent examples of this can be noted: hair length, style of dress, dance steps, music preferences, radicalism in antiwar activities, etc.

In our case, feminists are offering a new way to view relationships between the sexes. They are offering new ways to consider the personality and place of women. They are challenging old myths and offering new data about women's capabilities, emotions, physiology, and possibilities for leadership (Mednick, Tangri, & Hoffman, 1975). For women to take on leadership and competency roles, they must be trained. To expect that we can will or demand these roles is to set up double bind situations.

In a future conference, specific content that would deal with these issues would be helpful. Topics such as the difficulty women community psychologists experience in decision-making and power roles and assertiveness with male colleagues and/or supervisors would be a fine start. Support groups need to be set up with women community psychologists so that these issues can be discussed honestly and without coercion. (I have heard that within the Education and Training Committee of Division 27, a Task Force on Women is being considered. I heartily endorse an idea such as this.) Often to obtain support before moving on, women need to isolate themselves to find out that their professional/personal concerns are mutually shared.

Suggested topics for future conferences include:

1. What do women need or want? Within Division 27, women need a sense of community, a bit of "bonding," and role models.
2. How can women be helped in graduate schools of community psychology?
3. What are the women in communities facing?
4. Who should trainers be? (Can a traditionally conservative male, for example, supervise a female community psychology student and truly encourage and support her efforts toward more power and assertiveness? It must be remembered that not every trainer, male or female, is sensitive to women's issues.)
5. What changes might the establishment have to make if these issues were addressed?
6. Who are the feminists in Division 27? Feminists are usually the younger, politically oriented, and more radical of the women. Not all women are feminists.

Another proposal is to encourage articles on feminism in the Division 27 newsletter. These articles could sensitize members to the needs of students and women in the division and the needs of women in the communities.

Behavioral scientists, and especially community psychologists, can play an important role in remedying a situation feminists believe has created lost and depressed women, powerless and ineffective women, and women who desperately need to find their own potential. As community psychologists, we can elucidate the destructive effects of inequality and expose the paralyzing consequences of sexual discrimination. We can point out the positive advantages gained by people who have struggled for more equal human relationships.

REFERENCES

Bem, S., & Bem, D. Teaching the woman to know her place: The power of a non-conscious ideology. In M. Garskof (Ed.), *Roles women play.* Belmont, Calif.: Brooks/Cole, 1971.

Broverman, I., Vogel, R., Broverman, D., Clarkson, F., & Rosenkrantz, P. Sex role stereotypes: A current appraisal. *Journal of Social Issues,* 1972, *28,* 59–78.

Hacker, H. Women as a minority group. *Social Forces,* 1951, *30,* 60–69.

Iscoe, I. Community psychology and the competent community. *American Psychologist,* 1974, *29,* 607–613.

Itani, J. The society of Japanese monkeys. *Japan Quarterly,* 1961, *8,* 421–430.

Mednick, M. T. S., Tangri, S. S., & Hoffman, L. W. *Women and achievement.* Washington: Hemisphere, 1975.

D. Professional Concerns of Students in Community Psychology

Margaret L. Meyer

Students are actively concerned about professional issues in community psychology. This was readily apparent at the 1975 National Training Conference, where 41 graduate students, comprising 29% of all participants, took part in the sessions. They were a diverse group: 55% were women, 24% were members of ethnic minorities; their community orientation ranged from clinical to ecological psychology training programs; they were from regions throughout the country.

During the conference the students actively participated in work sessions and in describing training models; they served on panels and in discussion groups. They were catalysts for impromptu meetings after hours. Student involvement became an integral part of the conference, enhancing it by providing approaches, viewpoints, and questions not always heard at professional gatherings.

A number of issues of concern to students were discussed at the training conference. While some were settled, three principal ones remain unresolved: providing a variety of role models, implementing flexible training designs, and employing community psychologists.

ROLE MODELS

Providing role models for students entering a developing field is a complex problem. Students seek models on the basis of sex and race, for adaptation to settings, and for illustration of roles and skills. Minority and female students have particular difficulty in finding models, since few seasoned professionals are female or minority group members. While difficulty will diminish as present students become trainers, it is important currently for students and trainers, training programs, and professional groups to be resourceful in identifying minority and female role models and in considering other methods of providing role models for professional education.

Another role model of increasing importance to students is the practitioner-academic. For the graduate student whose major goal is applied work, it is essential to integrate university-based training with increasing amounts and varieties of field experience. The student's discovery that the task of integrating book learning and "real world" demands is one at which neither

The author wishes to thank Marge Rust, Bertha Holliday, and Brian Wilcox for their assistance in the preparation of this section.

professor nor field supervisor has been particularly successful surprises no one. The search for a role model is complicated by the fact that the student's home base is the university, and he or she is frequently unfamiliar, due to brief residence in the community, with professionals outside the university. This dichotomous professional reality is mirrored, to some extent, within Division 27, where academic-based community psychologists are more evident than field practitioners. In searching for role models, the student would be aided considerably by planned and extensive use of non-university-based supervision in training and through greater inclusion in professional groups of individuals whose principal employment is in both community application and academic training of psychology.

In addition to role models who successfully bridge town and gown, the fledgling community psychologist needs models who bridge traditional roles, such as counseling, research, and assessment, and newer roles, such as program design and administration. Here, again, the psychologist trainer may be a fledgling like the student; supervision in these roles might better be provided by a nonpsychologist manager, designer, or service provider. Those professionals—whether social workers, business managers, or whatever—who do best what the student strives to do should serve as models for these roles. The psychology trainee, however, needs the supplemental support of a psychologist during such experiences. The psychologist trainer, even when not proficient in a given role, has a clear sense of identity as a psychologist. The trainee, however, needs simultaneously to be a psychologist and to perform non-traditional roles. In the absence of one individual who embodies the personal characteristics (e.g., blackness), the professional identification (i.e., psychologist), and the specific skills (e.g., administration) desired in a role model, several individuals will be required to model different role dimensions.

Thoughtful students recognize that the "compleat" role model is an ideal type and perhaps not exemplified by any individual in faculty or field staff. Trainers, too, are aware of varying competencies among their own skills and role integrations. Many of the emerging community psychologist roles demand different combinations of skill and knowledge. Individual student career goals vary from research and teaching on a multitude of specialized topics to a wide range of applied roles. Such a diversity of role models will only be found in the next generation of trainers; current students have to seek many people to model multiple roles in varied settings. Identification of knowledge and skill components of successful functioning in specific dimensions of complex roles is a process beneficially shared by student and trainer. In this process each can develop a personal style as community psychologist and continue her or his professional development.

TRAINING DESIGNS

The working groups of the National Training Conference clarified and outlined a wide range of models for education, representing such diverse emphases as social change, community mental health, community development, and perspectives of social ecology and preventive intervention. This diversity reflects both current developments in training and the beliefs of conference participants. Students, for the most part, concur in the belief that a variety of training goals and models should be available to the prospective community psychologist. Linking specific training programs to one of the general models is helpful to applicants. Such linkages may be an important result of the conference.

Current graduate students, however, seek another type of diversity in training programs. Diversity between various educational sites is not enough; students committed to a particular university program want flexibility and diversity within that program. Variety in field settings and roles available to students for training is increasing; flexibility and variety in coursework is less widely available. Required coursework and departmental requirements minimize the flexibility of training opportunities. This situation is most common where community psychology is subordinated to other training, such as clinical practice. Many students prefer more flexible personalized education to rigidly standardized professional education. They seek adequate time to sample roles and settings or to specialize in one area of research and teaching. Maximizing individually guided education seems appropriate in a developing field whose major characteristic is diversity of training models and goals.

EMPLOYMENT

Community psychology education includes a variety of on-the-job experiences. Many trainees choose community psychology for its opportunities to impact social problems affecting individuals. They are interested in social change activities at many levels: in families, in schools, in governmental systems. Some community psychology trainees expect to work in universities, school districts, or community mental health centers. Others hope to be employed in less traditional settings.

Every student notices that many clinical and counseling and some social psychology training programs now offer a few courses in community mental health, program evaluation, community-based research, or social program administration. The concerned student also notices that job descriptions in traditional employment sites seldom require major training in policy analysis, program design, administration, and evaluation. How will this concerned student—the community psychologist—fare in competition with the clinical psychologist in obtaining jobs in these settings? Do employment realities make it desirable for community psychologists to meet licensure requirement for clinical service providers?

The interests and competencies of some community psychology trainees lead them to consider employment in planning agencies, local government, or other human service delivery organizations such as health, welfare, or justice departments. These students experience difficulty in uncovering job openings unless they remain as employees in agencies where they served as trainees. Even when they discover or create job opportunities, these trainees face the problem of selling themselves, as psychologists, into jobs viewed by the employer as roles for business graduates, social workers, or other professionals. These twin problems of identifying and obtaining jobs require creativity and attention in the immediate future.

Sophisticated students recognize that many academic jobs are obtained through the "old grad" system. Community based jobs are, to a lesser extent, advertised and obtained through this method. Can this personal referral and advertising system include more field-related jobs? Given that recent graduates often wish to move to new locations, would trainers familiar with those locations support them (on their trainers' recommendations, of course) for nonacademic jobs? Are trainers willing to work with field training sites to help them seek psychologists for job openings or define new jobs to include the skills of community oriented psychologists?

Professional group listings are another source of identifying job openings. Most psychologists use listings such as those in the American Psychological Association's newsletter, *APA Monitor*, or publications of special interest subgroups. Generalist graduate students may more closely fit jobs listed in a publication of another profession, such as social work or community planning. They may not, however, know of such materials.

Several issues related to employment of community psychologists have been mentioned: licensure, location, competition, sponsorship in new settings, and resource lists of job openings. Basic information about employment patterns of recent graduates would also provide current and prospective graduates guidelines in job hunting. These issues are of sufficient concern and timeliness to justify attention. A task force or committee constituted to investigate past employment patterns and resources for job applicants and to recommend procedures by which the professional community can assist employment of new community psychologists could meet this need.

Active student involvement in the conference has had consequences for Division 27 activities at both regional and national levels. An increasing number of students have become active in national committee work, particularly in committees concerned with graduate education, field training, and publications. Friendships begun in Austin have resulted in a national network of community psychologists. This network has facilitated sharing reports of regional actitivies and newsletters with information about workshops, job opportunities, and training events. Some campuses previously not identified with community psychology now have groups meeting to survey community-oriented education opportunities and resources and to provide mutual support for additional field experiences. Such activities may increase membership and interest in Division 27. A more important consequence, however, is the professional development of present and future community psychologists. Continuing involvement of new students and additional educational units in information sharing and role development can strengthen ties between students and former students who are now young professionals employed in academic and field settings. These ties potentially can improve the quality of education and practice in community psychology.

30 Applications of Community Psychology

A. "Community-Based" Community Psychologists

Karl A. Slaikeu

An important "unresolved issue" of the Austin Conference had to do with the role of nonacademic community psychologists in shaping the future of community psychology, including Division 27. Psychologists from non-academic settings were underrepresented at the conference, and implications of this low representation were raised in some of the discussion sections. The concern of many was that Division 27 not make the same mistake that Division 12 (Clinical Psychology) made in allowing itself to be too heavily weighted toward academic settings. Others stressed the irony of a field called *community* psychology attempting to plan its future with relatively little input or representation from those psychologists who work full time in community settings. This subchapter focuses on the problem, addresses the issue of what is lost if such underrepresentation of community-based psychologists continues, and suggests proactive measures to reverse the trend.

THE POPULATION

The population in question is community psychologists who take jobs in such settings as community mental health centers, hospitals, clinics, private nonprofit research and consulting organizations, and, increasingly, city, state, and federal government. Trained as behavioral scientists, these psychologists primarily identify themselves, not as teachers, but as practicing consultants, program designers, planners, administrators, evaluators, and researchers. Their main identifying characteristic is that they "do community psychology" in nonacademic settings. While many of them publish research reports and articles, these endeavors are not tied to a tenure track in an academic department. Many are involved in training of some sort, if not of practicum students and interns who choose to train in their agencies, then of fellow staff members. In sum, their professional life has more to do with applying

The author wishes to thank Drs. Rosie Cripps, Tom Cripps, and Mary Teague for their helpful comments in the preparation of this paper.

community psychology principles than with teaching them. Since these individuals have different constraints on their professional lives than do academics, it is predictable that their input to training programs (based on their experience in the field) will be different than that of academically-based community psychologists.

WHAT IS LOST?

Losses that grow from the exclusion of this group can be described from the viewpoint of those involved in the training programs, as well as from the viewpoint of the community-based community psychologists themselves. For the ones in training programs, the most important consideration has to do with the need for input from individuals who are presently functioning as community psychologists in the field. The question to be addressed is: "After your formal training, what have you found yourself doing professionally, and what are the implications for further refinement of our present training programs?" For example, this writer's experience as an administrator suggests a need for experience in such "practical" areas as dealing with the press, communicating with politicians, public speaking, negotiating agreement between conflicting parties, dealing with issues of staff morale, working with committees, and using time efficiently. In addition, theoretical/conceptual grounding in intergroup process (Tavistock), organizational psychology, and general systems theory have been most useful. Feedback from other community psychologists working in applied settings would suggest other important training focuses and might underline some of the areas mentioned here. There is clearly a need to refine training programs to elicit feedback from people who have completed formal training, have taken jobs in community settings, and are in a position to evaluate their training and offer suggestions for redirection of training programs.

A second half of the question of what is lost by the relative absence of community-based psychologists at Division 27's national gatherings concerns the need of these individuals for a reference group. Many simply do not see Division 27 as adequate or helpful in that role. They view themselves as experiencing different constraints on their work and different needs for continuing education than the academics experience. In the absence of Division 27 providing a reference group, they seem now to be looking toward people in other professions who are involved in similar activities, such as management consultants, planners, social workers, etc. Many feel more "at home" when attending national conferences on alcoholism, drug abuse, and juvenile delinquency (i.e., issues discussed at such gatherings are often more tied to their everyday work) than at APA's Division 27 gatherings. Steps need to be taken, then, to insure that Division 27 also becomes a reference group for these colleagues. This is not to in any way denegrate interdisciplinary affiliations, support, and activity. It is, rather, to suggest that community psychologists, once they leave university settings and involve themselves in work in the community, have a need and a desire to maintain ties with colleagues who also have roots in psychology.

PROACTIVE SUGGESTIONS

A number of fairly straightforward possibilities come to mind in an attempt to (1) make use of feedback from this group in the refinement of training programs as well as (2) provide an opportunity for Division 27 to serve as a reference group for community-based psychologists. Regarding the use of feedback, it seems essential that university psychology programs sponsor more workshops and symposia in their departments to allow individuals "in the field" to return to the academic settings and discuss issues. The suggestion here is simply to expand on that which already takes place in some training programs, namely, having community-based individuals speak to students and faculty. Questions addressed by these individuals should include: What was the nature of your training? What activities are you presently engaged in? What is your job description? Who else is presently doing what you are doing in your setting? To what extent do you identify yourself as a psychologist in your work? What was the most helpful part of your training in preparing you to do what you now do? What might we add to our training program to prepare our students to face the responsibilities you now face? How might such training be developed?

In addition to feedback loops for training, a possible outgrowth of these discussions might be a move by departments to face squarely the issue of "job slot" creation and placement. As things presently stand, few graduates of community psychology programs take jobs bearing the community psychologist title (other than academic positions). Such discussion might move toward clearer definition of community psychology job descriptions as an aid to employers. The larger issue, of course, has to do with increasing the marketability (in nonacademic settings) of "products" of community psychology training programs.

An exciting idea raised at the Community Psychology Training Conference in Austin was the suggestion that Division 27 sponsor preconvention workshops directed toward continuing education and skillbuilding for community-based individuals. The notion was that while paper sessions are conducive to meeting needs of academics, workshops might be more in line with the interests of other community people and might be the best way for individuals to interact with one another on a national level. (This would apply as well to meetings of regional psychological associations.) While this suggestion is in the service of continuing education, it also relates positively to the issue of Division 27 providing a reference group for these people. The topics could focus on any number of pressing and often value-laden concerns of community psychologists working in community settings, such as issues and strategies in putting together public boards, and psychological and social implications of forced school busing to achieve racial balance.

Another suggestion proposed at the conference dealt with Division 27's publishing, as a part of the *Newsletter* or the *American Journal of Community Psychology*, a section in which applied issues could be raised, not so much to report research results as to pinpoint important issues in applied work. This might take the form of a "consultant's notebook" in which cases or portions thereof could be presented for the edification of colleagues in other settings. The realization here was that there might well be a place in our literature for case experiences and specific procedures around such issues as management, staff evaluation, delivery of services, planning, and political negotiation. This would include failures of various community interventions as well as successes (assuming that the absence of certain conditions of success in one setting could be helpful to others facing similar issues in different settings). A "half-baked idea" from one community psychologist might well turn out to be just the stimulus needed by another colleague in another community.

Finally, it could well be that the most potent intervention on this set of issues would be to allocate a percentage of Division 27's executive committee slots for community-based community psychologists. This suggestion is based on the assumption that reshaping the destiny of an organization can best come about through solid participation in decision making at high levels. If we take into account our recommendations to other "disenfranchised" community groups, and if we recognize the need for changes on the issues discussed, then we need to face squarely issues of participation, power, and decision making in our own national organization. Interestingly enough, in attempting to determine what percentage of executive committee slots should go to community-based individuals, it becomes apparent that we do not yet know how many such people there are, that is, there is an absence of baseline data on which to make this decision. The very absence of these data underlines the importance of the issues raised, namely, that there is a need for participation of these individuals, and even prior to that there is a need to specify who they are, where they are, and what they are doing. The final proactive suggestion of this paper, then, is that Division 27 allocate a percentage of executive committee slots to community-based individuals, so that the committee can reflect the needs and interests of this group as well as those of university-based psychologists.

In explicating this unresolved issue of the Austin Conference, the issues in one sense are obvious and not peculiar to community psychology. It is hoped, however, that the commonness of the issues will not detract from their importance. Division 27's credibility as a shaper of the field will be questioned if the separation between academic and field community psychologists persists. The matter goes beyond field community psychologists being included in the activities of Division 27; the main issue has to do with their sharing equitably in its redirection.

B. The Private Practice of Community Psychology

A. Rodney Nurse

Psychology's services are (or should be) designed to meet the needs of the consumer, not those of psychologists or existing traditional institutions involved with service delivery. Full acceptance of the import of this principle leaves the psychologist open to consider new service delivery approaches in the context of contemporary trends, issues, and available data. This openness, it is suggested, needs to be furthered in light of recent professional developments.

DELIVERY OF PSYCHOLOGICAL SERVICES

A major guidepost in considering the delivery of psychological services is *Standards for Providers of Psychological Services*, developed by the Task Force on Standards for Service Facilities of the APA (1975). The Task Force report states that a single set of standards is needed to cover all service settings, taking into account providers (all psychological specialties), consumers, and sanctioners. This uniform set of standards should, of course, apply equally to what are now considered public and private sectors. Consumers of health services especially need the protection of law and choice of vendor provided when services are obtained on a private basis. And the private consumer needs the basis of peer review ordinarily considered to be available in the public setting.

In health settings the terms *public* and *private* are tending to meld in character. Consumers frequently pay community mental health centers on a sliding scale in relation to ability to pay. Consumers with private insurance ordinarily receive 50% to 80% reimbursement if they see a private, independent practitioner for psychodiagnostic or psychotherapeutic services.

With the anticipated advent of national health insurance, consumers will have more opportunity to choose private practitioners. Practitioners will most likely be associated with an Independent Practice Association, a type of Health Maintenance Organization (HMO), thus meeting professional review (PSRO) standards. If national health insurance becomes an actuality, there may be a demise of both public and private independent practice as they are known today (Dorken, 1975).

While these trends seem relevant to clinical psychology, some may argue that they have little importance for community psychology. If the emphasis of health service were to focus on reimbursement for illness and curative services in this developing Independent Practice Association model, consultation, education, and primary prevention activities would appear to be excluded. These activities, plus quality of life developmental efforts, would seem to be undertaken out of this fee-for-service model only minimally.

A HEALTH-MAINTENANCE MODEL

However, the traditional fee-for-service "illness" model is not the model for developing HMO's and Independent Practice Associations. On the contrary, the so-called Kaiser Model is the basis for these new trends. With this model an HMO contracts with groups to *maintain* health. The more effective the primary and secondary preventive efforts, the fewer the visits to any form of "curers" associated with the group. The financial base is a monthly fee for health.

Reports from Follette and Cummings (1968) have demonstrated that just one psychotherapeutic visit markedly lowers the utilization rates in "medical" clinics. This evidence suggests the efficacy of early secondary prevention and is compatible with the common observation that a high percentage of visits to physicians are psychogenic in motivational origin. What remains to be seen is the potential impact of various primary prevention measures, such as educational, consultative, and systems interventions with a focus on quality of life for the organizational, or covered, group. And here, of course, is the opportunity for community psychologists, particularly those with training stemming from clinical/community and community mental health, community development and systems, and intervention/preventive backgrounds.

Health Maintenance Organizations cannot hire psychologists to provide service; they must, instead, contract for services. This is true in California, at least, where it is based on the California Attorney General's ruling of 1975. Thus, community psychology services in the health field will come of necessity from private contracts with Independent Practice Associations of psychologists and related professionals, just as is the case with physicians.

OPPORTUNITIES FOR PRIVATE PRACTICE

Community psychologists apparently will have an opportunity to contribute in a significant way to a national health base rather than the anachronistic illness base of the present system, assuming trends in HMO proposals and proposed national health insurance laws continue in their present direction. Furthermore, escalating costs and more effective cost-effectiveness studies indicate that present public services need to be and are being contracted out already, for example in mental health, rehabilitation, and probation fields. Thus, these contemporary trends will reinforce the possibilities of private practice in community psychology. Even if they continue at a slow pace while the present trends in the health insurance and HMO areas continue as outlined, the size and weight of the health industry itself will be sufficient to bring along many of these services under the independent practice association banner.

Community psychologists must not be caught in the old fee-for-service practice, turning their backs on the developing approaches in the health area. The health area is not for clinical psychologists alone. On the contrary, there appear to be major possibilities in the primary and secondary areas of prevention for the community psychologist as well as for the clinical psychologist trained in community approaches.

REFERENCES

Dorken, H. National health insurance: Prospects for profound change. *American Psychologist*, December 1975, *30* 685–694.

Follette, W. T., & Cummings, N. A. Psychiatric services and medical utilization in a prepaid health setting (Part 2). *Medical Care*, 1968, *6*(1), 31.

Task Force on Standards for Service Facilities of the Board of Professional Affairs of the American Psychological Association. Standards for providers of psychological services. *American Psychologist*, June 1975, *30*, 1158–1160.

C. Ecological Perspectives in Community Ecology: A Tale of Three Cities

Charles J. Holahan

Kurt Lewin's maxim, "There is nothing so practical as a good theory," bears poignant legitimacy for those engaged in the practice of community psychology. For, while the social imperatives that generated the emergence of community psychology cannot be argued, neither can the reality that its mature development has been hindered by its failure to develop a sufficient theoretical foundation. Recent discussion among community psychologists of an ecological viewpoint may augur a fruitful direction for the evolution of a requisite conceptual basis for the area. Unfortunately, however, while ecology has been frequently invoked and praised, its meaning has often been clouded. Because the term lends itself to almost ubiquitious usage, it may be useful at the outset to agree on a focused definition. Ecology within community psychology may be characterized in terms of three basic postulates that define

From "The Role of Ecology in Community Psychology: A Tale of Three Cities" by C. J. Holahan, *Professional Psychology*, 1977, *8*(1), 25–32. Copyright 1977 by the American Psychological Association. Reprinted by permission.

The author expresses appreciation to Ira Iscoe, Robert Reiff, and David Todd for their suggestions in preparing this manuscript.

its major emphases: (1) it focuses on the environmental context of human behavior, (2) it adopts a social systems perspective in conceptualizing the environment, and (3) it views psychological adjustment in terms of the transactional relationship between the individual and the environment.

The purpose of this subchapter is to analyze from a historical perspective the evolution of the ecological viewpoint in community psychology. The initial impetus for the paper derives from insights fostered at the National Conference for Training in Community Psychology held in Austin, Texas, in the spring of 1975. However, while the Austin Conference provided a forum for the explicit discussion of ecology by community psychologists, a complete picture of the ecological perspective necessitates, in addition, a retrospective analysis of events associated with two other cities—Washington and Boston. In fact, the three postulates cited have evolved successively, and each is referable to one of the three cities of Washington, Boston, and Austin.

WASHINGTON: MENTAL HEALTH IN THE NATURAL ENVIRONMENT

The decade of the 1960s witnessed the most significant developments in the mental health field since the advent of psychoanalysis at the turn of the century. The repercussions of the community mental health philosophy presaged changes at all levels in the mental health field, from treatment tactics and professional training to the locus and timing of the delivery of services. A historically significant event was the publication in 1961 of the federally supported Joint Commission Report on Mental Illness and Health, assessing mental health needs and services on a national scale. Most significantly, the report stressed potential benefits implicit in shifting the treatment arena from clinic to community. Underlying the new philosophy was an awareness that mental illness was as much a community as a personal responsibility, and a conviction that the community offered a strategically more effective treatment realm in terms of both geographic and temporal accessibility. The ensuing Community Mental Health Act of 1963 represented a partial implementation of the report, and amid portentous enthusiasm it established the framework for a national network of community mental health centers.

The events that generated the new community emphasis were, however, pragmatically rather than conceptually based. Confronted with strong discouragement involving shortages in professional resources, growing evidence of the restricted success of psychotherapy, and blatant classism in service delivery and accessibility, mental health professionals turned to more innovative treatment tactics, such as the store-front clinic serviced by indigenous community members. However, as the new army of mental health workers moved into the community they brought with them a time-worn, though persistent, intrapsychic model of psychological adjustment.

The most disturbing consequence of the lack of conceptual innovation implicit in the early community mental health movement was not theoretical imprecision but practical disappointment. Initial evaluations of the new community mental health movement tended to afford a pessimistic picture. An in-depth review of the most advanced community mental health centers concluded with disillusionment that the treatment of choice remained traditional psychotherapy on a one-to-one basis, in a 50-minute hour (Smith & Hobbs, 1966). The new walk-in centers, which had promised an effective referral service to a wide array of human service agencies, had generally reverted to revolving-door, short-term psychotherapy (Reiff, 1968). In summary, this initial phase in the community mental health movement was characterized by an important change in the locus of delivery for mental health services without, however, confronting the more fundamental issue of whether the old, intrapsychic model offered a viable conceptual foundation for community-based interventions.

BOSTON: COMMUNITY AS SOCIAL SYSTEM

The beginning of a conceptual revolution in the community mental health field occurred in 1965 when clinical psychologists gathered near Boston, Massachusetts, ostensibly to discuss training for community mental health. However, as the underlying discontent associated with the initial failure of the community mental health thrust to achieve its established objectives became overt, the conference assumed a broader scope and purpose. Participants admitted that initial failures were in major part a function of the inherent inadequacies of the conceptual tools with which psychologists had approached the community. Reiff (1967) has commented pointedly on this situation:

Sometimes changes in tactics or techniques are necessary and sufficient to solve a problem. . . . However, frequently when professionals face the issue of ideology they escape into technology. But when the problem has ideological roots, changes in techniques without the necessary ideological innovation often result in nothing more than old wine in new bottles.

When psychologists from clinical backgrounds entered the community, they found themselves confronted with an array of situations for which they possessed neither language nor theory, and responded by falling back on the still accessible rhetoric and technology of psychodynamics. Based on the concerns voiced at the Boston Conference, attention shifted toward developing social systems theory as a more appropriate framework for conceptualizing community processes. The emerging perspective emphasized employing social system interventions to change individual behavior, along with a concern that interventions go beyond the individual client toward modifying the behavior of many people in the system (Reiff, 1970).

Social systems theory sensitized action-oriented psychologists to two cardinal properties of community settings—the interdependence of diverse elements and the process of temporal change. Community change agents were forced to engage in modes of intervention that recognized the interrelatedness and complexity of behavioral phenomena. Individually targeted treatment in the classroom succeeded only in shifting the problem behavior from one pupil to another as long as systemic issues such as ineffective administrative policy and low teacher morale remained unattended. Community psychologists were also compelled to deal with the historical and developmental themes inherent in community groups and settings. Granting only meager power to a mental health administrative board composed of minority members sharing a long history of political and economic disenfranchisement resulted in frustration and bitterness as often as in effective cooperation.

AUSTIN: PERSON-ENVIRONMENT TRANSACTION

The post-Boston period was characterized by increasing discussion of the role of social systems in community psychology. A major shortcoming of the systems perspective for the practicing community psychologist was that it lacked a thorough explication of the interrelationship of the individual and the social system. The conference in Austin offered a forum for extensive group discussion among community psychologists of an ecological perspective able to deal explicitly with the issue of person-environment transaction. The ecological theme recurred throughout the conference: in the principal addresses of James Kelly, Seymour Sarason, and Robert Reiff, in an "ecological model group," and in the conference summary at the end of the proceedings. While the ecological view was not initiated in Austin, the conference offered an opportunity for integrating in a single fabric the diverse threads spun during previous years. Special reference should be made, however, to the pioneering work of Kelly (1968, 1969) in laying the groundwork for considering ecology as a potential conceptual foundation for community psychology. The ecological theme of the Austin Conference bears important implications relevant to this contemporary stance in both theory and practice.

Theory

Two themes were prominent in the discussion of ecology in Austin: (1) a conceptualization of psychological adaptation in terms of person-environment congruence, and (2) a concern with effective coping. The ecological perspective views psychological adjustment in transactional terms. In contrast to defining adjustment exclusively on the basis of internal personality dynamics, adjustment is construed in terms of the transactional relationship between individuals and the environmental settings in which they function. Specifically, psychological adjustment may be defined as the state in which an individual's needs and proclivities for action are congruent with the demands and opportunities of the particular settings in which he or she operates. In addition, the ecological view emphasizes effective coping rather than maladjustment or pathology.

Rather than conceptualizing ecology as a tightly defined theoretical model, conference participants felt that ecology within community psychology represents essentially a perspective or a viewpoint. As a perspective it is relevant to a number of different content areas and problem types. The ecological viewpoint is appropriate to conceptualizing urban problems, analyzing the relationship between a community mental health center and its surrounding community, and investigating the internal forces operative in a regional school system. The ecological perspective is also applicable across different levels of problem analysis, including role relationships in an organizational setting, the effects of physical environment on behavior, and the pervasive influence of culture and history on community process. Despite the breadth of content that potentially can be synthesized beneath the ecological umbrella, the viewpoint serves a vital role as a conceptual backdrop for a number of important contemporary developments in community psychology, which share an underlying emphasis on the transactional relationship of person and environment.

Practice

The most immediate implication of an ecological model of adaptation for community psychology practice is that it vastly increases the armamentarium of available interventions for improving quality of life in the community. First, the community psychologist may choose to focus on enhancing an individual's level of functioning. However, the thrust will likely be toward improving the skills the individual needs to cope with particular institutional or environmental blocks to achieving desired objectives rather than toward personality integration per se. In addition, in the circumstances where psychologists discover a particular environmental setting that has precipitated severe psychological stress in a large number of individuals, they may shift the intervention strategy toward changing the characteristics of the environment that present serious obstacles to individual functioning. Further, they may identify and bolster those systems in the community that can perform effectively as restabilizers for the individual under stress. Most important, an ecological model allows psychologists to assume an innovative and vital role as participant conceptualizers (c.f., Spielberger & Iscoe, 1970) in the process of developing a range of new social systems designed specifically to effectively anticipate and accommodate the needs of community members.

The increased flexibility in professional practice encouraged through an ecological view should not be minimized. Caplan and Nelson (1973), in addressing the more general issue of psychologists' involvement in social problems, have observed that the tendency to emphasize deficits from past experiences has obscured psychologists' awareness of contemporary institutional blocks to the achievement of an acceptable quality of life for disenfranchised groups. Ryan (1971) has lamented the all-too-common circumstance whereby social analyses by well-meaning psychologists have concluded by "blaming the victims" of social problems for the conditions in which they find themselves.

Ecological Field Projects

Two examples of action research projects in community psychology incorporating an underlying ecological perspective may help to elucidate these issues. One example of the application of an ecological view in a field project can be found in the work of Kelly (1969) in Ohio. Kelly studied two high schools in the Columbus area that were highly discrepant environmentally. He predicted that if a congruence model of adaptation were valid, then two contrasting environments should support divergent types of effective coping behavior. The two high schools studied differed markedly in rate of population exchange, with one school (the flux environment) characterized by an excessively high turnover rate and the other (the constant environment) by a low rate of population exchange. As expected, Kelly discovered that the two schools differed dramatically in terms of prevailing social ethos. The flux environment was characterized by heterogeneity in its social structure, with broadly defined roles, flexible behavioral standards, and a normative structure encouraging innovation and exploration in creating a unique personal niche in the school society. The constant environment, in vivid contrast, was characterized by homogeneity in social life, with minimal distinctions between individuals in both dress and behavior and a normative structure demanding that individuals locate themselves appropriately within the school society. Predictably, adaptive and maladaptive behavior differed sharply over the two environments. In the flux environment, high adaptive individuals were creative, adventuresome, and exploratory, while poorly adaptive individuals were passive, receptive, and rule-oriented. In the constant environment, in contrast, high adaptive individuals were passive, responsive, good citizens, while poorly adaptive individuals were innovative and exploratory.

A further example of an action research project in community psychology reflecting an ecological orientation can be seen in a study currently in process at the University of Texas (Holahan & Wilcox, in press). The focus of the project is a systematic investigation of the relationship of environmental design and individual difference variables with living satisfaction in university dormitories. The study is focusing on differences in the social ecology of high-rise megadorms relative to low-rise residences. In addition, a particular emphasis of the project is the identification of adaptive social coping strategies within the living environment. Initial results have indicated that residents of low-rise dorms are significantly more satisfied than residents of megadorms, with the range of dissatisfaction in high-rise housing very broad, including feelings about social contact and support, the physical setting, and bureaucratic alienation. Especially interesting are preliminary findings that indicate that megadorm settings are most dissatisfying for more socially assertive individuals. It appears that in megadorms, less assertive students adapt to this situation by establishing more proximate and immediately available friendship networks. This particular coping strategy has proven especially effective, as a strong positive relationship has been observed between proximate friendship networks and living satisfaction.

THE FUTURE

What type of role is ecology likely to play in community psychology's future development? First, it will probably remain a broad and flexible perspective rather than solidifying as a tightly defined model. This is consistent with a thrust at the Austin Conference toward recognizing a diversity of social goals, intervention strategies, and institutional bases within community psychology. Second, the potential social policy relevance of the ecological view, in contrast to the intrapsychic position, augurs favorably for its ability to respond to an increased emphasis on social relevance in the current posture of federal funding. Third, the ecological perspective is congruent with community psychology's growing effort to train students for careers in fields other than mental health, such as community organizations, urban and regional planning, and public policy formulation and evaluation. Fourth, the facility of the ecological perspective in integrating a sound conceptual basis with social action will enhance its viability within prestigious departments of psychology. In fact, the current crisis of confidence in social psychology (Elms, 1975; Helmreich, 1975) may make ecology an attractive conceptual model to some social as well as community psychologists. Finally, and especially promising, at Austin the younger, future members of the Division of Community Psychology were particularly responsive to and resonant with the ecological viewpoint. This is probably based both on ecology's ability to be closely in tune with the social urgency and unrest of recent years, and on the fact that the younger members present at Austin reflected increased participation by women and racial and ethnic minorities, groups keenly aware of environmentally-based obstacles to change in their own experience.

REFERENCES

Caplan, N., & Nelson, S. D. On being useful: The nature and consequences of psychological research on social problems. *American Psychologist*, 1973, *28*, 199–211.

Elms, A. C. The crisis of confidence in social psychology. *American Psychologist*, 1975, *30*, 967–976.

Helmreich, R. Applied social psychology: The unfulfilled promise. *Personality and Social Psychology Bulletin*, 1975, *1*, 548–560.

Holahan, C. J., & Wilcox, B. L. Ecological strategies in community psychology: A case study. *American Journal of Community Psychology*, in press.

Kelly, J. G. Toward an ecological conception of preventive interventions. In J. W. Carter (Ed.), *Research contributions from psychology to community mental health*. New York: Behavioral Publications, 1968.

Kelly, J. G. Naturalistic observations in contrasting social environments. In E. P. Willems & H. L. Raush (Eds.), *Naturalistic viewpoints in psychological research*. New York: Holt, 1969.

Reiff, R. Mental health manpower and institutional change. In E. L. Cowen, E. A. Gardner, & M. Zax (Eds.), *Emergent approaches to mental health problems*. New York: Appleton-Century-Crofts, 1967.

Reiff, R. Social intervention and the problem of psychological analysis. *American Psychologist*, 1968, *23*, 524–531.

Reiff, R. The need for a body of knowledge in community psychology. In I. Iscoe & C. D. Spielberger (Eds.), *Community psychology: Perspectives in training and research*. New York: Appleton-Century-Crofts, 1970.

Ryan, W. *Blaming the victim*. New York: Vintage, 1971.

Smith, M. B., & Hobbs, N. The community and the community mental health center. *American Psychologist*, 1966, *21*, 499–509.

Spielberger, C. D., & Iscoe, I. The current status of training in community psychology. In I. Iscoe & C. D. Spielberger (Eds.), *Community psychology: Perspectives in training and research*. New York: Appleton-Century-Crofts, 1970.

D. Continuing Education for Community Psychologists

Francis T. Miller

Prior to 1975, the APA Division of Community Psychology (Division 27) was involved in continuing education and the professional development of its members and interested others through two primary channels. One channel consisted of addresses, paper sessions, and symposia sponsored and encouraged at national, regional, and state meetings. The other was through publications sponsored and/or encouraged by the division. That picture changed during the spring of 1975 when the division convened a National Conference on Training in Community Psychology at Austin, Texas.

An expressed need at the Austin Conference was for greater involvement by the division in continuing education. To explore that need and give it clearer definition, a questionnaire was quickly constructed and presented to the participants. Only 37 questionnaires were returned to comprise a response rate for this captive audience of less than 30%. However, the responders (though perhaps a biased sample of a biased sample of community psychologists) represented a cross-section of the experience levels of the conference participants: 8 were graduate students; 11 had had their doctoral degrees less than five years; 8 had been out of school more than 5 but less than 15 years, and 10 had been in the field more than 15 years; 25 were male and 12 were female.

Each participant was asked about past involvements in continuing education activities, the kinds of continuing education activities in which they might like to participate, and the kinds of roles they felt the division should play in continuing education. Only one respondent felt the division should not be involved in continuing education because "continuing professional development is a personal rather than a collective responsibility." All other respondents felt that the division should play some role. This result is in contrast to one obtained in a survey of industrial psychologists (Lawler, 1967) where 60% of the respondents indicated their professional organization should undertake responsibility for sponsoring continuing education. If Division 27 is to be more active in continuing education, is its own membership a likely consumer group? Surveys of psychologists in the southeast have indicated a high interest in continuing education (Katahn, 1970). However Division 12 (Hasazi, 1975) has reported that its members do not exactly beat down the doors to gain admission to the postdoctoral institutes. Therefore, we were particularly interested in community psychologists' reports of their recent involvement in continuing education.

When attendance at professional meetings was considered along with other categories of continuing education, all the respondents had participated in continuing education during the preceding year and at a fairly high frequency but with important differences based on experience levels. Graduate students reported an average of 6.5 experiences, the group with less than 5 years postdoctoral experience reported 8.36, the 5 to 15 year group reported 7.38, and the most experienced group reported 4.3. When professional meeting involvements were removed from the list of continuing education activities, the mean participation rates decreased by more than a half to 3.37, 3.09, 2.63, and 1.40 respectively for the four groups. Thus, there appears to exist a clear trend wherein more experienced professionals are less frequently involved in continuing education activities. This phenomena is in contrast to published information estimating the half-life of professional knowledge in psychology at 10 to 12 years (Dubin, 1972), which might lead one to postulate a greater need for continuing education on the part of older, more experienced psychologists. The data also indicated that offering continuing education experiences to others tended to be by the early and midcareer groups. Half in each group stated that they were actively involved in offering continuing education during the previous year, while less than a third of the more experienced group so reported.

Respondents were also asked to identify their most meaningful continuing education experiences during the previous three years. Again, there were differences attributable to experience levels. Those newer to the field reported skill development and technology mastery experiences as most meaningful, while the older group was more substantively focused. For example, the younger group reported as meaningful topics community evaluation, intervention strategies, grant writing, consultation skills, and legal issues in drug abuse. The older group listed the president's conference on human behavior, a conference on conflict resolution, the design of drug abuse prevention programs, mental health and urban problems, and a colloquium on social experimentation. The data suggest that the focus during early career may be on skill development and, in later career, on the nature of the settings where the skills might be applied.

That distinction, however, does not hold when one considers the responses to the question "given the best of all possible worlds, list the community psychology relevant continuing education areas in which you would like to be involved." The graduate students listed both knowledge and skill areas. Their list included health care systems, child care systems, architecture and psychology, political realities, epidemiology as a technique for identifying mental health needs, network mapping, and consultation as an intervention strategy. These were the areas the graduate students said they want to know more about.

The early career group placed different items on their "want-list." They expressed interest in social change, social policy analysis, the politics of mental health delivery, and planning for long term social change. That list also included skill areas such as prevention approaches, community needs assessment, grant writing, acting as a catalyst for advisory boards, and supervision of community students.

The midcareer group contained items from the previous lists, but included teaching, programming, and planning items. Their list included primary prevention methodology, CEP programming, organizational analysis, planning processes, data-based planning, training of human service deliverers, ecological psychology, constructing a community psychology course, and teaching evaluation.

The group with more than 15 years in the field listed some of the expected skill areas such as program evaluation, systems analysis, community needs assessment, and early detection and prevention of disorders, all of which are areas of rapidly developing technology. The list also included knowledge base for professional practice, system intervention versus experimentation issues, the university and social change roles, quasi-experimental field research designs, utilization of scientific knowledge, policy research methods, and applied ecological methods.

The lists of desired continuing education experiences include knowledge and skill areas from city planning, public policy, and administration as well as from psychology. It is obvious that psychology does not meet all of these interest areas, and that many of the areas are of interest to others than community psychologists. There is some agreement on the importance of particular areas such as program evaluation, community needs assessment, and prevention programming, but there is great diversity as well.

The final survey question focused on the role that Division 27 should play in the continuing education for its membership. There was a clear message that the division should become active in serving the training needs of the membership through developing and sponsoring continuing education programs and workshops in conjunction with state, regional, and national meetings. It was also felt that the division should become more active in facilitating communication about continuing education opportunities throughout the country.

The division is making some moves to meet the mandate offered by those responses. At the 1975 meeting of the APA, three workshops were offered. However, possibly because of lack of advance publicity and short lead time, only the one workshop was actually held. The other two were cancelled because of insufficient registration. During 1975-1976, attempts were made to generate workshops at regional meetings. Two workshops were offered and one held at the Southeastern Psychological Association meetings, and workshops were held at the Rocky Mountain and the Eastern Psychological Association meetings. A workshop proposal was submitted for the Midwestern Psychological Association meeting but declined by the program committee. A workshop was also held in conjunction with the meeting of the California Psychological Association. In process, at the time of this writing, were plans to offer three workshops in conjunction with the 1976 annual meeting of the American Psychological Association in Washington, D.C. Those workshops were publicized through the *APA Monitor*, the *Community Mental Health Journal*, the *Division 27 Newsletter*, and the APA program.

It is anticipated that the effort to develop workshops in conjunction with national and regional meetings will continue. However, for the division to move fully into continuing education, a number of other approaches might be considered. The division might develop and publicize a speakers bureau of members and others prepared to address topics indicated here and others as they become salient to community psychologists. Grants might be obtained to develop filmed or videotaped teaching modules that could be made easily available to local settings and universities. Such modules could be in the form of lectures or demonstrations or in the form of articulated learning experiences with prescribed exercises and tasks to accompany the filmed material. Alternatively, the division could encourage and sponsor the development of programmed learning materials based on skill or topical areas of interest to community psychologists in the field. Or the division might adopt

George Albee's (1975) recommendation to develop "a library of audio tapes or videotapes which could be rented at a reasonable rate to solitary or small groups of practitioners who want to listen to leaders and innovators in the field or to watch them in their actual practice of new techniques." However, for these and other developments to occur, the division needs to hear the voice and wishes of the membership. In the service of that need, a more comprehensive survey instrument is being developed and will be distributed at a later time to the Division 27 membership.

REFERENCES

Albee, G. W. Statement. In G. B. Dodrill (Ed.), Statements from the nominees for president-elect. *Continuing Professional Development*, 1975, *12*(1), 1–2.

Dubin, S. S. Obsolescence or lifelong education: A choice for the professional. *American Psychologist*, 1972, *27*(5), 486–498.

Hasazi, J. E. Postdoctoral institutes: Rationale and recent activities. *Continuing Professional Development*, 1975, *12*(2), 5–9.

Katahn, M. A survey of the interest in continuing education among mental health professionals in the southeastern states. *American Psychologist*, 1970, *25*(10), 941–952.

Lawler, E. Post-doctoral training for industrial psychologists. *The Industrial Psychologist Newsletter*, Spring 1976, *4*(2), 34–40.

31 Community Psychology in Puerto Rico

Meeting the Challenge of a Rapidly Changing Society

Jose J. Bauermeister, Celia Fernandez de Cintron, and Eduardo Rivera-Medina

Puerto Rican society at present faces serious problems in its development and day-to-day interactions. Evidence of these problems can be seen in the magnitude of psychosocial indicators such as the rate of violence, unemployment, drug addiction, crime, and family dissolution. The size and intensity of migratory movements has also been an important index of the stresses confronted by the Puerto Ricans.

After a painful process of soul searching and lengthy debates on how to meet the challenges posed by these alarming social statistics, the Department of Psychology of the University of Puerto Rico (Rio Piedras Campus) revised the training objectives of its master's degree program. Until recently, this program followed an academic, general-experimental orientation, with no attempt to provide for any applied specializations. Since its inception, the only major additions within the realm of applied psychology were limited to several courses in clinical and industrial psychology.

The present revision of the program stemmed from a process of analysis initiated during the academic year 1974-1975. In it the needs of community agencies, the degree of readiness and capability of the department, and the needs and interests of graduate students were taken into consideration. Manpower studies and the information available from government agencies (e.g., the Governor's Commission on Mental Health and the Health Department's Project on Mental Health Manpower Needs) underscored the need for professionals and paraprofessionals in the mental health area to have a broad service orientation. It soon became evident, however, that the traditional ways of offering mental health services in Puerto Rico have proved on many occasions to be insufficient and limited in their approaches. Toward the end of this process, after the Department of Psychology had endorsed the idea of establishing several areas of specialization, one of which was to be in social-

The authors are listed alphabetically. Further information on the ideas presented in this chapter can be obtained from the authors, Department of Psychology, Rio Piedras Campus, University of Puerto Rico, Rio Piedras, Puerto Rico 00931.

community psychology, the National Training Conference was held in Austin, Texas. Two of the new program's professors attended this conference and were able to discuss the objectives and format of the Puerto Rican project. Although the Puerto Rican program is tailored to meet and respond to the specific needs of a society immersed in the problems of rapid growth and change and a cultural setting that differs widely from the mainland U.S., the conference provided valuable assistance.

Participation in the conference was particularly useful in reaffirming the need and justification for the new social-community program. This new specialization had the advantage of being created in response to needs already expressed by the community. The program was conceived as an effort to use all the resources available to the university, including those that were beyond the boundaries of the Department of Psychology.

The Austin Conference facilitated the critical evaluation of plans by outside observers. Some of the difficulties expected were discussed, and the most glaring limitations of the proposed curriculum became evident. There were three additional results of Puerto Rican participation in the conference: (1) It became clear that the new program was part of an effort with at least 10 years of history and development; (2) in spite of the lack of prior formal communication with other programs, it was evident that the UPR was following basic general principles and trends that characterize the field of community psychology, and that resources of manpower, publications, materials, and overall experiences already developed in other areas were available to Puerto Rico; and (3) contacts and preliminary commitments were made with several participants at the Austin Conference for future consultations. Finally, the UPR department, at the time of the conference, was in the midst of submitting a proposal to NIMH for a training grant for the development of its graduate programs. The discussion and issues raised in the conference allowed the Puerto Rican participants to strengthen the presentation of the proposal to NIMH.

COMMUNITY PSYCHOLOGY TRAINING MODEL

The specific training model for community psychology at UPR is designed to provide an educational foundation to facilitate the growth, development, and functioning of communities and their components. It assumes that the community has within it certain resources, and that the task of the psychologist is to facilitate their discovery, development, and the best ways to use them. At the same time, this model also assumes that many of the needs of a community, particularly those instances that involve a need for fundamental social change, can and should be satisfied by resources of the community itself. This does not exclude optimal use of outside resources.

In terms of training, the general objective of the program is to help the students develop a conceptual framework to understand phenomena that influence psychosocial behavior and that serve as a basis for the development of skills for primary prevention in the communities. The following are specific objectives:

1. To train the students to identify, understand, and investigate the psychosocial processes and needs of communities in order to gain knowledge about attitudes, leadership, values, socialization processes, propaganda, social change, and planning.
2. To prepare the students so that they can identify and develop available community resources to meet the needs of the population.
3. To develop skills in primary prevention with groups, recognizing and showing due respect for the social forces that exist in the community. This does not preclude the community psychologist from influencing these forces.
4. To develop skills in consultation and in the evaluation of the mental health and social programs.

The student is expected to complete the training program in four semesters. In addition to formal courses, the curriculum includes a number of supervised practicum experiences and an internship. Following is a description of the proposed required and elective courses.

First Semester

The main objective of the courses offered during this semester is the acquisition of basic concepts. Although practicum experiences are not formally required, students are encouraged to become involved with ongoing research projects or other related activities. The following courses are required:

Statistics Applied to Psychology.
Theories of Personality. Selected theories of personality are discussed with particular emphasis on the effects of society and culture on personality development.
Advanced Social Psychology. The course attempts to develop a theoretical as well as a methodological orientation to help students understand the social construction of reality. Students are familiarized with major theories, particularly ethnomethodology and symbolic interaction, and focus on selected topics such as deviance and social control, attitudes, communication, attribution, social comparison, social movements, and ideology.
Community Psychology. The course is designed to familiarize the student with the history and issues of community psychology. It also attempts to develop skills in needs assessment and identification of resources available to Puerto Rican communities and organizations.

Second Semester

The objectives of this semester include an expansion of the conceptual framework and the development of skills in community psychology through participation in a practicum. The following courses are required:

Seminar: Methods in Psychological Research. An examination of the basic methods of research in social and community psychology.

Proseminar in General and Applied Psychology. The student must select three one-credit modules from the following: Principles of Supervision, Principles of Consultation, Epidemiology, Ethical Issues in Professional Psychology, Program Evaluation, and Decision-Making Processes.

Group Dynamics. The course concentrates study on the structure and function of groups, interaction within groups, and group leadership. Attention is given to force-field analysis and other skills in group intervention programs. (Two hours of lecture and three hours of laboratory per week.)

Seminar on the Psychological Analysis of Social and Cultural Change in Puerto Rico. The purpose of the seminar is to critically analyze the traditional indicators of social change and to help the student achieve an adequate understanding of the present situation in Puerto Rico. (This seminar may be substituted, with departmental authorization, by a course on theories of change and development offered by the Graduate School of Planning.)

Practicum in Community Psychology. The purpose of this practicum is to expand the theoretical framework discussed in the Community Psychology course. It also aims to develop skills in community interventions, systematic recompilation of data, and related aspects of field work. (Eight hours of practicum per week.)

Third Semester

The two objectives of this semester are development and, if possible, completion of thesis and the further acquisition of skills that will enable the student to participate fully during the following semester in a work setting internship. The following courses are required:

Thesis Seminar. Development of the thesis research and collection of data.

Analysis of Strategies for the Management of Conflicts and Crises. The course is designed to conceptualize and develop skills in the prevention and management of interpersonal, group, and community conflicts in Puerto Rican society.

Practicum in Analysis of Strategies for the Management of Conflicts and Crises. Supervised practicum experiences geared to the development of intervention skills needed for the prevention and management of

interpersonal, group, and community conflicts and crises. (Eight hours of practicum per week.)
Elective Course.

Fourth Semester

The objective of this semester is, basically, the application of the skills developed in an actual work setting. It also provides needed additional time for students to complete their theses.

Thesis Work. The course is designed to provide advice and assistance to students working on thesis research.
Internship in Social-Community Psychology. Supervised practicum experiences in community interventions at different levels; informal groups, organizations, institutions, and geographical and sociological communities. Emphasis will be given to the development of skills in primary and secondary prevention. (Twenty hours of work experience per week.)

The field practica and internships are carried out in different institutions, such as the Center for Interdisciplinary Practice of the Rio Piedras Campus, psychiatric hospitals, mental health centers, preventive and counseling school centers, and in geographical communities. For example, during the past two years two communities located in socioeconomically deprived areas have been used as practicum sites. In one of them coordinated efforts have been made with a preventive and counseling school center. This center is collecting data on the population served and conducting primary prevention activities with the families of the students enrolled in the school system of the community. For the other, which is a "rurban" community (both rural and slum characteristics are present), data have been gathered and primary preventive activities designed and implemented. An example of the activities are group discussions about effects of social change, the organization of groups of teenagers and their parents, and anticipatory guidance with mothers of first- and second-graders.

The social-community program is clearly not clinically oriented. It is geared to training psychologists capable of organizing and participating in primary prevention efforts, general program development, and evaluation. Nevertheless, the curriculum revision allows for a subspecialization that combines social-community psychology with clinical skills. It is expected that students choosing this subspecialization will work primarily in community mental health settings, while the graduates of the social-community program will pursue careers in other agencies as well. The Departments of Education, Addiction Services, Social Services, and the Youth Action Administration also have programs that will require the skills of this new professional.

The social-community program is firmly committed to an interdisciplinary approach and attempts to use those resources that are available beyond the boundaries of the Department of Psychology. Specifically, courses offered by the Graduate School of Planning are recommended as complementary to the curriculum. Faculty members of the Sociology and Anthropology Department, as well as researchers from the Social Science Research Center of the Rio Piedras Campus, have been participating in meetings and seminars sponsored by the new program. To broaden the scope and perspective of the work, there is a deliberate effort to recruit all the resources available within the academic community. This effort extends beyond the walls of academia, as the program emphasizes the "learn by doing" approach, which requires close liaison with agencies and professionals in the Puerto Rican community.

CENTER FOR INTERDISCIPLINARY PRACTICE

The National Training Conference in Community Psychology also contributed to the further development of a University Center for Interdisciplinary Practice (CIP), which is one of the most important field training sites for the Department of Psychology clinical and social community students. The CIP was recently created through joint efforts of the Psychology Department, the Social Work Graduate School, the Graduate Program in Rehabilitation Counseling, and the Department of Sociology and Anthropology. The center provides psychosocial services to the community that surrounds the Rio Piedras Campus and promotes the understanding of an interdisciplinary, integrative approach to the delivery of psychosocial services and the development of creative and innovative models of professional intervention.

The center is especially directed toward dealing with the problems of communal living and functioning in the area of Rio Piedras, and it is attempting to develop a model for interdisciplinary training and intervention that corresponds with a dynamic urban society. This model considers, among other issues, the relationship between individual and city, between the city's spatial and social organization, and interactions among the different social sectors.

The CIP is organized in three training units: (1) preventive and remedial interventions, which offers psychological and social services mainly to the low-income inhabitants and families in the CIP catchment area; (2) organizational and community design and intervention, which is responsible for the identification of needs, resources, and situations that require professional intervention; and (3) socioanthropological research, which aims to carry out a socioanthropological study of the catchment area. The goal of this study is to identify and develop social indicators of mental health. It will also identify those social and cultural variables affecting dysfunctional behavior as well as those that promote social integration and solidarity.

Students of both the social-community and the clinical program participate in the three units of the CIP with students from the other participating disciplines. This interdisciplinary collaboration in training, research, and the rendering of services should result in the development of a community psychologist capable of acknowledging and meeting the challenges of contemporary Puerto Rican society.

32 Conferences, Program Models, and Accreditation in Community Psychology

Louis D. Cohen

I had an old public health administrator friend who would advise that we follow the biblical admonition and go up the mountain for an overview whenever we came to working on a really difficult problem. Such a course is helpful for seeing the broad patterns, for details become obscure—and it was my preferred course when I was asked to reflect on some of the major themes in a comparison of the Austin and Swampscott community psychology meetings. Having participated in the Swampscott Conference, where I had the opportunity to present one of the position papers, and having also attended other training conferences that hit on similar themes, I looked for some major trends among them. I was particularly reminded of the Palo Alto Conference on mental and public health in 1955, when Robert Felix, then director of the National Institute of Mental Health, introduced Eric Lindemann, professor of psychiatry at Harvard, who electrified that conference with his public health/mental health synthesis. Dr. Lindemann sketched a broad reconceptualization of the posture appropriate to mental health practice and advocated an active outreach, which in that period and climate seemed most visionary and even impractical.

Ten or so years later at Swampscott, the conference on community mental health again developed a vision of where community programs might go and vibrated to an exciting charisma of hope and inspiration. The climate of the mid-1960s was more activist and revolutionary, and Lindemann's vision of only 10 years earlier now seemed quite possible to achieve.

The '60s and early '70s of this century have seen enormous changes in the basic human rights that American society is prepared to recognize as inalienable. It is only a little more than 50 years since women got the right to vote, but the past 15 have seen revolutionary achievements in privileges and expectations for the rights of women. But not only for women; similar changes have taken place in the area of eliminating racial, religious, income, age, and other types of discrimination. There is still much to be done to attain equal opportunity for all citizens, but when a minority-group citizen elects to risk prison in America rather than "freedom" in a foreign country, we can believe that the American scene is beginning to respond. From the perspective of someone born early in this century, an incredible set of changes has taken place.

Community psychology has gained much zest because of these social changes, and much enthusiasm derives from the expectation that change is possible and probable. But there have also been frustrations, many born from an impatient expectation of sudden, permanent social changes. The climate of change in America over the past 15 years has given reassurance to a change orientation, but for permanent or deep changes much more time and persistent attention seem necessary.

At the Swampscott meeting in 1965 a description of community psychology was articulated, although it was not specifically spelled out. In the intervening years a number of meetings have been held to sharpen a single, strong position to describe community psychology. This aim has been regularly defeated, and it has proved to be impossible to get a neat and comprehensive statement of what community psychology is. The Procrustean bed of a single definition has defeated attempts at consensus in the past. Interestingly, the Austin meeting overcame the difficulty by accepting the notion of different training models of which I personally was able to resonate to three. By adopting a multimodel format the conference was able to provide an umbrella under which the diverse emphases of community psychology might be considered.

At Austin there seemed to be a large group of participants who affiliated with the community/clinical emphasis, whose base of operations was the clinic, the mental health setting, or the university and whose concern was to intervene in a social setting as it might impinge upon and create behavior difficulties for citizens. A second group at Austin emphasized a concern with social psychology and community program evaluation in which the method was the analysis of social systems and the evaluation of effectiveness of systems in meeting the social, health, education, and welfare needs, or for meeting some other significant aspect of the community's human rights concerns. A third group at Austin seemed to cluster around an interest in social system analysis with a view to articulating social criticism and sharpening advocacy goals; this group was also concerned with developing sophisticated change-agent skills.

Getting these three, and other models, under one definition has proved to be impossible, but nonetheless the acceptance of multiple models provided a way for all the different emphases in community psychology to come together in peace.

There was another major development, and that was the acceptance that an ideological integration was not necessary and probably not possible at this time. Providing a longer period of time for the field of community psychology to develop its knowledge base, to explore its constancies, to experiment with its action, will probably make it possible for the field to substitute experience for the present rhetoric. The fact that the conference was prepared to accept a more relaxed time framework and was prepared to develop its definitions made working and living together much simpler.

Another question has arisen. It is now 10 years since the Swampscott meeting. Is this a good time to deal with accreditation of training programs? The question was put to me, since I happen to be involved currently with the relevant APA committees. As you might guess, there are both positive and negative aspects to becoming involved in accreditation of training programs at this time.

One of the major concerns with accreditation processes in new areas is that of premature closure on the field. It is obvious that in an area like community psychology, where technology and ideology are still being actively forged, early codification may be harmful to development. Thus, the problem involves an estimate of when the field has developed sufficient stability and consensus to permit a statement of modal criteria.

Since the process of accreditation involves the setting of standards, specifying criteria, and identifying regularities, the process compels some conformity in the programs and on the behavior of individuals and organizations. APA in its accrediting process has shown remarkable flexibility, encouraging individuality and self-determination for programs. But, inevitably, an accreditation process provides a yardstick against which a performance may be measured, and if there is a yardstick some uniformity will emerge.

When a specific program area is accredited, such as community psychology, there is need to spell out the content, the activities, the skills, the knowledge, the settings, and the faculty experience that would be necessary as a minimum set of attributes of a program. As one reviews the Austin Conference for signs of a necessary consensus to identify these minimum sets of attributes, one becomes aware that the conference might have been successful primarily because it could tolerate diverse orientations. The conference did and could contain different passions and could provide a forum for varied postures.

It could well be that moving toward accreditation of training programs in community psychology at this time is premature. If there is need to select one model, one would find that the conference itself could not do this. If two or more models are required, one may find that the selections would be arbitrary. It could be that the reasonable posture would be to develop a consensus of training experiences throughout the field that at some appropriate time would have reached such a stage of acceptance as to be recognized as modal and appropriate for the field. And, perhaps, the best way to test this consensus is to take readings at frequent intervals.

It is an exciting vista from the mountain. One sees the variety of ideas that are common in community psychology today. There are concerns with the quality of life, with social indicators of well-being, concerns with environmental quality, with the well-being of communities, both natural and intentional, which suggest that the field has come a long way in making practical the vision of Lindemann, Felix, and a host of Swampscott veterans. The Austin Conference was reassuring in showing the progress that had been made. But perhaps it was also sobering in the realization that progress was only beginning to be made. There is much more to be done, but we seem to be at the threshold.

VII EPILOGUE

33 Community Psychology in Transition

Reflections on the Austin Conference

Charles D. Spielberger and Ira Iscoe

The National Conference on Training in Community Psychology represents the culmination of the individual and collective efforts of many people. The goals of the conference were to bring together a broadly-representative cross-section of community psychologists with strong commitments to training. The historical context for the conference was examined in Chapter 1 of this volume, in which previous national training conferences in other fields of psychology were also described. Details of the planning process and the preconference preparations were discussed in Chapter 2.

In selecting conference participants, inputs were actively sought from leaders in the field of community psychology, directors of training programs, national organizations concerned with training in psychology, and individual community psychologists working in academic and community settings. The people invited to attend consisted of approximately equal numbers of community psychologists who were recognized as leaders in the field, younger community psychologists who had received their Ph.D.'s within the past five years, and graduate students.

The Conference Planning Committee also endeavored to obtain a balance in the number of participants from academic institutions and field training settings, and to insure that representation within each of these constituencies included substantial numbers of women and minority groups. In addition, observers were invited from the National Institute of Mental Health, which was the primary source of funding for the conference, the APA Boards for Education and Training and Professional Affairs, and other national and regional organizations concerned with mental health training.

The conference participants began to converge on the Thompson Center of the University of Texas at Austin on a beautiful, balmy Sunday afternoon. By the opening conference session on Monday morning, the winds had intensified, the skies had become overcast, and the temperature had dropped more than 20 degrees. At the end of the first session, the rain began to descend in a most inhospitable manner, and continued for two full days.

However, by the end of the final session, the sun burst forth in time to dry the terrain for the Texas-style barbecue that culminated the conference activities.

The mood and progress of the conference seemed to parallel the vicissitudes in the Austin weather. Initial conviviality among old acquaintances and the pleasure of making new friends gave way to frustration as the participants were confronted with the complex task that lay before them. Each participant was assigned to two different types of groups, one concerned with conceptualizing a particular model or approach to training in community psychology, and the other devoted to evaluating a central issue in the training of community psychologists. Despite much initial turmoil and confusion, the commitment and dedication of conference participants to the task was clearly reflected in the fact that many of them worked long into the evenings to prepare presentations on topics to be discussed the following day.

This volume has provided detailed descriptions and cogent analyses of what went on at the Austin Conference. While it is not possible to convey adequately the complex deliberations on which this report of conference proceedings is based, it should be noted that initial frustration with the complexity of the task that confronted the participants was subsequently replaced with a sense of satisfaction and achievement. By the final plenary session, in which the reports of the training models and special interest groups were presented, most participants were agreed that much had been accomplished. There was also considerable optimism about the future of community psychology.

In this brief epilogue, we can only endeavor to highlight some of the important issues that emerged at the Austin Conference. For a fuller appreciation of the range and scope of the topics that were considered, and for a more comprehensive understanding of the conclusions that emerged, it is essential for the reader to examine carefully the entire contents of this volume.

AN OVERVIEW OF THE CONFERENCE PROCEEDINGS

The Austin Conference began with presentations by distinguished contributors to the field of community psychology who were invited to present keynote addresses. These keynotes served to clarify the ideology of community psychology, and to identify and delineate critical issues and problems in training. Three papers based on keynote addresses are included in Part II and one in Part III of this volume. The remaining papers reported in Part III are based on the deliberations of the groups that considered specific training models, and those in Part IV are concerned with critical issues in training. Recent surveys of trends in training and in the practice of community psychology that were reported at the conference are included in Part V. In addition, reflections of individual participants were solicited by the editors on a number of issues and problems not fully considered at the conference, and these are included in Part VI.

The Ideology of Community Psychology

In the initial keynote address, Seymour Sarason set the tone for the conference by challenging community psychology to establish an identity that was separate and distinct from clinical psychology. Rather than limiting ourselves to concerns about mental illness and mental health, Sarason stressed the importance of building communities that would be better equipped to meet human needs. He also emphasized the vital role of "networks" of communication and power that must be understood and utilized if one wishes to work successfully in community settings.

Robert Reiff's keynote address recognized the legitimacy of what he termed the healing, developmental, and social systems approaches to meeting human needs. Reiff observed that community psychology still lacks a clear conceptual framework and a consistent value base. In Reiff's view the future of community psychology is "inextricably linked to the welfare of the people in our society." For Reiff, the continued growth and development of community psychology will depend on how well we come to understand critical social issues, and on our ability to develop theories, research methods, and modes of practice that contribute to effective community interventions at the social systems level.

James Kelly's keynote address reviewed issues related to levels of training and the varied educational settings in which training takes place. Kelly emphasized the need for an open-systems approach in which there is continuing communication among university faculty, community leaders, and psychologists who work in community settings. Thus, Kelly joined Sarason and Reiff in advocating a social-systems orientation to solving human problems as the most meaningful and appropriate conceptual framework for community psychology.

In the final keynote address, which is included in Part III, John Glidewell commented on training models in community psychology. He identified a continuum of human problems, ranging from "pain-distress" through "life-enhancement," and cited specific examples of community interventions that are appropriate for particular clients. Glidewell also noted the complexity of the field, reviewed the skills and qualifications that are required for different types of community interventions, and warned that community psychologists must recognize their limitations by selecting problem areas within which they can work competently and effectively.

Training Models and Approaches

The complexities noted by Glidewell were reflected in the deliberations of the conference groups that considered various training approaches. Whereas the scientist-professional model was adopted for clinical psychology at the Boulder Conference, and the Vail Conference recently recommended a professional training model for psychologists primarily concerned with clinical practice, the participants at the Austin Conference accepted the reality and the need for multiple, diverse models and approaches to training in community psychology.

At the present time, training in community psychology takes place in a variety of settings in which many different combinations of resources are used by practitioners with varied backgrounds. Since lack of agreement with respect to any single approach is an accurate reflection of the present status of the field, premature crystallization with respect to training models and modes of practice seems unlikely. While some community psychologists deplore the prevailing heterogeneity among training programs, others note that diverse approaches to training permit a wide range of experimentation and innovation, as well as flexibility in designing training programs that are uniquely suited to particular settings. Clearly, educational programs in community psychology are free to explore new approaches and methods in meeting a wide range of community intervention and research needs.

Even though there is great diversity among individual models and approaches to training, there are also important commonalities in most community psychology training programs. For example, there was general agreement at the Austin Conference on the desirability of moving away from a mental illness model, and focusing instead on broader social-systems problems that relate to the enhancement of coping skills and competencies. Another commonality was a strong preference for indirect services, such as working with community agencies and institutions, rather than working directly with individual clients. The need for community-based research to establish a cohesive body of knowledge was also stressed in the groups that considered the different models and approaches, and there was substantial agreement with regard to the importance of maintaining a solid academic base to facilitate the integration of theory, field work, and research.

Each of the six models considered at the Austin Conference represents a different approach to the integration of theory and practice in community psychology. Each model also reflects salient features of existing training programs, and may be viewed as providing guidelines for the development of new programs. The ultimate viability of any training approach will depend on how well individual programs that follow this particular model are able to deal with the critical issues of central importance to community psychologists.

Critical Issues in Community Psychology

A major goal at the Austin Conference was to examine important conceptual issues in the field of community psychology. Five training issues were identified as critical: (1) entry levels and subprofessional personnel; (2) field training and placement; (3) future conceptual directions; (4) the knowledge and research base; and (5) alternative conceptual models. Emory Cowen was given the primary responsibility for extracting data relating to these issues from the conference deliberations. To assist him in this task, Cowen recruited five young community psychologists on the basis of a unique set of guidelines that are delightfully described in the introduction to Part IV. Each of these psychologists was assigned a critical training issue and the responsibility for clarifying this particular issue. They also met at the conference with special interest groups, and participated in a symposium devoted to further discussion of critical training issues, held at the 1975 APA meeting. The papers reported in Part IV reflect deliberations that took place during the Austin Conference and inputs from the APA symposium.

In his comments on issues relating to entry levels and subprofessional personnel, Steven Danish recommends that people engaged in the delivery of human services should be judged, not by the degrees that they hold, but by their basic competencies. He proposes a developmental framework for the delivery of human services in which the enhancement of human functioning is emphasized, in contrast to the traditional focus on the remediation of clinical symptoms. Within the context of this developmental approach, Danish suggests specific procedures and methods that are appropriate for people at various levels of training in community psychology.

David Stenmark observes in his paper in Part IV that lack of conceptual focus has been a serious detriment to formulating the goals of field training in community psychology. In stressing the need for community psychologists to develop evaluative and administrative skills, Stenmark proposes a sequential, step-by-step progression through four levels of training experiences: (1) observer of community service delivery systems; (2) program evaluator; (3) intervenor and social change agent; and, (4) conceptualizer and designer of community programs. The general competencies required for effective performance in each of these areas are related by Stenmark to each of the six models and approaches to training in community psychology that were considered at the conference.

With respect to future conceptual directions for community psychology training programs, Julian Rappaport notes that existing paradigms, such as the clinical intervention model, are neither adequate nor appropriate for the types of activities in which community psychologists are engaged. Stressing the importance of relating conceptual analysis to the strategies and tactics that are employed in social interventions, Rappaport provides specific examples of conceptual frameworks that are appropriate for particular types of community-based intervention procedures.

Trickett and Lustman contend that community psychology must embrace a wide range of research methods and procedures in order to understand relationships between individuals and social settings, as well as ecological research procedures that clarify the structure and functions of institutions and neighborhoods. In planning and conducting research in community settings,

Trickett and Lustman emphasize the importance of agreement between citizens and scholars with regard to establishing priorities and defining research problems.

Jack Chinsky was initially assigned the responsibility of formulating alternative conceptual models to those considered at the Austin Conference, but this proved to be an impossible task. Instead, he identified "nine coalescing themes" that reflected the major concerns of the conference participants. In evaluating these themes, Chinsky counsels community psychologists to examine their personal ties to their own communities, and to endeavor to integrate their professional work with their own personal experiences.

Collectively, the analyses of major training issues in community psychology in the papers reported in Part IV reflect current priorities and future aspirations of the field. Evidence bearing on the degree to which these priorities are presently being met is provided by the survey results described in Part V, and in the discussions of problems of vital concern to community psychologists reported in Part VI.

Current Trends in Community Psychology

The results of four recent surveys of interest to community psychologists are reported in Part V. Three of these surveys provide information with regard to current trends in the practice of community psychology from the perspectives of training program directors, members of APA Division 27, and professional staff associated with community mental health centers. The fourth survey samples the interests and aspirations of advanced graduate students in applied psychology programs.

In comparing the rhetoric of community psychology with the reality of the trends reflected in the surveys, Bloom observes a marked disparity between the ideology and the practices of community psychologists. The ideology of community psychology emphasizes crisis-oriented services in preference to long-term treatment, primary prevention and the enhancement of coping skills instead of remediation, and the modification of social systems to meet human needs rather than dealing with casualties of these systems. But most community psychologists who are currently associated with mental health centers continue to spend the bulk of their time in activities related to clinical practice, and many training program directors and Division 27 members continue to place strong emphasis on the development of clinical skills.

The survey of advanced graduate students conducted by Zolik, Sirbu, and Hopkinson also reveals some interesting disparities between student desires and aspirations, and the training experiences that are currently available to them. Apparently, many graduate students in applied psychology programs espouse the ideology of community psychology, and are greatly dissatisfied with academic courses and practicum training experiences that continue to emphasize traditional approaches to the delivery of mental health services. While some disparity is to be expected between the interests and aspirations of graduate students and the training that is available to them, it is hoped that the deliberations at the Austin Conference will provide productive guidelines for bridging the gap between student expectations and current training practices.

It should be noted that three of the four surveys that are reported in Part V were sponsored by, and received financial support from, the Division of Community Psychology. The support of these surveys provides tangible evidence of the division's commitment to obtaining information that will serve to stimulate and upgrade community psychology training programs. Since the surveys reflect feedback from the consumers of training efforts, they provide data that should prove useful in helping to close the gap between the ideology of community psychology and current approaches to training.

It was obviously not possible within the context of a three-day conference for detailed consideration of all of the many issues and topics related to training in community psychology. Although one conference session was devoted entirely to the discussion of topics not otherwise considered, there were nevertheless significant gaps in the coverage. In order to obtain additional input with regard to some of the topics that were not fully considered at the conference, the editors invited participants who expressed concern about these topics to contribute position papers to this volume. Invited position papers on social change, on the professional concerns of minority groups, women, and students, and on applications of community psychology in a variety of settings are included in Part VI. Other papers in Part VI examine the growing importance of community ecology, the need for continuing education for community psychologists, and the advantages and disadvantages of accrediting community psychology training programs.

One direct and immediate outcome of the Austin Conference was the establishment of a community-social psychology training program at the University of Puerto Rico. In this masters level program, which is described in Chapter 31 of this volume, students will be trained to identify and develop community resources that can be utilized in primary prevention programs to be implemented in a rapidly changing social environment, with tremendous problems of poverty and limited professional resources.

COMMUNITY PSYCHOLOGY IN TRANSITION

Community psychology has evolved out of clinical psychology and continues to be strongly tied to the mental health movement. While many community psychologists continue to be engaged in some clinical work, most of the participants at the Austin Conference were actively involved in community-related activities such as program evaluation, primary and secondary prevention, social-systems analysis, and community planning. When these community activities are contrasted with the results of the recent surveys reported in Part V, it would seem that a large gap exists between ideology and practice in community psychology. It is also apparent that the field of community psychology is currently in a state of rapid transition.

Granted the transitional status of community psychology, what is in store for the future? Predictions are hazardous in these uncertain times, especially for community psychology, which, by its very nature, must take into account a broad range of social forces and policies at the local, state, national, and even the international level. These difficulties are compounded by the rapidity with which social changes occur, and the relative paucity of solid information upon which to base predictions. Nevertheless, despite the hazards, the present status and future directions of community psychology must be evaluated if we are to develop effective training programs.

In the decade that followed the Boston Conference, community psychology gained increasing acceptance within academia. This acceptance is clearly reflected in the proliferation of courses and training programs with community content at the graduate and undergraduate level, and, especially, in the emergence of doctoral programs. The establishment of three major journals devoted primarily to community psychology, the publication of numerous books and monographs, and the increasing availability of academic positions for people with community psychology training provide additional tangible evidence of the growth and vitality of the field.

The development of community psychology will continue to be influenced by public policy regarding community mental health, national health and welfare programs, and support for higher education. The quality of life in most communities seems to be declining as evidenced by mounting dissatisfaction with public schools, increases in violence, and uncertainty and anxiety on the part of both young and old. Evidence of societal uncertainty and change was frequently noted in the present volume.

There are numerous indications that the delivery of traditional mental health services does not occupy the same priority of funding that was the case ten years ago, and that strategies for the delivery of human services are undergoing enormous change. Furthermore, despite commendable successes, community-based mental health centers have not fulfilled the promise of dealing more effectively with mental health problems, and have only begun to deal with alcoholism and drug abuse. These failures may well reflect a lack of understanding by community mental health center professionals of the communities that they serve.

In preference to clinical approaches to solving human problems, the majority of the participants at the Austin Conference espoused active interventive roles based on research in the social and behavioral sciences. A number of different community psychology training models and approaches were discussed, and some perspective about the future can be gained by an examination of what has been accomplished thus far. In an earlier symposium on training and research in community psychology, we identified five areas of concern: "(1) the definition and conception of community psychology; (2) the relationship between clinical and community psychology; (3) new roles for psychologists in institutional and community settings; (4) the academic foundations that seem essential for training programs in community psychology; and (5) the kinds of field training experiences that are needed to prepare psychologists to work effectively in community settings" (Spielberger & Iscoe, 1970, p. 227). The discussions at the Austin Conference suggested that training issues in these five areas are no less timely today. Although a detailed analysis of each of these issues is beyond the scope of this volume, a brief examination of their current status may help us to determine how much progress has been made, and what might be accomplished in the future.

The Definition of Community Psychology

The multiple models emerging from the Austin Conference and the establishment of training programs labeled *community, clinical-community,* and *community-clinical* psychology indicate that no single definition of community psychology exists. Community psychology overlaps with applied social psychology, developmental psychology, clinical psychology, human ecology, and other behavioral sciences. While there is some comfort in the fact that older and better established areas of psychology also have difficulty with defining themselves, it is apparent that community psychology is continuing to struggle with an identity problem.

With regard to the definition of community psychology, there now appears to be less concern with reaching a consensus on this topic. Community psychology *is* what community psychologists *do*, and it is apparent that community psychologists are presently engaged in a wide variety of professional activities. While some of these activities might just as easily be carried on under more traditional labels, the proliferation of training programs with a community orientation suggests that the "community concept" in psychological training, however vaguely defined, is now widely accepted. This evolving community emphasis in psychology training programs reflects a growing recognition of the significance of social-psychological and environmental factors in human adjustment in contrast to the earlier emphasis on intrapsychic factors.

Separation of Community from Clinical Psychology

Community psychology developed in part as a protest against the lack of effectiveness of the clinical approach in dealing with many behavioral problems. But community psychology continues to be closely tied to the community mental health movement, and a significant portion of the energies of many people who identify with community psychology is presently invested in the delivery of more or less traditional clinical services. While some community psychologists have begun to fulfill their hopes for intervention and prevention through mental health consultation and educational programs, such activities occupy at best a very small part of the total energy investment of most psychologists who are presently employed by community mental health centers.

The separation of community psychology from clinical psychology was strongly recommended by a number of participants at the Austin Conference. Some contended that unless this separation was carried out community psychology would never be able to proceed with the types of activities that are needed to solidify its identity. While many feel that divorce from clinical psychology is inevitable, others recommended marital counseling. The advantages of clinical and community psychology continuing to live together may be seen in the complementarity of professional roles, and in the greater employment opportunities for community psychologists with clinical skills.

Community psychology must face the issue of whether or not training in clinical skills is essential. As previously noted, a powerful argument for providing clinical training is that clinical skills are often required in the delivery of community mental health services, and this results in broader employment opportunities. An argument against clinical training is that the practice of community psychology is necessarily different from clinical practice, and it is not possible to provide training in the practice of both clinical and community psychology without unduly lengthening the period of training.

The recent establishment of training programs specifically labeled *community psychology* provides tangible evidence of a trend toward separation from the clinical approach. Several community psychology doctoral programs have been established, and other programs with strong community emphasis are now operating at both the Ph.D. and the master's level. The support that is received by community psychology programs, the degree to which they are accepted by academic colleagues, and the type of work that the graduates perform will eventually clarify the question of the optimal relationship between community psychology and clinical psychology.

New Roles and Employment Opportunities for Community Psychologists

Considerable frustration was voiced by participants at the Austin Conference concerning current roles and opportunities for employment. It was noted, for example, that there are many opportunities for psychologists to work as consultants and planners, and that clinical psychologists with community skills appear to be in strong demand in both academic programs and human service settings. However, as recent surveys have indicated, most of the roles played by community psychologists are still based on traditional approaches to the delivery of mental health services.

Within the job market itself, there are relatively few positions specifically available for community psychologists, and these are primarily at the academic level where there is now open advertising for psychologists with community skills. This state of affairs is in marked contrast to the evolution of clinical psychology where graduates of clinical training programs were eagerly sought, and there was a fairly direct relationship (at least at the beginning) between the diagnostic and therapeutic skills that were acquired in graduate training programs and applications of these clinical skills in employment settings.

It seems unlikely that new positions for community psychologists will be created in community mental health centers, or in other existing human service settings. However, training in community psychology provides meaningful preparation for a wide range of positions relating to the design, delivery, and evaluation of human services. Just as lawyers need not practice in law offices, nor engineers build bridges, people with community psychology training can find meaningful employment in a number of areas; for example, as evaluators of mental health and human service delivery systems, as urban planners and city managers, and in state and federal agencies concerned with human welfare.

Community psychologists will need to convince employers that they have something constructive to offer. The fact that community psychologists are not likely to be completely equipped for the job should not impede their contributions. Other professionals, if employed in responsible agencies, are generally expected to spend considerable time in getting to know the specific requirements of the positions they fill. The future employment opportunities for community psychologists will, therefore, depend on their ingenuity and their ability to find ways of "selling" their professional services.

Academic Foundations for Training in Community Psychology

There was no clear consensus at the Austin Conference with respect to the academic foundations most essential for training in community psychology, but there was strong agreement that community psychology must develop its own knowledge and research base. Since community psychology cannot "go it alone," it must draw on advances in the social and behavioral sciences. In 1970 we remarked on the difficulty of the transition from the laboratory of the university to the laboratory of the community, and we noted the need to establish agreement between citizen and scholar with regard to priorities for community-based research (Iscoe & Spielberger, 1970), a need that was discussed by Kelly in this volume in his comments on multiple methods for studying social systems.

Lack of correspondence between existing knowledge in the social and behavioral sciences, and validated applications to the problems of human beings underlies the issue of the appropriate academic foundation for community psychology. Until there is sufficient feedback from community-based research, there will be no way to resolve the question of the optimal academic preparation for community psychologists. It is encouraging to note, however, that there was substantial agreement at the Austin Conference concerning the importance of training in field research methodology and the need for intensive practicum experience in community settings. Given the acceptance of multiple training models by the participants at the Austin Conference, it seems likely that community psychology training programs will continue to have different goals that will require different academic inputs.

Field Training in Community Psychology

Appropriate field settings for practicum and internship training in community psychology continues to be a matter of significant concern. At the Austin Conference, there was substantial agreement that field training experiences should be more varied and broader in scope than is presently the case. A promising approach to field training in community psychology is described by Stenmark in Chapter 18 of this volume.

The need for a closer relationship between academic training and field work in community psychology was emphasized at the Austin Conference. It was also acknowledged that mutually-rewarding working relationships between university and human service agencies must be developed, and it will take time for such associations to be established. The success or failure of community psychology training programs may very well hinge on how successful program directors are in arranging for community internship and practicum placements, and for support for students from nontraditional, community-based sources.

Authentic field training in community psychology will require that people in field settings be welcome in academic departments, and there must be adequate two-way communication. Indeed, one of the most frequent complaints at the Austin Conference was the failure to include a sufficient number of field-based community psychologists as participants at the conference, and as instructors and supervisors in training programs. The process by which knowledge is put to work in field settings and, more importantly, the process through which appropriate field training settings are created, would seem to be a top priority for community psychology in the years ahead.

It seems to us that community psychology has made substantial progress with regard to the training issues that we identified in 1970. In bringing these issues into contemporary perspective, and attempting to extrapolate observable trends, we confidently predict that an effective community psychology will emerge from the current state of transition. This will require that new theories and practices be tested in community settings in order to add to the knowledge base. While community psychology has the potential to facilitate future applications of behavioral science knowledge to the benefit of society, the realization of this potential will critically depend on the development of effective training programs.

REFERENCES

Iscoe, I., & Spielberger, C. D. The emerging field of community psychology. In I. Iscoe & C. D. Spielberger (Eds.), *Community psychology: Perspectives in training and research.* New York: Appleton-Century-Crofts, 1970.

Spielberger, C. D., & Iscoe, I. The current status of training in community psychology. In I. Iscoe & C. D. Spielberger (Eds.), *Community psychology: Perspectives in training and research.* New York: Appleton-Century-Crofts, 1970.

APPENDIXES

A National Conference on Training in Community Psychology

Committees

DIVISION 27 EXECUTIVE COMMITTEE 1974–1975

Charles D. Spielberger, President, Department of Psychology, University of South Florida

Emory Cowen, President-Elect, Department of Psychology, University of Rochester

J. Wilbert Edgerton, Past President, Department of Psychiatry, University of North Carolina Medical School

Betty L. Kalis, Secretary/Treasurer, San Francisco, California

Morton Bard, Representative to APA Council of Representatives, Graduate Center, City University of New York

Barbara Dohrenwend, Member-at-Large, The Graduate School and University Center, City University of New York

J. R. Newbrough, Member-at-Large, George Peabody College

Melvin Zax, Member-at-Large, Department of Psychology, University of Rochester

Thomas Glynn, Graduate Student Representative, Catholic University

Margaret Meyer, Graduate Student Representative, University of Texas at Austin

CONFERENCE PLANNING COMMITTEE

Ira Iscoe, Chairman, Department of Psychology, University of Texas at Austin

Bernard Bloom, Cochairman, Department of Psychology, University of Colorado

Barbara Dohrenwend, Graduate School and University Center, City University of New York

Dorothy Fruchter, private practice, Austin, Texas

Meg Gerrard, Social Work Research Institute, University of Texas at Austin

Joseph Aponte, Department of Psychology, University of Louisville

Charles Holahan, Department of Psychology, University of Texas at Austin

Bertha Holliday, Department of Psychology, University of Texas at Austin

James Kelly, School of Community Service and Public Affairs, University of Oregon

Tim Kuehnel, Psychiatric Research Unit, University of California at Los Angeles

Margaret Meyer, Department of Psychology, University of Texas at Austin
Robert Reiff, Center for the Study of Social Intervention, Albert Einstein College of Medicine of Yeshiva University
Karl Slaikeu, Counseling-Psychological Services Center, University of Texas at Austin
Charles D. Spielberger, Department of Psychology, University of South Florida
Edison Trickett, Department of Psychology, Yale University
Brian Wilcox, Department of Psychology, University of Texas at Austin

B National Conference on Training in Community Psychology

Preconference Materials— Table of Contents

I. Background Documents and Preconference Statements and Reports
    A. Anderson, L., Cooper, S., Hassol, L., Klein, D., Rosenblum, G., and Bennett, C. Community Psychology: A Report of the Boston Conference on the Education of Psychologists for Community Mental Health—Introduction and Summary, 1966.
    B. Spielberger, C., and Iscoe, I. Graduate Education in Community Psychology. In Golann and Eisdorfer (Eds.) *Handbook of Community Mental Health.* New York: Appleton-Century-Crofts, 1972.
    C. Bard, M., and Dohrenwend, B. Community Psychology: An Alternative to Community Mental Health.
    D. Cowen, E. Suggestions for Division 27 Training Conference Foci.
    E. Kaswan, J. Some Modest Proposals for the 1975 Community Psychology Conference.
    F. Murrell, S. Directions and Priorities for Community Psychology.
    G. Rhodes, W. Untitled Statement.
    H. Vail Conference Community Psychology Recommendations.
    I. Zolik, E., Sirbu, W., and Hopkinson, D. Graduate Student Perspectives on Training in Community Mental Health—Community Psychology.
    J. Meyer, M., and Ford, J. Psychology in Action: Training for the Future—Conference Report and Recommendations.

II. Community Psychology Training Program Descriptions:

Reader Note: All contributors were asked to describe their programs or models along seven dimensions, i.e., ideology and value base, goals and objectives, units of study, knowledge and research base, technology and skills required, content areas, format or organization. The programs described represented a valuable assemblage of information about existing training programs in community psychology. The analysis of these programs constitutes the basis of Glidewell's keynote address in Section III of the present volume.

Descriptions were submitted from Boston College, California School of

Professional Psychology, University of California—Irvine, University of Colorado, University of Connecticut, DePaul University, Federal City College, George Peabody College, University of Illinois, University of Louisville, University of Maryland, University of Massachusetts, University of Michigan, The Graduate Center—City University of New York, Richmond College of the City University of New York, Ohio State University, University of Oregon, Pennsylvania State University, University of Texas, Wheaton College, University of Wisconsin—Green Bay, and Yale University.

III. Community Psychology Academic and Field-Training Issues
    A. Presser, N., and Dietz, A. An Interschool Placement Program for Broad-Based Graduate Training in Community Psychology.
    B. Rappaport, J., Davidson, W., Wilson, M. and Mitchell, A. Alternatives to Blaming the Victim or the Environment: Our Places to Stand Have Not Moved the Earth.
    C. Swift, C. The Role of the Community-Based Professional in Peer Training.
    D. Todd, D. Our Concepts, Ourselves: Implications of Person-Environment Interaction Concepts for Training in Community Psychology.
    E. Tyler, F., and Gatz, M. If Community Psychology Is So Great, Why Don't We Try It?

IV. Ethics of Social Intervention
    A. Code of Ethics of the Society for Applied Anthropology.
    B. Hassol, L. Freedom to Choose: An Ethical Basis for Social Intervention.
    C. Simon, G. Is Professional Training a Barrier to Social Responsibility?

V. Subdoctoral Training in Community Psychology
    A. Kalafat, J. The Paraprofessional Movement as a Paradigm Community Psychology Endeavor.
    B. Kuppersmith, J., Blair, R., and Levin, H. Description of a Community Mental Health MA Program Designed Especially for an Ethnic Working Class Community.
    C. Rossi, A. Community Psychology at the Undergraduate Level.

VI. Community Psychology and Social Action
    A. Liberman, A., Nelson, H., Amidon, R., and Retish, P. Politics in Mental Health—A New Measured Response.
    B. Price, R., and Cherniss, C. Training for a New Profession: Research as Social Action.

C National Conference on Training in Community Psychology

Conference Agenda

SUNDAY, APRIL 27

Afternoon and evening—Registration and continuous informal reception for conference participants.

MONDAY, APRIL 28

Morning

Opening remarks and welcome: Ira Iscoe, Chairman, Conference Planning Committee.

Goals and scope of the conference and introduction of representatives from other divisions and organizations: Charles Spielberger, President, Division 27.

Greetings and informal remarks: W. H. Holtzman, Ph.D., President, Hogg Foundation for Mental Health.

Invited Address: Community Psychology, Networks, and "Mr. Everyman"—Seymour B. Sarason; introduced by Emory Cowen.

Invited Address: Critique of Training Models and Approaches Submitted in Preconference Materials—John G. Glidewell; introduced by Faye Goldberg.

Afternoon

First meeting of working groups to organize and begin discussion on models and approaches to training in community psychology and participation in one of six groups:

Clinical/community and community mental health models
Community development and systems approaches
Intervention and prevention approaches
Social change models and approaches
Social ecology approaches
Applied social psychology approaches

Late Afternoon

Meeting of special interest groups:

Conceptual Directions, Julian Rappaport, Chairman
Knowledge and Research Base, Edison Trickett, Chairman
Field Training, David Stenmark, Chairman
Entry Levels, Steven Danish, Chairman
Alternative Models, Jack Chinsky, Chairman

Evening

Dinner. Invited Address: "Varied Settings for Education in Community Psychology," James G. Kelly; introduced by Wayne H. Holtzman.

TUESDAY, APRIL 29

Morning

Invited Address: Robert Reiff, "Ya Gotta Believe." Introduced by Charles Holahan.
The State of the Art—Brief Reports on Important Facets of Community Psychology

Graduate Students View Their Training—Edwin Zolik
Similarities and Differences in Community Psychology—Joseph Aponte
Southern Regional Education Board and Community Psychology Training—Louis Ramey
Employment and Community Psychology—Carolyn Suber
Fellowship Support for Ethnic Minorities—Dalmas Taylor
Problems and Prospects for Chicanos in Community Psychology Training—Manuel Ramirez
Panel of Reactors: Barbara Dohrenwend, Steven Hobfoll, Maurice Korman, Richard Price, N. Dickon Reppucci, Stanley Sue, Meg Meyer

Afternoon

Continuation of consideration of models and approaches, deadlines and responsibility and completion to be decided by groups.

Late Afternoon

Second meeting Special Interest Groups.

Evening

No formal meetings scheduled. Spontaneous meeting of groups to discuss matters of mutual interest and concern.

WEDNESDAY, APRIL 30

Morning

Chairmen of Models Report to Full Session—John Newbrough, Chairman.
Other Issues Not Discussed at Conference—Bernard Lubin, Chairman.

Afternoon

Reports of Leaders of Special Interest Groups—Emory Cowen, Chairman
Panel of Respondents: Karl Slaikeu, Brian Wilcox, Kemba Young plus keynote
    speakers.

Late Afternoon

Plenary Session—Recommendations of the Conference—Charles Spielberger
presiding.

Evening

Texas style barbecue.

THURSDAY, MAY 1

Meeting of Conference Planning Committee and Division 27 Training Committee—Charles Spielberger, Chairman.

D National Conference on Training in Community Psychology

Roster of Participants and Observers

PARTICPANTS

Adelson, Dan, University of California, San Francisco

*Andrade, Sally, University of Texas at Austin

Andrulis, Dennis, Community Psychiatry, School of Medicine, University of North Carolina

Aponte, Joseph, University of Louisville

Attkisson, C. Clifford, Langley Porter Institute, University of California, San Francisco

Bailey, Bruce, Stephen F. Austin University

Barton, Keith, Community Psychiatry, University of North Carolina

*Bell, Keith, University of Texas at Austin

Blair, Rima, Richmond College, City University of New York

Bloom, Bernard, University of Colorado at Boulder

Brennan, George, University of Massachusetts

Bugen, Larry, University of Missouri, Columbia

Callahan, Robert, National Institute of Mental Health

Carman, Roderick, University of Wyoming

Cherniss, Cary, University of Michigan, Ann Arbor

Chinsky, Jack M., University of Connecticut, Storrs

Cintron, Celia F., University of Puerto Rico

Cohen, James K., Albert Einstein College of Medicine

Cohen, Louis, University of Florida

Cowen, Emory, University of Rochester

Cripps, Rosalie, Bexar County MH/MR Center, San Antonio, Texas

Cripps, Tom, Bexar County MH/MR Center, San Antonio, Texas

*Cuellar, Israel, University of Texas at Austin

Culler, Ralph, University of Texas at Austin

Czeh, Robert, National Institute of Mental Health

D'Augelli, Anthony, Pennsylvania State University

*Davis, Linda, University of Texas at Austin

*Community Psychology Training Program, University of Texas at Austin.

Danish, Steven J., Pennsylvania State University
*Dean, Ben, University of Texas at Austin
Delworth, Ursula, Western Interstate Commission on Higher Education
Derby, Nancy Jo, University of Texas at Austin
Dohrenwend, Barbara, City University of New York
Dorr, Darwin, Washington University
*Doty, Sue, University of Texas at Austin
Escoffrey, Aubrey, Norfolk State College
Esparza, Ricardo, University of Michigan
Fleischer, Kristine, New York University
Fruchter, Dorothy, private practice, Austin, Texas
Gallessich, June, University of Texas at Austin
Garcia, Sandra Anderson, University of South Florida
Gatz, Margaret, University of Maryland
Gaudreault, Cheryl, University of South Carolina
Gerrard, Meg, School of Social Work, University of Texas at Austin
*Gilius, Terry, University of Texas at Austin
Glidewell, John C., University of Chicago
Goldberg, Faye, University of Chicago
Gonzales, Humberto, University of Houston
Gonzales, José, University of Texas Health Science Center, San Antonio, Texas
Goodman, Gerald, University of California, Los Angeles
Gottlieb, Benjamin, University of Guelph, Ontario, Canada
Haas, Leonard, University of Colorado at Boulder
Hassol, Leonard, Wheaton College
Haywood, Charles, Crisis Intervention Institute, Buffalo, New York
Helge, Swen, Texas Christian University
*Hilbertz, Regina, University of Texas at Austin
*Hill, Gayle, University of Texas at Austin
Hobfoll, Stevan E., University of South Florida
Hodges, William F., University of Colorado at Boulder
Hoffman, David B., University of California, Los Angeles
Holahan, Charles J. (Josh), University of Texas at Austin
*Holliday, Bertha, University of Texas at Austin
Iscoe, Ira, University of Texas at Austin
James, Leonard, Texas Technological University
James, Sherman, University of North Carolina
Kalafat, John, Florida State University
Katkin, Edward S., State University of New York at Buffalo
Kelly, James G., University of Oregon
Key, Martha, Long Beach VA Hospital
Klass, Tobey, Albert Einstein College of Medicine
Korman, Maurice, University of Texas Health Science Center, Dallas, Texas
Kramer, Judy, Red Bank Community Mental Health Center, New Jersey
Kruger, Bruce, Corpus Christi, Texas

*Community Psychology Training Program, University of Texas at Austin.

Kuehnel, Tim, University of Texas at Austin
Larcen, Stephen W., University of Connecticut, Storrs
Lehmann, Stanley, New York University
Leidig, Margie W., University of Colorado at Boulder
Liem, Ramsay, Boston College
Lorion, Raymond, Temple University, Philadelphia
Lubin, Bernard, University of Houston
McLean, Christine, Marist College
*Meyer, Margaret, University of Texas at Austin
Miller, Francis T., University of North Carolina
Monahan, John, University of California, Irvine
Moore, Thom, University of Illinois
Mulvey, Anne, City University of New York
Munoz, Ricardo, Psychological Clinic, Eugene, Oregon
Myers, Ernest R., Federal City College
Nelson, Sherman, National Institute of Mental Health
Nesbit, Mimi, University of Texas at Austin
Newbrough, John R., Peabody College
Newmark, Justin, University of Texas at Austin
Nottingham, Jack A., Georgia Southwestern College
Nurse, Rodney, California School of Professional Psychology, San Francisco
Padesky, Christine Anne, University of California, Los Angeles
Payne, Sherry, Fort Worth Public Schools System, Fort Worth, Texas
Perez, Manuel S., Community Mental Health Center, Watsonville, California
Phillips, Beeman, University of Texas at Austin
Pierce, Maureen, Brooklyn College
Pitts, Henry, Howard University
Price, Richard H., University of Michigan
Raffaniello, Eileen M., University of Texas at Austin
Ramey, Louis, Southern Regional Education Board
Ramirez, Manuel, University of California, Santa Cruz
Rappaport, Julian, University of Illinois
Reiff, Robert, Albert Einstein College of Medicine
Reiss, Maxine, Florida State University
Reppucci, N. Dickon, Yale University
Rivera, Eduardo, University of Puerto Rico
Roehl, Carol, West Virginia University
Rooney, William, University of Houston
Roquemore, Gwendolyn Johnston, Morehouse College
Rust, Margaret, University of Michigan
Rutherford, Brenda, Dillard University
Sarason, Seymour, Yale University
Sarata, Brian, University of Nebraska
Schneider, Stanley, National Institute of Mental Health

*Community Psychology Training Program, University of Texas at Austin.

Schoenfield, Lawrence, University of Texas Health Science Center, San Antonio, Texas
Semler, Ira, Austin Child Guidance Center, Austin, Texas
Silverman, Wade, Illinois Mental Health Institutes, Chicago, Illinois
Sirbu, William, DePaul University
Slaikeu, Karl, University of Texas at Austin
*Smith, David, University of Texas at Austin
Smith, James, Washington University
Smith, Lynette, University of Houston
Spielberger, Charles, University of South Florida
Stenmark, David, University of South Carolina
Suber, Carolyn, American Psychological Association
Sue, Stanley, University of Washington
Swartz, Jon, University of Texas Permian Basin, Odessa, Texas
Taylor, Dalmas, American Psychological Association
Teague, Mary, University of Texas at Austin
Tefft, Bruce M., University of Rochester
Terrell, David L., Meharry Medical College, Nashville, Tennessee
Todd, David M., University of Massachusetts
Tomes, Henry, Meharry Medical College, Nashville, Tennessee
Trickett, Edison, Yale University
*Turner, Neomia, University of Texas at Austin
Tyler, Forrest, University of Maryland
Van Hoose, Tom, University of Texas Health Science Center, Dallas, Texas
Whitley, Jeffrey, University of Texas Medical Branch, Galveston, Texas
*Wilcox, Brian, University of Texas at Austin
Williams, Robert, Washington University
Young, Carl, Pennsylvania State University
Young, Kemba, University of Maryland
Zolik, Edward, DePaul University

Individuals listed above engaged in all of the activities of the conference. Some also were acting in the role of observers and representatives as noted below.

OBSERVERS AND OFFICIAL REPRESENTATIVES

Robert Callahan, Training Branch, National Institute of Mental Health
Louis Cohen, Education and Training Board, American Psychological Association
Robert Czeh, National Institute of Mental Health
Ursula Delworth, Western Interstate Commission on Higher Education (WICHE)
Wayne Holtzman, Hogg Foundation for Mental Health
Sherman Nelson, National Institute of Mental Health
Rodney Nurse, California School of Professional Psychology
Beeman Phillips, Division 17, American Psychological Association

*Community Psychology Training Program, University of Texas at Austin.

Louis Ramey, Southern Regional Education Board (SREB)
Stanley Schneider, Training Branch, National Institute of Mental Health
Carolyn Suber, American Psychological Association
Dalmas Taylor, Ethnic Minority Scholarship Program, American Psychological Association
Forrest Tyler, Board of Professional Affairs, American Psychological Association

Author Index

Subject Index